Rapid Review of

Clinical
Medicine
for MRCP Part 2

Sanjay Sharma
BSc (Hons) MRCP (UK) MD
Specialist Registrar in Cardiology and Internal Medicine
St George's Hospital Medical School
London, UK

Rashmi Kaushal
BSc (Hons) MRCP (UK)
Research Fellow in Endocrinology and Diabetes
St George's Hospital Medical School
London, UK

MANSON
PUBLISHING

Reprinted 2001, 2002, 2003, 2004

ISBN 1–874545–99–5

For full details of all Manson Publishing titles, please write to:
Manson Publishing Ltd
73 Corringham Road
London NW11 7DL, UK
Tel: +44 (0)20 8905 5150
Fax: +44 (0)20 8201 9233
Email: manson@mansonpublishing.com
Website: www.mansonpublishing.com

Project manager	**Paul Bennett**
Sub-editor	**William H. Down**
Design and layout	**Paul Bennett**
Illustration	**MTG**
Colour reproduction	**Tenon & Polert Colour Scanning Ltd, Hong Kong**
Printer	**Grafos SA, Barcelona, Spain**

Contents

Preface

Passing specialist examinations in internal medicine is a difficult milestone for many doctors, but is a mandatory requirement for career progression. Pass rates in these examinations are generally low due to 'high standards' and 'stiff competition'. Thorough preparation is essential and requires a broad knowledge of internal medicine. The pressures of a busy clinical job and nights 'on call' make it almost impossible for doctors to wade through heaps of large text books to acquire all the knowledge that is required to pass the examinations.

The aim of this book is to provide the busy doctor with a comprehensive review of the most popular cases and data interpretation questions in examinations in internal medicine. The questions are based on topics encountered in the MRCP (UK) and similar examinations in adult medicine over the past decade. In most instances, the level of difficulty of each question is of the same standard as the college examination. However, some cases are deliberately more difficult for teaching purposes.

A broad range of subjects is covered in 178 questions ranging from metabolic medicine to infectious diseases. Precise answers and detailed discussion follow each question. Where appropriate, important differential diagnoses, diagnostic algorithms and up-to-date medical lists are presented. Many questions comprise illustrated material in the form of radiographic material, electrocardiograms, echocardiograms, blood films, audiograms, respiratory flow loops, histological material, and slides in ophthalmology,

dermatology and infectious diseases. Over 180 commonly examined illustrations are included.

Tutorials are included at the end of the book to aid the interpretation of illustrated material as well as important, and sometimes difficult, clinical data, such as respiratory function tests, cardiac catheter data and dynamic endocrine tests. Some questions have multiple-choice type answers in accordance with the increasingly popular format adopted in the MRCP Part 2 and similar examinations. As well as broadening medical knowledge, the book concentrates on examination technique. Answers to difficult questions are presented in order of those scoring the best marks at the top and those scoring lower marks at the bottom. The book will prove invaluable to all those studying for higher examinations in internal medicine, and to their instructors.

Sanjay Sharma
Specialist Registrar in Cardiology and Internal Medicine
Senior Lecturer for Medipass Intensive Courses for the
    MRCP Part 2

Rashmi Kaushal
Research Fellow in Endocrinology and Diabetes
Senior Lecturer for Medipass Intensive Courses for the
    MRCP Part 1

November 1999

Acknowledgements

We are grateful for the help of several colleagues who helped provide slides for the book:

Dr L Wilkinson, Ms S Gowrinath, Ms H Derry, Mr P Radomskij, Dr J Waktare, Ms A O'Donoghue, Dr S Rosen, Dr A Mehta, Dr L Shapiro, Professor M E Hodson, Dr G Rai, Dr A Ghuran, Professor C Oakley, Ms F Goulder, Dr J Axford, Dr S Jain, Dr M Stodell, Dr B Harold, Dr D Seigler, Dr C Travill, Dr G Barrison, Dr D Hackett, Dr J Bayliss, Dr R Lancaster, Dr R Foale, Dr W Davies, Professor D Sheridan, Professor W McKenna, Professor G MacGregor, Dr A Belli, Dr Adams, Dr J Joseph, Dr M Impallomeni, Dr D Banerjee, Dr N Essex, Dr S Nussey, Dr S Hyer, Dr A Rodin, Dr M Prentice.

We are also grateful for the assistance of the Audio-visual Departments at Luton and Dunstable Hospital, St Mary's (Paddington) Hospital and St George's Hospital Medical School and the ECG, Echocardiography and Radiology Department at St George's Hospital Medical School.

Dedication
For Seema, Anushka and Shivani

Classification of Cases

Abbreviations

5-HIAA	5'-hydroxyindole acetic acid	Hb	haemoglobin
AAFB	acid-alcohol fast bacilli	HCC	hydroxy-cholecalciferol
ACE	angiotensin-converting enzyme	HCM	hypertrophic cardiomyopathy
ACTH	adrenocorticotrophic hormone	HCV	hepatitis C virus
ADH	antidiuretic hormone	HIV	human immunodeficiency virus
AIDS	acquired immune-deficiency syndrome	HS	hereditary spherocytosis
AIP	acute intermittent porphyria	HSMN	hereditary sensorimotor neuropathy
ALA	aminolaevulinic acid	INR	International Normalized Ratio
ALT	alanine transaminase (SGPT)	IVP	intravenous pyelogram
AMP	adenosine 5'-monophosphate	JVP	jugular venous pressure
ANCA	anti-neutrophil cytoplasmic antibodies	KCO	corrected carbon monoxide transfer factor
APCKD	adult polycystic kidney disease		
APTT	activated partial thromboplastin time	LBBB	left bundle branch block
ARDS	adult respiratory distress syndrome	LDH	lactate dehydrogenase
ASD	atrial septal defect	LFT	liver function tests
AST	aspartate transaminase (SGOT)	LH	luteinizing hormone
AZT	zidovudine	LHRH	luteinizing hormone releasing hormone
BCG	bacille Calmette-Guérin	LQTS	long QT-syndrome
BT	bleeding time	LVEDP	left ventricular end-diastolic pressure
CAH	chronic active hepatitis	MAHA	microangiopathic haemolytic anaemia
CFA	cryptogenic fibrosing alveolitis	MAOI	monoamine oxidase inhibitor
CFTR	cystic fibrosis transmembrane regulator (protein)	MCH	mean cell haemoglobin
		MCHC	mean cell haemoglobin content
CMV	cytomegalovirus	MCV	mean cell volume
CRP	C-reactive protein	MEN	multiple endocrine neoplasia
CSF	cerebrospinal fluid	MGUS	monoclonal gammopathy of undetermined significance
CT	computed tomography		
CVA	cerebrovascular accident	MPO	myeloperoxidase
CVP	central venous pressure	MRI	magnetic resonance imaging
DC	direct current	NADPH	nicotinamide adenine dinucleotide phosphate (reduced)
DHCC	dihydroxy-cholecalciferol		
DIC	disseminated intravascular coagulation	NAPQI	N-acetyl-p-benzoquinoneimine
DIDMOAD	diabetes insipidus, diabetes mellitus, optic atrophy and deafness	NSAID	non-steroidal anti-inflammatory drug
		PAS	periodic acid–Schiff
EBV	Epstein–Barr virus	PBC	primary biliary cirrhosis
ECG	electrocardiogram	PBG	porphobilinogen
EEG	electroencephalogram	PCOS	polycystic ovary syndrome
ELISA	enzyme-linked immunosorbent assay	PCR	polymerase chain reaction
EMF	endomyocardial fibrosis	PCT	porphyria cutanea tarda
ERCP	endoscopic retrograde cholangiopancreatogram	PCV	packed cell volume
		PCWP	pulmonary capillary wedge pressure
ESR	erythrocyte sedimentation rate	PEFR	peak expiratory flow rate
FBC	full blood count	PNH	paroxysmal nocturnal haemoglobinuria
FEV_1	fixed expiration volume in 1 second	PRL	prolactin
FSH	follicle stimulating hormone	PT	prothrombin time
FTA	fluorescent treponemal antibody	PTH	parathormone or parathyroid hormone
FVC	forced vital capacity	RBBB	right bundle branch block
GBM	glomerular basement membrane	RMAT	rapid macroagglutination test
GFR	glomerular filtration rate	RTA	renal tubular acidosis
GH	growth hormone	RV	residual volume
GHRH	growth hormone releasing hormone	SIADH	syndrome of inappropriate antidiuretic hormone
GPI	glucophosphatidylinositol		
GT	glutamyltransferase	SLE	systemic lupus erythematosus

Abbreviations (*continued*)

SROS	Steele–Richardson–Olszewski syndrome
TB	tuberculosis
TIBC	total iron-binding capacity
TLC	total lung capacity
TLCO	total lung carbon monoxide transfer factor
TPHA	treponema pallidum haemagglutination test
TRH	thyrotrophin releasing hormone
TSH	thyroid stimulating hormone
TT	thrombin time
U&E	urea and electrolytes
US	ultrasound
VDRL	Venereal Diseases Research Laboratory test
VIP	vasointestinal polypeptide
VMA	vanilyl mandelic acid
VSD	ventricular septal defect
WCC	white cell count

Cases

Question 1

A 41-year-old female was admitted to hospital with acute confusion. She had been generally unwell for two days. A worried neighbour looked through her letter box when she failed to answer the door bell, and found her lying on the floor. There was no other history of note.

On examination, she was confused. She had a wide-spread rash (1a). Her left eye is shown (1b). The heart rate was 120 beats/min; the blood pressure was unrecordable. There was no evidence of nuchal rigidity, and Kernig's sign was negative. There was no focal neurological deficit. Examination of the cardiovascular, respiratory and gastro-intestinal tract was normal.

Investigations are shown.

FBC	Hb 11 g/dl
	WCC 24×10^9/l
	Platelets 30×10^9/l
Biochemistry	Sodium 135 mmol/l
	Potassium 5 mmol/l
	Creatinine 156 µmol/l
Clotting	PT 48 s (control 13 s)
	Fibrinogen degradation products >25,000

1. Which single investigation would you perform next?
2. List three therapeutic steps in her immediate management.

Question 2

A 36-year-old woman is seen in the accident and emergency department after having taken 40 paracetamol tablets with a quarter-bottle of vodka six hours earlier, following an argument with her husband. She was nauseous, but had not vomited. There was no past medical history of note. A physical examination was normal.

Investigations are shown.

Biochemistry	Sodium 138 mmol/l
	Potassium 3.9 mmol/l
	Urea 5.1 mmol/l
	Bicarbonate 18 mmol/l
PT	15 s (control 15 s)
Serum paracetamol level 200 mg/l	

1. What is the immediate management (two steps)?
2. Which three tests would you perform the next day to assess her prognosis?

Answer 1

1. Blood cultures.
2. i. Intravenous benzyl penicillin and cefotaxime (until results of blood cultures available).
ii. Restore circulation with intravenous fluids and possibly inotropes.
iii. Correct clotting with fresh-frozen plasma.

The eye demonstrates a conjunctival haemorrhage and conjunctival suffusion. The rash is a necrotic purpuric rash which is typical of meningococcal septicaemia. The patient has septic shock and requires immediate therapy. The recognition that she has meningococcal septicaemia is important for the choice of antibiotics which you will use. In medical emergencies, the reader must be familiar with the drugs which are used in that particular emergency, but not necessarily the dosage as this can be found in the *British National Formulary* or the equivalent. Although most *Neisseria meningitidis* strains are sensitive to benzyl penicillin, it is prudent to cover the patient with additional cephalosporin or aminoglycoside antibiotic therapy until the sensitivities of the organism are known. The circulation must be restored to prevent hypoperfusion of vital organs, particularly the kidneys. The presence of low platelets, high fibrinogen degradation products and abnormal clotting is suggestive of DIC, which should be treated with fresh-frozen plasma to prevent haemorrhage.

Neisseria meningitidis, the causal Gram-negative diplococcus, can be cultured from the CSF in over 80% of cases with evidence of neurological involvement. However, the presence of very low platelets and DIC is contra-indicated because of the dangers of bleeding into the spinal canal, particularly because the yield is just as high in the blood and nasal swabs. It is also possible to isolate the meningococcal antigen from blood before blood culture results are available. This test is particularly useful if antibiotics have been given before the patient is brought to hospital (negative blood cultures).

Meningococcal meningitis and septicaemia are caused by serogroups B and C. Septicaemia is associated with widespread petechial haemorrhage. Conjunctival haemorr-hage may be the first physical manifestation. Shock is common due to the production of a circulating endotoxin. DIC is a commonly recognized complication which may result in adrenal haemorrhage (Waterhouse–Friedrichson syndrome). Meningitis is often characterized by a myalgia, headache, photophobia, neck stiffness, nausea and vomiting. In the absence of DIC, the diagnosis is made rapidly by performing a Gram stain on the CSF. Blood cultures are positive in the majority of patients with menin-gitis. Focal neurological signs are less common than in pneumococcal meningitis.

Note: individuals in contact with affected patients must receive rifampicin chemoprophylaxis.

Answer 2

1. i. Activated charcoal given orally. Gastric lavage is useful if performed within 1 hour of the overdose.
ii. Intravenous acetylcysteine should be given within 8–10 hours of ingestion of the overdose, and continued while the liver function is abnormal. It is useful because it replenishes cellular glutathione stores and reduces oxidative damage caused by the toxic metabolite, NAPQI. An alternative to this is methionine.
2. Serum creatinine, blood pH, PT.

The patient has taken 20 g of paracetamol. An ingestion of 15 g is considered potentially serious in most patients. The toxicity of paracetamol is related to the production of a toxic metabolite of paracetamol. This is NAPQI, which usually is immediately conjugated with glutathione and

excreted. In paracetamol overdose, the toxic metabolite is produced in excess and depletes cellular glutathione. The liver is unable to deactivate NAPQI, which is responsible for massive hepatic necrosis and hepatic failure. Patients may have nausea, anorexia or vomiting on the first day. After 72 hours, features of liver and renal failure may ensue.

A rise in serum creatinine due to renal failure is a bad prognostic sign. A level of over 300 µmol/l is associated with over 70% mortality. Systemic acidosis (due to the failure of clearance of lactate by the liver) more than 24 hours after the overdose is associated with a poor prog-nosis. A pH of below 7.3 is associated with only 15% chance of survival. The PT is usually the first liver test to become abnormal. A PT of >20 s at 24 hours after overdose is suggestive of significant hepatic damage. A peak PT of >180 s is associated with a 90% mortality.

Question 3

A 52-year-old female was brought into the accident and emergency department after being found collapsed outside a public house. There was no one accompanying her, and there was no information regarding her next of kin.

On examination, she was very drowsy and had a Glasgow coma score of 6 out of 15. Her pupils were 10 mm each and reacted very sluggishly to light. On attempting to examine her fundi, she was noted to have coarse nystagmus, but a clear view of her fundi did not demonstrate any abnormalities. The tone in all her limbs was increased and her reflexes were brisk. The plantars were both upgoing. The heart rate was 135 beats/min, and regular. The blood pressure was 105/60 mmHg. The respiratory rate was 20/min. Examination of the precordium and lung fields was normal, but examination of the abdomen revealed a firm palpable mass 4 cm above the symphysis pubis.

The patient was catheterized and drained 2 litres of urine.

Investigations are shown.

Shortly after the lumbar puncture, the patient had a generalized seizure which lasted 30 s. The attending nurse raised concerns about an arrhythmia on the cardiac monitor, and a 12-lead ECG was performed (**3**).

1. Calculate the plasma osmolality.
2. Explain the discrepancy between the calculated plasma osmolality and the measured plasma osmolality.
3. Give two possible explanations for the low urine osmolality.
4. What is shown on the ECG?
5. Which diagnosis best fits all the information given above?
6. Which three investigations would you perform to help in this patient's management?
7. Give six immediate management steps.

FBC	Hb 14 g/dl
	WCC 12×10^9/l
	Platelets 221×10^9/l
	MCV 88 fl
Biochemistry	Sodium 144 mmol/l
	Potassium 4.0 mmol/l
	Urea 13 mmol/l
	Creatinine 100 µmol/l
	Bicarbonate 20 mmol/l
	Chloride 108 mmol/l
	Calcium 2.4 mmol/l
	Phosphate 1.3 mmol/l
	Bilirubin 12 µmol/l
	AST 33 u/l
	Gamma GT 28 u/l
	Alkaline phosphatase 120 u/l
Plasma osmolality	333 mOsm/l
Urine osmolality	120 mOsm/l
Blood glucose	6 mmol/l
Chest X-ray	Normal-sized heart and clear lung fields
Skull X-ray	Normal; no fractures seen
Brain CT scan	Normal
Lumbar puncture	CSF pressure 100 cm H_2O
	Cells 3/mm^3
	Protein 0.35 g/l
	Glucose 3 mmol/l
ECG	Sinus tachycardia; right axis deviation

Answer 3

1. The plasma osmolality is calculated by the formula $2([Na] + [K]) + [Urea] + [Glucose]$. In this case, the calculated plasma osmolality is 315 mOsm/l.

2. The measured plasma osmolality is higher than the calculated one suggesting that the patient has ingested something which has not been measured, but has an effect of increasing the plasma osmolality. The most likely possibility in this case is alcohol ingestion. Although lithium contributes to plasma osmolality, it would be very unusual for the lithium concentration to be high enough to increase the plasma osmolality by 18 mOsm/l, considering that a serum lithium concentration of 2.5 mmol/l causes dangerous toxicity.

3. Nephrogenic diabetes insipidus from lithium therapy or inhibition of ADH secretion as a result of alcohol ingestion.

4. There is a broad-complex tachycardia with extreme axis deviation and concordance of the QRS complexes in the chest leads. These findings are suggestive of ventricular tachycardia.

5. Tricyclic antidepressant drug overdose with alcohol.

6. **i.** Arterial blood gases.
ii. Serum lithium level.
iii. Blood alcohol level.

7. **i.** Protect the airway, and give oxygen via a mask.
ii. Gastric lavage under anaesthetic supervision (within 12 hours of ingestion) followed by activated charcoal via a nasogastric tube.
iii. Monitor on a high-dependency unit.
iv. Correct hypoxia.
v. Correct acidosis.
vi. Intravenous fluids to improve blood pressure.
Acidosis should be corrected with sodium bicarbonate. Arrhythmias usually settle on correction of hypoxia and acidosis. Administration of class I antiarrhythmic agents may paradoxically worsen arrhythmias, with the exception of phenytoin. Status epilepticus should be corrected with intravenous diazepam.

Epileptic seizures and ventricular arrhythmias in a patient found collapsed should raise the suspicion of tricyclic antidepressant drug overdose. The low urine osmolality suggests that the patient has probably taken the overdose together with alcohol, and it is possible that she may have also taken lithium. The normal CT scan of the brain and normal CSF are against pathology in the central nervous system. She has dilated pupils, which is against narcotic abuse. Indeed, the combination of dilated pupils, tachycardia and urinary retention are all suggestive of the anticholinergic side effects of tricyclic antidepressants. Severe lithium toxicity is associated with seizures, coma and ventricular arrhythmias, but anticholinergic effects are not a feature. In addition, lithium toxicity is associated with ataxia and dysarthria. Chronic lithium ingestion may cause hypothyroidism. Sodium-depleting drugs such as diuretics lead to excess absorption of lithium by the kidney, and predispose to toxicity.

The arterial blood gases are an important investigation because they will identify hypoxia and acidosis, both of which precipitate ventricular arrhythmias in patients with tricyclic antidepressant overdose. The serum lithium level will be useful to determine whether lithium has been ingested, and will help decide whether the patient should have forced diuresis. In general, patients with a serum lithium of >3 mmol/l should have forced diuresis. Haemodialysis is recommended if serum lithium exceeds 4 mmol/l.

The management of the patient is outlined in the response to part 7 of the question.

Question 4

A 76-year-old male presented with a three-month history of anorexia, weight loss and fever. Apart from sweating excessively at nights and feeling very thirsty, he did not have any other symptoms. He was a non-smoker and had been a school teacher for 40 years before retiring.

On examination, he was thin. The finding on inspection of his hands is shown (**4a**). The heart rate was 100 beats/min and the blood pressure 180/105 mmHg. His temperature was 37.8°C (100°F). Examination of the cardiovascular system and the respiratory system was normal. Abdominal examination revealed minimal tenderness and some fullness in the right loin. Examination of the genitalia revealed some oedema of the scrotum. The lower limbs were oedematous.

Investigations are shown.

FBC	Hb 18 g/dl
	WCC 10×10^9/l
	Platelets 300×10^9/l
ESR	110 mm/h.
Biochemistry	Sodium 140 mmol/l
	Potassium 3.1 mmol/l
	Creatinine 120 µmol/l
	Calcium 2.6 mmol/l
	Albumin 36 g/l
Chest X-ray (**4b**)	
CT scan of abdomen (**4c**)	
Urinalysis	Blood +++
	Protein +
	Bilirubin 0

1. Give two explanations for the serum calcium level.
2. What is the most probable diagnosis?
3. List three important tests you would perform to help achieve a diagnosis.
4. What is the management?

Answer 4

1. i. Bone metastases.
ii. PTH-related peptide secretion from a right-sided renal carcinoma.
2. Right-sided renal carcinoma.
3. i. Renal angiography.
ii. Renal venography and inferior vena cavogram.
iii. Bone scan to detect bony metastases.
4. Surgical removal of the right kidney if his general health will allow.

This patient presents with anorexia, weight loss, and a fever which may represent sepsis or malignancy. The right loin tenderness and haematuria are suggestive of renal involvement. The chest X-ray reveals a large opacity in the right lung which represents a cannon-ball metastasis from the right kidney to the lung in this case. CT scan of the abdomen reveals a carcinoma of the right kidney which is invading the inferior vena cava; hence the scrotal and lower-limb oedema. Hypernephroma characteristically presents with a triad of haematuria, loin pain and swelling. Haematuria is present in 50% of cases, but pain and swelling are less frequent. Non-specific symptoms such as anorexia, weight loss and fatigue may be present for several months before the diagnosis is made. The neoplastic cells often produce peptide hormones such as erythropoietin, renin, ADH, PTH-related peptide. This patient has a relative polycythaemia, hypercalcaemia, hypokalaemia and hypertension which reflect erythropoietin, PTH-related peptide and renin secretion, respectively. Fever is present in approximately 20% of patients and is probably secondary to the secretion of a pyrogen by the tumour. Hypertension is present in approximately 30% of patients. Metastases usually occur via the bloodstream, although direct invasion of the renal veins or the inferior vena cava is relatively common. Some 10% of hypernephromas are bilateral, so close attention is given to the contralateral kidney when reviewing the CT scan. Venography and arteriography allow assessment of invasion of the veins and the vascularity of the tumour, respectively. Urine cytology may reveal malignant cells but the diagnostic yield is low. Removal of the hypernephroma (even when distant metastases are present) improves survival and causes regression of the metastases in many, but not all, patients. Radiotherapy and chemotherapy have been used in the treatment of this tumour, but the results are not very encouraging. The overall survival rate is 30–50%.

Question 5

An 84-year-old female was referred to clinic with increasing forgetfulness. Her general practitioner had commenced her on a small dose of haloperidol for agitation eight months ago. According to the staff at the nursing home where she resided, she had become increasingly confused over the past few months and more recently had developed odd movements affecting her face, arms and legs. Her general practitioner had reviewed her two weeks previously and stopped the haloperidol; however, she remained confused and the movement disorder had become much more pronounced. She was not taking any other medication.

On examination, she had a mental test score of 4/10.

Her vital parameters were normal. She exhibited intermittent yawning motions of the mouth, with occasional tongue protrusion. There were semi-purposeful movements of her arms and legs. There was also clinical evidence of increased tone and cog-wheel rigidity on neurological examination of her limbs.

A CT scan of the brain revealed generalized cerebral atrophy and calcification of the basal ganglia.

1. What is the cause of her movement disorder?

Question 6

A 33-year-old Iranian male was investigated for a six-month history of general malaise, weight loss, fever, pain in his knees, ankles and wrists, and a sore mouth. On systematic enquiry, he gave a two-year history of a recurrent sore mouth which made it difficult for him to eat. Just before the onset of all his symptoms he had experienced an attack of abdominal pain and bloody diarrhoea which resolved after a week. He was seen by a gastroenterologist shortly afterwards, who diagnosed an inflammatory colitis, possibly secondary to infection. A rectal biopsy was performed by the gastroenterologist, and this was reported as a non-specific colitis. The patient had never experienced any abdominal symptoms after this, but had several episodes of soreness affecting the mouth. In addition, he developed painful eyes and pain on intercourse and on voiding urine. There was no history of urethral discharge. Shortly afterwards he was admitted to hospital with a femoral vein thrombosis

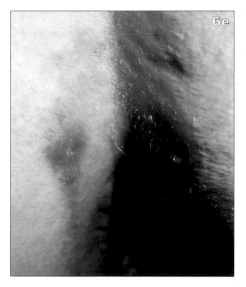

which was treated with anticoagulants and thought to be secondary to dehydration and immobility from his diarrhoeal illness. During the past six weeks his health had deteriorated. He had arthralgia and a fever.

He had been married for five years. He denied extramarital sex. His wife was well, and had not experienced any similar symptoms.

On examination, the patient appeared unwell. Examination of his oral cavity revealed an abnormality (**6a**). His eyes were sore (**6b**). He had submandibular lymphadenopathy. His ankle, wrist and knee joints were tender, and the joint movements were restricted. In addition, he had painful lesions on his legs (**6c**). Examination of his genitalia and anal areas are shown (**6d, 6e**). He also pointed out an erythematous lesion approximately 2 cm in diameter which had developed at the site of venepuncture during a blood test performed by his general practitioner two days earlier. All other aspects of the physical examination were normal.

Investigations are shown.

1. What is the most probable diagnosis?
A. Crohn's disease.
B. Ulcerative colitis.
C. Reiter's syndrome.
D. Behçet's syndrome.
E. Gonococcal septicaemia.
F. Stevens–Johnson syndrome.
G. Pemphigus.

FBC	Hb 9.8 g/dl
	WCC 13 × 10⁹/l
	Platelets 450 × 10⁹/l
	MCV 82 fl
CRP	200 g/l
Rheumatoid factor	Absent
Anti-nuclear antibody	Absent
Radiology of painful joints	Normal

Answer 5

1. Extrapyramidal side effects of haloperidol.

The woman has clinical evidence of dyskinesia and parkinsonism. The most common cause of her neurological signs is drug-induced extrapyramidal disease. Neuroleptic drugs which include haloperidol are extensively used in treating agitation in the elderly. By blocking dopamine receptors in the basal ganglia, these drugs can offset extrapyramidal side effects which include tremor, dystonia, akathisia, parkinsonism and tardive dyskinesia. Acute dystonic reactions appear within the first few hours or days, and consist of oculogyric crises, torticollis or trismus. Fortunately, they are uncommon, and resolve as soon as the drug is withdrawn. Chronic tardive dyskinesias are the most serious complication and affect 20% of patients on chronic neuroleptic therapy. They usually occur after a patient has been on treatment for at least three months, and can be made worse in the first few weeks after stopping the offending drug. In 60% of cases the dyskinesia resolves over three years after drug withdrawal; however, in the remainder of patients the movement disorder persists and is very difficult to treat. Characteristic features involve lip smacking, tongue protrusion, orofacial mouthing, trunk rocking and distal chorea of the hands and feet. A combination of any of these features may be present.

Cerebral calcification is an incidental finding in 0.5% of CT scans in the elderly. About 20–30% of patients with widespread calcification of the basal ganglia exhibit neurological signs which include parkinsonism, chorea, epilepsy, ataxia and dementia. There is an association between calcification of the basal ganglia and hypoparathyroidism or pseudohypoparathyroidism. Rare causes of basal ganglia calcification (**5**, arrowed) are cerebral irradiation and mitochondrial diseases.

Answer 6

1. D. Behçet's syndrome.

The patient has oral, genital and anal ulcers (**6a**, **6d** and **6e**, respectively), conjunctivitis (**6b**), arthritis, erythema nodosum (**6c**) and features of a systemic illness. There has been a single episode of bloody diarrhoea and a previous femoral vein thrombosis. The differential diagnoses include Crohn's disease, Reiter's syndrome and Behçet's disease (*Table*). Reiter's syndrome is classically a triad of conjunctivitis, urethritis and arthritis 1–4 weeks after an episode of bacterial dysentery or a sexually transmitted urethritis. Other features include plantar fasciitis, achilles tendinitis, keratoderma blenorrhagica, circinate balanitis, stomatitis, hepatitis, cardiac and neurological involvement, and occasionally amyloidosis. It is possible that the diarrhoeal illness may have been dysenteric and offset the reactive features of Reiter's disease. There is no history of promiscuity or urethral discharge. Venous thrombosis affects about 4% of patients with Reiter's disease and occurs early in the disease. Mouth ulcers are common in Reiter's disease and are painless. Erythema nodosum is not a feature of Reiter's syndrome. Arthritis is asymmetrical and usually affects the knee and ankle joints. The most common joint to be affected in the upper limb is the wrist, as in this case; however, joint involvement occurs early, whereas in this case the disease has been present for two years. Crohn's disease is a chronic granulomatous inflammatory disease of the gastrointestinal tract of unknown cause, and is a strong possibility in this case. Bloody diarrhoea is a recognized feature of Crohn's colitis. Colonic disease is associated with perianal disease in just over 30% of patients. A seronegative reactive arthritis is a recognized complication of Crohn's disease. Erythema nodosum occurs in some cases. Genital ulcers are rare, as is deep-vein thrombosis. Urethral involvement and dysuria only occur when an inflammatory fistula develops between the colon and the ureter. Recurrent urinary tract infections due to faecaluria can cause urethral stricture.

Behçet's disease is the most probable diagnosis. Behçet's disease is a recurrent multifocal disorder which persists over many years. It is characterized by recurrent mouth and genital ulcers, ocular lesions, skin, joint and neurological involvement. The incidence is high in Japan and in countries bordering the Mediterranean. Oral and genital ulcers are present in most patients, and can be painful. Ulcers can affect the pharynx and cause dysphagia. Genital ulcers can cause dysuria and dyspareunia. Ocular lesions are the most serious development. Recurrent uveitis and iridocyclitis, retinal vascular lesions and optic atrophy can lead to loss of vision in 50% of patients with ocular involvement. Erythema nodosum is a recognized feature. Other skin manifestations include a diffuse pustular rash affecting the face, erythema multiforme. The pathergy is a useful diagnostic sign. Pricking the skin can lead to erythema around the affected part within 24–48 hours, which is a relevant feature in our patient. A seronegative arthritis also affects about 40% of patients and most commonly involves the knees, ankles and wrists. Recurrent thrombophlebitis of the legs is a significant feature of Behçet's syndrome, leading to venous thrombosis. Less frequently, superior or inferior cava thrombosis may occur. Abdominal pain and bloody diarrhoea have been documented in some patients. Asymptomatic proteinuria is a recognized feature, but on a few occasions may reflect renal amyloidosis. Neurological complications occur in 20% of patients. Organic confusional states, meningoencephalitis, transient or persistent brainstem syndromes, multiple sclerosis and parkinsonian-type disorders are all recognized.

Causes of orogenital ulcers	
Behçet's syndrome	Syphilis
Crohn's disease	Gonococcal infection
Herpes simplex virus	HIV
Ulcerative colitis	Pemphigus pemphigoid
Reiter's syndrome	Stevens–Johnson
Lichen planus	syndrome

Causes of orogenital ulcers and venous thromboses	
Behçet's syndrome	Ulcerative colitis
Crohn's disease	Reiter's syndrome

Behçet's syndrome is a clinical diagnosis. There is no specific diagnostic test. HLA-B51, B12, DR2, DR7 and Drw52 are associated with the syndrome. Acute-phase proteins are elevated and immune complexes are present. The pathergy test is a simple useful test.

Genital ulcers and oral complications are treated with topical steroids. In severe cases, systemic steroids become necessary, together with azathioprine which acts as a steroid sparing agent. Colchicine, cyclosporin and levamisole have also been used in the management of this condition.

The causes of orogenital ulceration are tabulated above.

Question 7

A 16-year-old female was admitted with a six-month history of myalgia, loss of weight and night sweats. Over the past six weeks she had started to become breathless on exertion. On admission to hospital she had a temperature of 38.1°C (100.6°F). On auscultation of the precordium, there was an early diastolic murmur at the left lower sternal edge. Examination of the chest, abdomen and central nervous system was normal, with the exception of her fundi, one of which is shown (7a). An echocardiogram was performed to investigate the murmur (7b).

1. What is the abnormality on inspection of the fundi?
2. What is the abnormality on the echocardiogram?
3. What is the diagnosis?
4. Which important investigation would you perform to confirm the diagnosis?

Answer 7

1. Roth spots. These are haemorrhagic areas with a pale centre, and are usually due to a vasculitis. They are occasionally seen in chronic cases of infective endocarditis. Causes of Roth spots and other stigmata of endocarditis are tabulated below (*Table A*).
2. There is an echogenic mass attached to the aortic valve suggestive of a bacterial vegetation. (See Echocardiography, page 223.)
3. Infective endocarditis.
4. Serial blood cultures.

The diagnosis is infective endocarditis. Blood cultures are the single most important investigation in the diagnosis of infective endocarditis, and are positive in 90% of cases. Serial blood cultures should be performed, because a single set of blood cultures may not necessarily reveal the culprit organism. Although echocardiography is extremely useful in confirming the presence of vegetations, the absence of vegetations does not exclude endocarditis as vegetations less than 3 mm will not be seen on a transthoracic echocardiogram. In approximately 10% of cases no organism is discovered on repeated blood cultures. This is either because the patient has received antibiotics before culturing the blood, or has endocarditis due to a fastidious organism with respect to blood culture media. In patients who are immunosuppressed, blood cultures may be due to fungi which may be difficult to culture, and in very rare circumstances endocarditis may be a manifestation of SLE (Libmann–Sacs endocarditis) or a manifestation of malignancy, when it is termed marantic endocarditis. (See *Tables B* and *C*.)

Table A. Causes of Roth spots and othe stigmata of endocarditis

Causes of Roth spots	*Clinical features of endocarditis*
Infective endocarditis	Pyrexia
SLE	Cardiac murmur
Polyarteritis nodosa	Splinter haemorrhages
Severe anaemia	Osler's nodes; small; painful
Leukaemia	Janeway lesions; macular; painless
	Roth spots
	Splenomegaly
	Microscopic haematuria/nephritis

Table B. Causes of culture-negative endocarditis

Infective	*Non-infective*
Brucella	SLE (Libmann–Sacs)
Coxiella burnetti	Marantic endocarditis
Chlamydia spp.	
Mycoplasma	
Legionella	
Histoplasmosis	
Trophoryma whipelli	
Fungi	

Table C. Common causes of culture-positive endocarditis

Streptococcus viridans
Staphyloccus aureus
Streptococcus faecalis (associated with carcinoma of the colon)
Enterococci

Question 8

A 51-year-old accountant presented with a six-month history of persistent dull right upper quadrant pain and fever. The pain did not radiate elsewhere, but was exacerbated on lying on his right side. During this period she had intermittent pale bulky stool which was difficult to flush, and episodic dark urine. More recently, her appetite was reduced and she had lost approximately 1 kg in weight during the past month. Over the past week she had difficulty sleeping due to itching all over her body, and her colleague at work commented on a yellowish pigmentation in her eyes. Six months before this, she had been relatively well. She had a past history of a cholecystectomy for cholesterol stones at the age of 32 and subsequently had an ERCP and removal of sludge from the common bile duct six years ago. She consumed 10 units of alcohol per week. She was married with two sons aged 20 and 18, respectively. Three months ago she had been on holiday in Scotland. She was not taking any regular medication.

On examination, she was slightly icteric. Inspection of her hands is shown (**8**). There were spider naevi on her arms neck and face and scratch marks around her trunk and lower limbs. She had a temperature of 39°C (102.2°F). Her heart rate was 120 beats/min and blood pressure 140/80 mmHg. There were a few inspiratory crackles on auscultation of the right lung base. Abdominal examination demonstrated firm, slightly tender hepatomegaly 4 cm below the costal margin, and a moderately enlarged spleen. There were no other abdominal masses, and there was no evidence of shifting dullness. Rectal examination was normal.

Investigations are shown.

LFT	AST 60 u/l
	Alkaline phosphatase 360 u/l
	Bilirubin 82 μmol/l
	Albumin 25 g/l
	Total protein 93 g/l
INR	1.49
Chest X-ray	Normal

1. What investigation would you perform to ascertain the cause of her illness?
A. Blood cultures.
B. Liver biopsy.
C. ERCP.
D. Ultrasound of the biliary tract.
E. α-fetoprotein level.
2. What is the cause of her current presentation?
A. Sclerosing cholangitis.
B. Secondary biliary cirrhosis.
C. Primary biliary cirrhosis.
D. Cholangiocarcinoma.
E. Recurrent cholangitis.

Question 9

A 75-year-old male was seen by his general practitioner with a five-day history of wheeze and ankle swelling. He was prescribed some medication, but continued to deteriorate and was admitted to hospital.

Investigations are shown.

1. What is the acid–base disturbance?
2. Suggest two possible causes for this metabolic picture.

Arterial blood gases	pH 7.33
	pO$_2$ 7 kPa
	pCO$_2$ 6.5 kPa
	Bicarbonate 20 mmol/l
Biochemistry	Sodium 133 mmol/l
	Potassium 5 mmol/l
	Urea 28 mmol/l
	Creatinine 200 μmol/l

Answer 8

1. A. Blood cultures.
2. E. Recurrent cholangitis.

The key in this question is a prior history of cholelithiasis affecting the gallbladder and the biliary tree. Stones in the bile duct are a nidus for infections, particularly when there has been instrumentation, as in this case. Cholangitis is characterized by the triad of right upper quadrant pain, jaundice and fever. This patient has had previous episodes suggestive of cholangitis, and the best answer for the presenting complaint is recurrent cholangitis. She also has evidence of cirrhosis which is almost certainly secondary to chronic cholestasis. Although cholangiocarcinoma may rarely complicate biliary cholestasis, this is unlikely given the mode of presentation. Cholangiocarcinoma characteristically presents with intermittent jaundice, and causes duct obstruction before the onset of biliary cirrhosis. Primary sclerosing cholangitis is very uncommon. The aetiology is thought to be autoimmune, but the trigger factor is unknown. More usually, it is associated with ulcerative colitis, but may occur in patients with HIV either as a direct insult from HIV or due to opportunistic CMV, cryptosporidial and Entamoeba infection. Although it may lead to secondary biliary cirrhosis, it is unlikely in this question, given the history of chronic cholestasis. Primary biliary cirrhosis (PBC) is usually insidious. It is much more common in females and usually presents with pruritis and jaundice. Stones are not a recognized feature of PBC.

The investigation of choice is blood cultures which have high positive yield in cholangitis. The most common organism isolated is *Escherichia coli*. Hepatic ultrasound should be performed in all cases to exclude a secondary hepatic abscess, and to assess the common bile duct. ERCP and sphincterotomy may be therapeutic. There is no role for α-fetoprotein and liver biopsy in this case. α-Fetoprotein is often modestly elevated in cirrhosis of the liver, but may be in the thousands in hepatocellular carcinoma. The presentation here is of cholangitis. A liver biopsy should never be the first line of investigation in a jaundiced patient with a fever.

Answer 9

1. Combined respiratory and metabolic acidosis.
2. i. Acute cardiac failure.
ii. Severe exacerbation of obstructive airways disease and pre-renal failure from diuretics.

The patient has a respiratory acidosis which is characterized by a pCO_2 of 6.5 kPa or more, and a pH below 7.35, and is hypoxic. In the acute situation, respiratory acidosis is not compensated by the kidney but after 3–5 days the kidneys retain bicarbonate ions to compensate, which results in normalization of the pH at the expense of a relative metabolic alkalosis. In this patient, the bicarbonate is slightly low, suggesting a metabolic acidosis. This may be due to coexistent renal disease which prevents adequate compensation, or to another factor causing metabolic acidosis. The serum urea and creatinine are elevated, but there is a relatively larger increase in the serum urea, suggesting dehydration in this case. It is possible that he was prescribed a diuretic for symptoms of chronic obstructive airways disease which have precipitated renal failure by causing dehydration.

An alternative suggestion is that he has developed severe cardiac failure leading to pulmonary oedema causing hypoxia and respiratory acidosis and hypoperfusion of the kidneys, resulting in metabolic acidosis from renal failure. Other causes of combined respiratory and metabolic disorders is shown (*Table*).

Other causes of combined respiratory and metabolic acidosis

Aspirin poisoning
Severe pneumonia with renal failure due to septicaemia or interstitial nephritis (Legionnaire's disease)
Septicaemia from any cause complicated by ARDS
Malaria complicated by pneumonia
Acute renal failure and fluid overload
Renal pulmonary syndromes: anti-GBM disease, Wegener's granulomatosis, microscopic polyarteritis nodosa
Acute massive pulmonary embolism
Cardiac arrest (before ventilation)

Question 10

A 14-year-old male presented with joint pains, polydipsia and polyuria.

Respiratory function tests are shown.

1. What is demonstrated by the respiratory function tests?

2. In the context of the history, what is the diagnosis?

3. How would you confirm the diagnosis?

4. If these were the respiratory function tests of a young male with recurrent respiratory tract infections, which diagnosis would you consider?

	Actual	Predicted
FEV_1 (l)	2.0	4.5
FVC (l)	4.0	5.6
FEV_1/FVC	50%	80%
TLC (l)	4.9	7.0
Residual volume (l)	1.7	2.2
KCO (mmol/min/kPa)	5.0	10

Question 11

A 64-year old patient who had been attending the cardiology clinic for 15 years presented with increasing breathlessness on exertion and a reduced appetite. Examination of the face is shown (**11a, b**).

Investigations are shown.

FBC	Hb 13 g/dl
	WCC 7×10^9/l
	Platelets 190×10^9/l
	MCV 80 fl
Biochemistry	Sodium 135 mmol/l
	Potassium 4.1 mmol/l
	Urea 8 mmol/l
	Creatinine 100 µmol/l
	Bilirubin 48 µmol/l
	AST 160 u/l
	Alkaline phosphatase 180 u/l
	Albumin 39 g/l
Thyroid function tests	Thyroxine 190 nmol/l
	TSH <0.1 mu/l
ECG	Atrial fibrillation
	Ventricular rate 80/min
Echocardiogram	Enlarged left atrium
	Normal-sized left ventricle with good function
	Normal valves

1. Give one possible explanation for the breathlessness and all the abnormalities on the blood tests.

2. Which investigation would you perform to investigate the breathlessness further?

Answer 10

1. A mixed obstructive and restrictive defect with a reduced KCO.
The low FEV_1/FVC ratio is in keeping with an obstructive defect; however, the low residual volume also suggests a restrictive pattern.
2. The combination of polydipsia and polyuria with respiratory involvement is suggestive of diabetes insipidus. In a young patient with a mixed restrictive and obstructive defect the most likely diagnosis is histiocytosis X.
3. Transbronchial lung biopsy/liver biopsy/trephine aspirate may all show histiocytes and small round cells.
4. Cystic fibrosis.

Histiocytosis X is a benign disorder of unknown aetiology. It generally affects many systems, but only one system may be involved in up to 25% of cases. The peak age of presentation is between 2–4 years, and the condition affects males more than females. The skin, bones, ears, lungs, eyes, and the reticuloendothelial and central nervous systems are most often affected. A skin rash is common. Individual histiocytomas are pinkish brown papules of 1–5 mm in diameter. Respiratory manifestations include lung fibrosis, bullae and large airway obstruction by histiocytomas. Therefore, both restrictive and/or obstructive respiratory function patterns may occur. Bone involvement with marrow infiltration may be associated with pancytopenia. Any bone may be involved, but there appears to be a special predilection to the skull bones which manifests as large radiolucent lesions. Otitis externa and a troublesome aural discharge occurs in some patients. Ocular involvement is usually characterized by a retro-orbital mass, resulting in proptosis. Hepatosplenomegaly and lymphadenopathy may be present. Occasionally, lymphadenopathy may be massive. One-third of patients develop diabetes insipidus due to histiocytic infiltration of the pituitary stalk. Spinal cord compression may occur in exceptional cases.

The diagnosis is based on the demonstration of histiocytes and small round cells in histological specimens of affected tissues. Management is with steroids, but in some cases cytotoxic drugs such as vincristine or etoposide may be useful. In some cases spontaneous regression may occur.

Answer 11

1. Amiodarone toxicity.
2. Formal lung function tests including a KCO estimation.

The patient has biochemical evidence of hepatitis and hyperthyroidism. In a patient who has been attending the cardiology clinic for several years, and has underlying atrial fibrillation, it is highly likely that these abnormalities are due to the toxicity of amiodarone which was prescribed to control the atrial fibrillation. Amiodarone is a class III anti-arrhythmic agent which is very effective in the management of ventricular and supraventricular arrhythmias; however, it is associated with several side effects and complications (*Table*). Lung fibrosis is an important complication and almost certainly accounts for the patient's breathlessness. Early interstitial fibrosis may not be apparent on chest X-ray, but is suggested by a low KCO on respiratory function tests. Both hyperthyroidism and hypothyroidism are recognized due to the iodine content of the drug. Asymptomatic biochemical hepatitis may occur and some patients may progress to cirrhosis of the liver. Patients on amiodarone should have an annual thyroid test, an LFT and a KCO estimation. Photosensitivity is common, and long-term use is associated with slate-grey skin pigmentation (**11a, b**). Corneal microdeposits are universal and may cause night glare; however, these resolve on withdrawal of the drug.

Side effects and complications of amiodarone	
Side effects	*Complications*
Nausea	Optic neuritis
Metallic taste in the mouth	Peripheral neuropathy
Nightmares	Myopathy
Tremor	Hepatitis/cirrhosis
Headaches	Alveolitis
Rashes including phototoxicity	Hyper/hypothyroidism
	Epididymitis
	Conduction tissue disturbances

Question 12

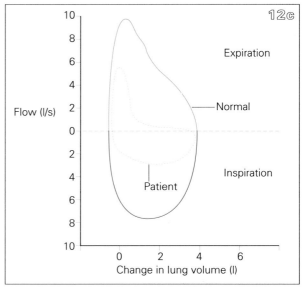

A 66-year-old retired plumber was seen in the accident and emergency department with progressively increasing dyspnoea and left-sided chest discomfort which was worse on inspiration. He was seen by his general practitioner one week previously, and treated with antibiotics for a chest infection. According to his wife, his appetite had been reduced and he had lost at least 6.5 kg in weight over six weeks. He stopped smoking five years previously, but before this was smoking 30 cigarettes per day for over 40 years.

On examination, he appeared thin and tachypnoeic. There was no clinical evidence of cyanosis, but he had early clubbing. His voice was hoarse. Respiratory examination revealed reduced chest expansion of the left hemithorax and dullness to percussion with reduced air entry affecting the left anterior hemithorax.

A chest radiograph taken in accident and emergency is shown (**12a**).

The patient was given oral amoxycillin and erythromycin for one week, and asked to return for repeat chest X-ray in two weeks. However, only four days later he was admitted as an emergency with increasing confusion. According to his wife, he had been extremely thirsty and was waking several times each night to pass large volumes of urine!

Investigations on this occasion are shown.

1. What is the probable underlying diagnosis?
2. What are the two abnormalities on the flow loop curve?
3. Give five possible reasons for his confusion.
4. What are the most likely reasons for his polydipsia and polyuria?
5. Give two reasons why this man is incurable.

FBC	Hb 10.8 g/dl
	WCC 14.2×10^9/l
	Platelets 80×10^9/l
	MCV 91 fl
U&E	Sodium 133 mmol/l
	Potassium 3.9 mmol/l
	Urea 18 mmol/l
	Creatinine 179 µmol/l
Glucose	8.1 mmol/l
Urinalysis	Glucose Nil
	Ketones +
Blood film (**12b**)	
Flow loop curve (**12c**)	

Answer 12

1. Bronchial carcinoma affecting the left lung.
2. i. Severely reduced expiratory flow consistent with obstructive airways disease.
ii. Reduced inspiratory flow limb consistent with upper airways obstruction. In this case it is probably due to a laryngeal nerve palsy causing vocal cord paralysis. (See Interpretation of Respiratory Flow Loop Curves, page 222.)
3. i. Hypercalcaemia.
ii. Cerebral metastases.
iii. Hypoxia.
iv. Concurrent respiratory tract infection.
v. Dehydration.
4. i. Hypercalcaemia.
ii. Cranial diabetes insipidus.
5. i. Local and distant metastases: (recurrent laryngeal nerve, bone and brain).
ii. Poor respiratory reserve.

The chest X-ray (**12a**) demonstrates a large mass arising from the left hilum which is complicated by left upper lobe collapse. The risks for developing bronchial carcinoma are smoking and the possibility of asbestos exposure during his occupation as a plumber.

The excessive thirst and polyuria reflects diabetes insipidus. Cerebral metastases may infiltrate the hypothalamus or posterior pituitary to cause cranial diabetes insipidus by affecting the production and release of ADH, respectively. Hypercalcaemia may render the distal renal tubules refractory to the action of ADH and produce a nephrogenic diabetes insipidus. In this case, the hypercalcaemia is probably due to bony metastases because the blood film demonstrates a leucoerythroblastic picture suggesting marrow infiltration (**12b**); however, in squamous cell bronchial carcinoma the hypercalcaemia may also be due to ectopic secretion of a PTH-related peptide.

The main contraindications to surgery include local and distant metastases and poor respiratory reserve.

Question 13

A 76-year-old Polish male was found collapsed in the toilet by the home help. He had been generally unwell for the past five months and was easily fatigued. His appetite was reduced because he felt constantly nauseous. He was seen in the accident and emergency department one month ago with abdominal pain, and was diagnosed as having constipation for which he was prescribed senna. He had not been out of bed for four days. He had a past history of hypertension and osteoarthritis. He lived alone and was becoming increasingly dependent on the social services as his health deteriorated. He smoked 10 cigarettes per day.

On examination, he was confused and agitated, and appeared pale. He was malnourished and clinically dehydrated. There was no evidence of cyanosis or lymphadenopathy. His temperature was 39°C (102.2°F) The heart rate was 110 beats/min and blood pressure 105/50 mmHg. The JVP was not raised. Examination of his tongue is shown (**13a**). On examination of the cardiovascular system, he had a fourth heart sound. Respiratory examination revealed a respiratory rate of 30/min. Movement of the right hemi-thorax was reduced. Percussion note was dull from the right mid-zone to the base. The abdomen was thin. A liver edge was palpable 3 cm below

the costal margin. Examination of the central nervous system was difficult due to his confusion and agitation, but there was no evidence of paralysis. He was clutching his right forearm and seemed to be in severe pain on the slightest movement of his right arm. The knee and ankle jerks were absent, but the plantar response was normal. Examination of the left fundus revealed an abnormality (**13b**). Inspection of his legs is shown (**13c**).

Investigations are shown.

FBC	Hb 8 g/dl
	WCC 25×10^9/l
	Platelets 90×10^9/l
Blood film (**13d**)	
ESR	148 mm/h
Biochemistry	Sodium 130 mmol/l
	Potassium 4 mmol/l
	Urea 16 mmol/l
Total protein	50 g/l
	Albumin 18 g/l
Alkaline phosphatase	220 u/l
AST	26 u/l
Bilirubin	13 µmol/l
Arterial blood	O_2 pH 7.4
gases (40%)	pO_2 9 kPa
	pCO_2 5 kPa
	Bicarbonate 18 mmol/l
Chest X-ray (**13e**)	
X-ray, right arm (**13f**)	
Bone marrow aspirate	Dry tap
Urinalysis	Protein +++
	No organisms

1. What is the diagnosis?
2. What is the cause of the abnormality in the left fundus?
3. Why does the patient have a painful right arm?
4. Comment on two abnormalities seen on his legs and give an explanation for each one.
5. List five complications of the disease which are evident in this patient.

Answer 13

1. Multiple myeloma.
2. Branch retinal vein occlusion.
3. He has a pathological fracture affecting his right ulna.
4. i. Oedema due to nephrotic syndrome.
ii. Bruising secondary to thrombocytopenia or amyloid related capillary fragility.
5. i. Sepsis affecting the right lung as a result of immunoparesis. Bronchopneumonia and renal failure are the most common causes of death in multiple myeloma.
ii. Amyloidosis. The tongue is enlarged due to amyloid infiltration. The patient is oedematous, hypoalbuminaemic and has marked proteinuria suggesting nephrotic syndrome which is a manifestation of renal amyloid. Amyloid often affects the heart in myeloma, and is an important cause of death. Skin deposits, a peripheral neuropathy and massive hepatic infiltration are all recognized features of amyloidosis associated with multiple myeloma.
iii. Bony involvement. There are numerous lytic lesions affecting the right humerus and a consequent pathological fracture. The blood picture (**13d**) reflects a leucoerythroblastic picture which, in this case is probably due to marrow infiltration of myeloma cells, although severe sepsis is also a recognized cause. The typical appearance of plasma cells is shown in the marrow (**13g**). The cell nuclei sit at the edge of the cytoplasm and are well defined.
iv. Hyperviscosity leading to venous thrombosis in the retinal vein. Hyperviscosity occurs when the paraprotein level is very high. Venous and arterial thrombosis can occur almost anywhere.
v. Renal failure. The raised urea suggests renal failure. There are several recognized causes of renal failure in myeloma which are shown (*Table*). Myeloma is also a recognized cause of proximal RTA, however, this does not cause renal failure *per se*.

Recognized causes of renal failure in myeloma

Tubular obstruction by light chain deposits
Infiltration of plasma cells in the kidney ('myeloma kidney')
Hypercalcaemia
Hyperuricaemic nephropathy
Amyloidosis
Recurrent pyelonephritis secondary to immunoparesis
Renal vein thrombosis secondary to hyperviscosity
Renal failure secondary to analgesics, such as non-steroidal anti-inflammatory drugs
Renal failure secondary to contrast agents, e.g. for an IVP

Question 14

A 60-year-old female presented with a four-month history of headaches and general malaise. Over the past three weeks she had developed nausea and epigastric pain following meals. She was restless at night and had noticed occasional palpitations, but attributed these symptoms to fear of illness. She also complained of episodic diarrhoea. On examination, she appeared anxious. She had an irregular swelling in her neck which moved vertically with swallowing. Her heart rate was 120 beats/min, and regular; blood pressure was 180/105 mmHg. Examination of all the major systems was normal.

Investigations are shown.

FBC	Hb 17 g/dl
	WCC 9×10^9/l
	Platelets 300×10^9/l
Biochemistry	Sodium 135 mmol/l
	Potassium 3.4 mmol/l
	Urea 10 mmol/l
Biochemistry	Creatinine 120 µmol/l
	Calcium 2.8 mmol/l
	Phosphate 0.6 mmol/l
Blood glucose	10 mmol/l
TSH	3 mu/l

1. What is the cause of this patient's epigastric pain?
2. Give two explanations for the diarrhoea.
3. What is the most likely cause for the hypertension?
4. How would you explain her haemoglobin?
5. What is the complete diagnosis?
6. List two tests you would perform to investigate the thyroid swelling.

Question 15

M-mode echocardiograms of two women (A and B) who were investigated for breathlessness in a busy cardiology clinic (**15a, b**).

1. What is the diagnosis in female A?
2. What is the diagnosis in female B?

Answer 14

1. Hypercalcaemia (peptic ulcer disease, pancreatitis).
2. i. Raised calcitonin levels.
ii. Phaeochromocytoma.
3. Phaeochromocytoma.
4. Secondary polycythaemia in association with phaeochromocytoma.
5. Multiple endocrine neoplasia type 2 (MEN 2).
6. i. Fine-needle aspiration of the thyroid.
ii. Serum calcitonin.

The patient has hypercalcaemia and hypertension associated with palpitations. She has an irregular swelling in the neck which is consistent with a thyroid goitre. The TSH is normal, indicating that she is euthyroid. The low serum phosphate and high calcium indicate that primary hyperparathyroidism is the most likely cause for the raised calcium. Although primary hyperparathyroidism by itself is a recognized cause of hypertension, it does not account for the palpitations and restlessness, which are best explained by a coexisting phaeochromocytoma. The combination of primary hyperparathyroidism and phaeochromocytoma should lead one to consider the possibility of MEN 2. In the context of this question it is very probable that the thyroid goitre represents a medullary cell carcinoma.

MEN 2 consists of tumours arising from thyroid C cell carcinoma, the parathyroid gland and the adrenal medulla. The latter is the most common expression of the disorder. It is rare below the age of 20, and becomes more common from there onwards. One-third of cases occur in patients aged over 70 years. The genetic abnormality is within the RET proto-oncogene on chromosome 10. The gene encodes a transmembrane glycoprotein receptor tyrosine kinase.

Medullary cell carcinoma develops in 80% of cases and is usually the first presentation; however, MEN 2 accounts for only 10–20% of all medullary cell carcinomas. Management is with surgery. Persistently elevated calcitonin levels after surgery suggest that the patient is not cured. Phaeochromocytomas occur in 50% of cases and are usually bilateral and may be asymptomatic; therefore annual screening with urinary catecholamine measurements is advised. Hyperparathyroidism occurs in only 5–10% and is restricted to certain families.

Screening in families with known disease is by genetic testing. Patients who are gene-positive should have a prophylactic thyroidectomy at a young age, and should then be screened annually with serum PTH, and urinary catecholamine estimation. In those families in whom a genetic abnormality has not been demonstrated, annual serum calcitonin should also be performed, and fine-needle aspiration of the thyroid is indicated if a goitre appears, or if the calcitonin becomes elevated.

Answer 15

1. Mitral valve prolapse.
2. Atrial myxoma.

Female A (**15a**): the mitral valve has a normal appearance in diastole. In systole, both the anterior and posterior leaflets appose normally in the beginning; however, in mid systole there is posterior movement (prolapse) of both leaflets, but predominantly the posterior leaflet. This is characteristic of mitral valve prolapse and is responsible for the mid-systolic clicks and/or the mid-systolic murmur of mitral regurgitation. Mitral valve prolapse is present in 2–5% of the general population. It is generally benign but may be associated with symptoms of sharp inframammary chest pain, breathlessness even with normal ventricular function, palpitation and odd neurological symptoms. There is a risk of infective endocarditis in patients with consequent mitral regurgitation, in whom prophylactic antibiotics during dental work are recommended, and supraventricular arrhythmias. Mitral valve prolapse has been implicated as a cause of sudden cardiac death in highly trained athletes, but its significance as the only finding at post-mortem is controversial because the high prevalence of the condition may mean the finding is coincidental, rather than causal. It is more likely that death may have been caused by the association of mitral valve prolapse with the Wolff–Parkinson–White syndrome causing atrial fibrillation which degenerates to ventricular fibrillation, or the LQTS which causes polymorphic ventricular tachycardia.

Female B (**15b**): there is echogenic shadowing in the mitral valve orifice which is typical of atrial myxoma. The condition is discussed in Answer **75**, page 102. (See also Echocardiography, page 223.)

Question 16

A 15-year-old Nigerian female was admitted with right upper quadrant abdominal pain. She had a history of sickle cell anaemia, and had several admissions with hand and foot crises. During the last two admissions she complained of abdominal pain. She was born in England. She was the only child of a middle-class family.

On examination, she was distressed with pain. The temperature was 37.6°C (99.7°F). She was mildly jaundiced. The pulse was 105 beats/min, and blood pressure 100/75 mmHg. On examination of the respiratory system there was dullness to percussion on the anterior aspect of the right lung. Abdominal examination revealed tenderness in the right upper quadrant. The liver was palpable 3 cm below the costal margin.

Investigations are shown.

FBC	Hb 6 g/dl
	WCC 12×10^9/l
	Platelets 200×10^9/l
Urea/Electrolytes	Normal
LFT	AST 50 u/l
	Alkaline phosphatase 150 u/l
	Albumin 34 g/l
Urine osmolality	120 mOsm/l/kg
Urinalysis	Urobilinogen +++
	Blood 0
	Protein 0
	Bilirubin 0
Chest X-ray	Opacification in the right upper zone

1. What is the cause of the abdominal pain?
2. What investigation would you request next?
3. What is the cause of the girl's respiratory and chest X-ray findings?
4. Explain the urine osmolality.

Question 17

A 25-year-old female presented with a right calf deep-vein thrombosis.

Blood results are shown.

FBC	Hb 12 g/dl
	WCC 7×10^9/l
	Platelets 140×10^9/l
Clotting	PT 13 s (control 12 s)
	APTT 59 s (control 40 s)
Anti-nuclear antibody factor	Not detected
Double-stranded DNA	Not detected

1. What is the diagnosis?
2. List three tests you would perform to confirm the diagnosis.
3. Apart from thrombotic tendencies, list other manifestations of this condition.

Answer 16

1. Acute cholecystitis.
2. Ultrasound of the liver.
3. Right upper lobe pneumonia.
4. Chronic tubulointerstitial nephritis or renal papillary necrosis leading to impaired concentrating ability.

Sickle cell anaemia is discussed in detail in Answer **102**, page 134. This question tests the reader's knowledge of complications secondary to sickle cell anaemia.

The story is typical of cholecystitis which, in this case, is secondary to pigment gall stones. Hepatic infarction due to a sickling crisis in the liver is unlikely because it would be associated with a higher AST. Sequestration is also unlikley because it is very rare in older patients with sickle cell anaemia. The shadowing on the chest X-ray is most probably secondary to streptococcal pneumonia. Patients with sickle cell anaemia are hyposplenic as a result of autosplenic infarction. As a result, they are predisposed to bacterial infections by capsulated organisms such as *Streptococcus pneumoniae*, *Neisseria meningitidis* and *Haemophilus influenzae*. Pulmonary infarction may also cause pulmonary shadowing on the chest X-ray but is less likely in the absence of pleurisy, and severe breathlessness.

Sickle cell anaemia is inherited as an autosomal recessive condition. A point mutation in the β globin gene leads to the substitution of glutamine by valine at position 6. In the deoxygenated state, this leads to sickling of cells. Chronic low-grade haemolysis is common and predisposes to pigment gall stones. Painful sickle cell crises are due to occlusion of small vessels, producing severe pain from affected organs. The bones are most commonly involved, particularly those of the digits of the hands and feet. Other crises include haemolytic, aplastic and sequestration crises (*Table*). An aplastic crisis may complicate infection with parvovirus B17. Sequestration crises are fatal and usually occur in young patients.

Precipitating factors for sickling include hypoxia, infection, dehydration, and pain.

Sickle cell crises
Thrombotic (hand foot syndrome, abdominal pain, pulmonary infarction and strokes)
Haemolytic
Aplastic
Sequestration

Answer 17

1. Antiphospholipid syndrome.
2. i. Antiphospholipid antibodies (these may result in a false positive VDRL test).
ii. Failure of APTT to improve after addition of normal plasma.
iii. Lupus anticoagulant.
3. Any of the following:
i. Recurrent abortions.
ii. Livedo reticularis.
iii. Pulmonary hypertension.
iv. Transient ischaemic attacks.
v. Chorea.
vi. Migraines.
vii. Valvular heart disease.
viii. Thrombocytopenia.

The antiphospholipid syndrome usually affects young women and is characterized by arterial and venous thromboses and recurrent abortions. In addition, there may be evidence of thrombocytopenia. The condition is caused by circulating antiphospholipid antibodies, which are IgG and IgM immunoglobulins directed against phospholipid molecules. They were first described in SLE, but may be present in a wide variety of autoimmune conditions and have also been associated with multiple sclerosis, acquired immunodeficiency syndrome (AIDS) and carcinomatosis. The antibodies may occur in isolation – the antiphospholipid syndrome. Cross-reaction with other antiphospholipid antibodies produces a false-positive Wassermann (VDRL) test. Some antibodies have an anticoagulant effect on coagulation tests *in vitro*, characterized by a prolonged APTT (with or without a minor prolongation of the PT time) which fails to correct after addition of normal plasma, suggesting the presence of a coagulation inhibitor. These antibodies are termed the 'lupus anticoagulant'. Despite the *in vitro* effect, the presence of the lupus anticoagulant has the opposite effect *in vivo*, and predisposes affected individuals to recurrent thrombotic events. Recurrent abortions are thought to be due to placental infarction. Other recognized associations of the antiphospholipid syndrome have been mentioned (see Answer **3**, page 12). The diagnosis is made by detection of antiphospholipid antibodies in the serum. Specific tests for detection of the lupus anticoagulant antibodies are also available. A negative VDRL and absence of circulating lupus anticoagulant does not exclude the presence of antiphospholipid antibodies. Management is with prophylactic anticoagulant therapy.

Question 18

A 35-year-old male was seen in clinic with a 12-year history of back ache. He was a keen football player, but for over 11 years had not participated in sport due to the disabling pain. He had been seeing an osteopath for almost 10 years. His back pain was originally controlled, but had now become unbearable. He had pain in his lower and upper back which was worsened by movement of the spine. Over the past two years he had noticed intermittent pain and swelling in both his knees which had responded to ibuprofen. There was no history of diarrhoea, skin rashes or mouth ulcers. He experienced transient dysuria after a trip to Amsterdam at the age of 21, but this cleared after a course of penicillin from his doctor. There was no family history of back pain.

On examination, he was in pain. He had lost his lumbar lordosis. Examination of his eyes and ear are shown (**18a, b**). His knee joints were swollen, with bilateral effusions; examination of the rest of his joints was normal. Cardiovascular, respiratory, abdominal and neurological examinations were all normal.

Investigations are shown

FBC	Hb 15 g/dl
	WCC 10×10^9/l
	Platelets 230×10^9/l
ESR	30 mm/h
Biochemistry	Calcium 2.3 mmol/l
	Phosphate 0.8 mmol/l
	Alkaline phosphatase 90 u/l
	Albumin 40 g/l
X-ray of spine (**18c**)	
Urinalysis	Glucose ++
	Protein 0

1. What is the diagnosis?
2. How would you confirm the diagnosis?
3. How would you account for the result of urinalysis?

Answer 18

1. Alkaptonuria.
2. Urinary homogentisic acid level. Urine becomes dark on standing.
3. Homogentisic acid is a reducing substance and therefore gives a positive reaction to glucostix (Clinistix). Other substances which produce a false-positive glucostix test are shown (*Table*). Glucose oxidase (Clinitest) sticks do not give this false-positive reaction.

Alkaptonuria is inherited as an autosomal recessive trait. There is a deficiency in the enzyme, homogentisic oxidase, leading to accumulation of homogentisic acid in the urine and increased pigmentation (ochronosis) in cartilage and connective tissue. Urine becomes dark on standing due to oxidation and polymerization of homogentisic acid. Freshly voided urine appears normal in colour, so these patients do not often report dark urine. Abnormal pigmentation is found in the ear and sclerae (**18a**, **18b**) as well as articular cartilage (at surgery).

Premature arthritis predominantly affecting the back, and later the large joints, is the most serious manifestation of the disorder. Intervertebral disc calcification is characteristic of alkaptonuria and is seen on the spinal X-ray (**18c**). The knees are commonly affected. The sacro-iliac joints are spared. Calcification of the aorta is often seen on the chest X-ray.

A low-protein diet is recommended to reduce the amount of homogentisic acid, which is a breakdown product of tyrosine; however, this does not prove very effective.

Causes of a false-positive Clinistix test

Fructose
Pentose
Lactose
Salicylates
Ascorbic acid
Homogentisic acid

Question 19

An 18-year-old male was referred to the respiratory outpatient clinic with a three-year history of progressively increasing breathlessness. Until the age of 15 years he was able to participate in school sports, but since then he had noticed increasing fatigue and breathlessness on exertion. He was diagnosed as having exercise-induced asthma and was prescribed salbutamol and beclomethasone inhalers, with initial relief of his symptoms until he was 16 years of age when his symptoms started to deteriorate. At this stage he was seen by a hospital specialist who felt that he had resistant asthma and started him on a two-week trial of oral steroids, which proved to be successful. Subsequently, the dose of inhaled steroid was increased. Three months before coming to clinic his symptoms had deteriorated considerably. He was breathless on walking less than 200 metres on the flat at a slow pace. His appetite was reduced, and he had noticed that his ankles were swollen towards the end of the day.

He was a non-smoker, and had never consumed alcohol. He was currently at a college attempting to do his GCSE examinations, but was having considerable difficulty because of his illness. He was an only child. Both parents were well and had a shared business. They were non-smokers. The family had a pet budgerigar.

On examination, the patient was thin. He was below the 10th centile for weight, and on the 50th centile for height. He appeared very slightly jaundiced, but was not cyanosed or clubbed. His heart rate was 120 beats/min and regular. The blood pressure was 110/65 mmHg. The JVP was not elevated. The respiratory rate was 28/min. Chest expansion was symmetrical, but moderately reduced. The percussion note was resonant and auscultation revealed reduced breath sounds in the lungs, particularly at both bases. On examination of the abdomen, the liver edge was palpable 3 cm below the costal margin. In addition, the tip of the spleen was just palpable. There was no clinical evidence of ascites; however, there was pitting ankle oedema to the shins.

Investigations are shown.

FBC	Hb 17 g/dl	Chest X-ray (**19**)	
	WCC 9×10^9/l	Lung function	PEFR 200/min (predicted 550/min)
	Platelets 130×10^9/l		FEV$_1$ 2.0 l (predicted 4.2 l)
	MCV 100 fl		FVC 4.1 l (predicted 5.6 l)
Biochemistry	Sodium 135 mmol/l		TLC 7.5 l (predicted 6.4 l)
	Potassium 4.1 mmol/l		KCO 0.7 (predicted 1.6)
	Urea 3 mmol/l	Arterial blood gases	pH 7.34
	Creatinine 60 μmol/l		pO$_2$ 8.4 kPa
	Calcium 2.1 mmol/l		pCO$_2$ 5.6 kPa
	Phosphate 1.0 mmol/l		Bicarbonate 32 mmol/l
	Total protein 66 g/l		Base excess +10
	Albumin 31 g/l		
	Bilirubin 58 μmol/l		
	AST 49 u/l		
	Alkaline phosphatase 600 u/l		

1. What does the chest X-ray demonstrate?
2. What do the respiratory function tests reveal?
3. What is the cause of the abnormal liver function tests?
4. What is the unifying diagnosis?
5. Which single test would you request to confirm the diagnosis?
A. Sweat sodium concentration.
B. Liver biopsy.
C. Transbronchial lung biopsy.
D. Serum immunoglobulins.
E. Measurement of serum α-1 antitrypsin and its electrophoretic mobility.

Question 20

A 48-year-old baker presented with a right deep-vein thrombosis affecting the right calf. Apart from a swollen right calf, physical examination did not demonstrate any other abnormality.

Investigations are shown.

1. What is the haematological abnormality?
2. List at least three investigations you would perform to investigate the underlying cause.

Hb	18 g/dl
PCV	0.57
MCV	89 fl
WCC	9×10^9/l
Neutrophils	92%
Lymphocytes	8%
Monocytes	4%
Platelets	388×10^9/l
Blood film	Normal

Answer 19

1. Hyperinflated lung fields with significantly reduced lung markings at both lung bases.
2. An obstructive defect and markedly reduced KCO.
3. Cirrhosis of the liver.
4. α-1 antitrypsin deficiency.
5. E. Measurement of the serum α-1 antitrypsin and its electrophoretic mobility.

The combination of chronic lung disease and cirrhosis of the liver in a young patient should raise suspicion of two important diagnoses: α-1 antitrypsin deficiency; and cystic fibrosis. In this case, the chest X-ray is against the diagnosis of cystic fibrosis (**19**). Furthermore, the absence of cough productive of sputum is also against the diagnosis of cystic fibrosis.

α-1 antitrypsin deficiency is a rare autosomal recessive disorder due to a genetic abnormality on chromosome 14. The absence or reduced levels of this protease inhibitor leads to alveolar and liver damage. There are several different abnormal alleles for the gene. 'M' is the normal allele, and 'Z' and 'S' are the most frequently encountered abnormal alleles. The expression of each phenotype is suffixed by the letters 'Pi', which stand for protease inhibitor.

PiZZ and Pi null null are associated with a high risk of premature emphysema, but only the PiZZ genotype is associated with cirrhosis.

The majority of patients with α-1 antitrypsin levels of less than 20% present with emphysema in the fifth decade. Cirrhosis usually occurs at a young age, and patients with the PiZZ genotype may present with neonatal jaundice. The diagnosis is confirmed by measuring the levels of α-1 antitrypsin.

The respiratory manifestations are treated with some success by using synthetic α-1 antitrypsin, but the hepatic manifestation of this condition requires liver transplantation.

Genotype	α-1 antitrypsin levels
PiMM	Normal
PiSS	>50%
PiZZ	<10%
PiSZ	20%
Pi Null null	Nil

Answer 20

1. Secondary polycythaemia.
2. i. Red cell mass estimation.
ii. Arterial blood gases.
iii. Abdominal ultrasound with particular reference to the kidneys and the liver.
iv. α-fetoprotein.
v. Erythropoietin level.

The patient has an elevated haemoglobin and a raised PCV. The differential diagnosis is between pseudo-polycythaemia, primary polycythaemia (polycy-thaemia rubra vera) or a secondary polycythaemia. In pseudopoly-cythaemia, the Hb and the PCV are raised due to haemoconcentration resulting from any cause of reduced extracellular volume (dehydration, diuretics). Pseudopolycythaemia can be differentiated from true polycythaemia by red cell mass estimation, which will reveal a normal red cell volume to extracellular fluid volume ratio in pseudopolycythaemia, and a raised ratio in true polycythaemia. A popular cause of pseudo-polycythaemia in the MRCP and similar examinations is Gaissbock's syndrome, which occurs in middle-aged men who are usually obese and have a smoking history. In this case, the red cell volume is normal, but the plasma volume is reduced. True polycythaemia is divided into primary polycythaemia and secondary polycythaemia. The former is a result of a myeloproliferative disorder causing erythroid hyperplasia independent of raised circulating erythropoietin, and is better known as polycythaemia rubra vera. In addition to a raised Hb and red cell count, the white cells are also increased in 70% and the platelets in 50% of cases, and physical examination may demonstrate a palpable spleen. In contrast, secondary polycy-thaemia is due to raised levels of circulating erythro-poietin, either due to a physiological reason, for example, living at high altitude, chronic lung disease, or cyanotic heart disease, or due to inappropriate secretion of ery-thropoietin from various sources (*Table*). In this condition, the white cells and platelets are unaffected, and the spleen is not palpable.

When faced with a patient with raised Hb and PCV who also has raised white cells, platelets and a palpable spleen, the diagnosis is polycythaemia rubra vera. The investigation required to confirm the diagnosis is a bone marrow aspirate, which will show erythroid hyperplasia and increased megakaryocytes. The leucocyte alkaline phosphatase concentration is also increased. When the white cell and platelet counts are normal, and there is no evidence of splenomegaly, then secondary causes must be sought. The investigation of secondary causes is shown (**20**).

Important note: in polycythaemia rubra vera there is a

tendency to bleed. Many patients have occult bleeding from the gastrointestinal tract, and have normal Hb and a high red cell count, but microcytic red cell indices. In these patients, the clue that they may have polycythaemia rubra vera comes from the elevated white cell and platelet counts (see 87, page 114).

Causes of polycythaemia

Pseudopolycythaemia
Dehydration
Gaissbock's syndrome

Primary
Polycythaemia rubra vera

Secondary
1. Physiological increase in erythropoietin (due to chronic hypoxaemia):
Chronic lung disease
Living at high altitudes
Cyanotic heart disease
Smoking (carboxyhaemoglobin)
Familial (HbM)

2. Inappropriate increase in erythropoietin:
Renal cell carcinoma, polycystic kidneys, transplant kidney
Adrenal tumours (phaeochromocytoma)
Hepatocellular carcinoma
Ovarian fibroma
Cerebellar haemangioblastoma (part of Von Hippel–Lindau)

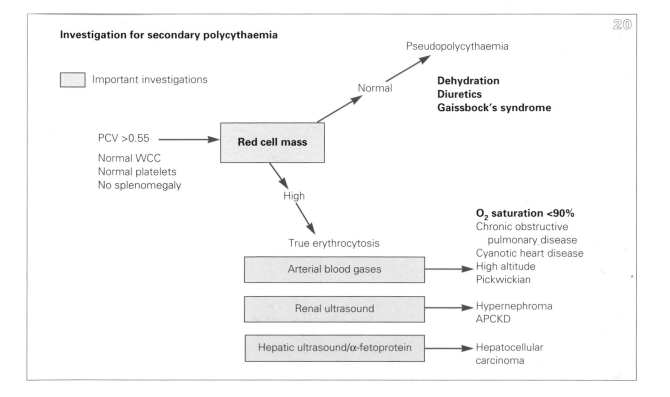

Investigation for secondary polycythaemia

20

☐ Important investigations

PCV >0.55 → **Red cell mass**

Normal WCC
Normal platelets
No splenomegaly

Normal → Pseudopolycythaemia
**Dehydration
Diuretics
Gaissbock's syndrome**

High → True erythrocytosis

Arterial blood gases → **O_2 saturation <90%**
Chronic obstructive pulmonary disease
Cyanotic heart disease
High altitude
Pickwickian

Renal ultrasound → Hypernephroma
APCKD

Hepatic ultrasound/α-fetoprotein → Hepatocellular carcinoma

Question 21

A 62-year-old former insurance broker presented to the cardiology out-patient clinic with a five-week history of increasing breathlessness and ankle swelling which started while on a three-week holiday in Spain. Over the past three days he had become breathlessness at rest, and was having to sleep propped up on four pillows to help his symptoms. His general practitioner had commenced him on a small dose of diuretic, which had not made any difference. There was no history of chest pain and no coryzal illness over the past few months. Eight months previously he was diagnosed as having diabetes mellitus which was not well controlled on oral hypoglycaemic agents, and he had recently started insulin injections. The only other past medical history to note was intermittent pain and swelling in both knees which was helped by taking a NSAID. He was married and had three sons. He had never smoked, and consumed a very occasional glass of wine. There was a strong family history of diabetes and ischaemic heart disease. His father had died from 'heart failure'.

On examination, he was slightly tanned. He was breathless on mild exertion. His heart rate was 110 beats/min and regular. His blood pressure was 100/60 mmHg. Examination of the neck is shown (**21a**). The apex was displaced in the 6th intercostal space and anterior axillary line. On auscultation of the precordium there was a loud third heart sound, and a soft systolic murmur in the mitral area. Auscultation of the lung fields demonstrated basal inspiratory crackles bilaterally. The ankles were swollen. Abdominal examination revealed a palpable liver edge 4 cm below the costal margin, but there was no other palpable organomegaly.

Initial investigations are shown below.

The patient was treated with intravenous diuretics, and made a good recovery. He underwent invasive investigation (**21f, g**), and was discharged on an ACE inhibitor, frusemide and digoxin. He was reviewed in the cardiology clinic three months later when he complained of some right upper quadrant discomfort and that he had experienced three hypoglycaemic episodes following discharge. The examining cardiologist detected a palpable liver edge, but there was no obvious evidence of cardiac failure. Plans were made for him to have a liver ultrasound and to be reviewed again in three months. However, one week before his clinic appointment he was admitted with increasing right upper quadrant pain, abdominal distension and ankle oedema.

On examination, he had a heart rate of 100 beats/min and a blood pressure of 100/65 mmHg. The JVP was not raised and the heart sounds were normal. The abdomen was distended from ascites, and the ankles were swollen. Urinalysis was normal. The dose of his diuretics was increased and his ascites started to resolve. An abdominal ultrasound was performed. The ultrasound appearance, with the probe in the left lower costal margin, is shown (**21h**). A liver biopsy was also performed (**21i**).

FBC	Hb 14 g/dl
	WCC 10×10^9/l
	Platelets 158×10^9/l
	MCV 90 fl
Biochemistry	Sodium 134 mmol/l
	Potassium 3.5 mmol/l
	Urea 11 mmol/l
	Creatinine 110 µmol/l
	AST 100 u/l
	ALT 110 u/l
	Alkaline phosphatase 130 u/l
	Albumin 38 g/l
Blood glucose	6 mmol/l
ECG (**21b**)	
Chest X-ray (**21c**)	
Echocardiogram	Parasternal long-axis view(**21d**);
	four-chamber view (**21e**)

1. What was the original cause for this patient's admission?
2. What is shown on the chest X-ray?
3. What is the abnormality on the 12 lead ECG?
4. What does the echocardiogram demonstrate?
5. Which invasive investigation was performed during the initial hospital admission, and what did it demonstrate?
6. What is the most probable cause for the pain in his knees?
7. What was the cause of his second admission?
8. What is demonstrated on the abdominal ultrasound?
9. What is the stain used on the liver biopsy, and what is its significance?
10. What is the unifying diagnosis?
11. Suggest one therapeutic management step.
12. Suggest one non-therapeutic management step.

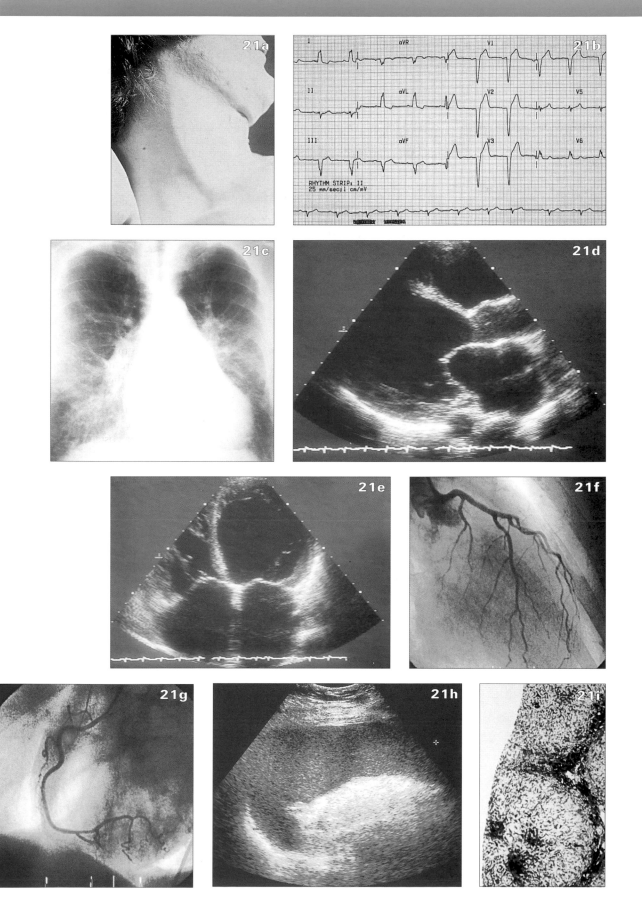

Answer 21

1. Congestive cardiac failure.
2. Cardiomegaly and pulmonary oedema.
3. LBBB (*Table A*).
4. Dilated left ventricle. The upper limit of normal size for the left ventricular end-diastolic dimension is 54 mm. Each white line on the scan represents 10 mm.
5. Coronary angiography which demonstrates a normal left and right coronary artery. See diagrammatic representation of the coronary anatomy (**21j**).
6. Chondrocalcinosis (*Table B*).
7. Cirrhosis of the liver complicated by portal hypertension.
8. Enlarged spleen which, in the presence of ascites, would be consistent with the diagnosis of portal hypertension in the context of this history.
9. Perl's stain, which is used to demonstrate the presence of iron. In the presence of iron, Perl's stain produces a dark blue/black colour.
10. Idiopathic haemochromatosis.
11. Weekly venesection until the serum ferritin is normal.
12. Screen his sons for the genetic disorder. This could be done genetically, or with iron studies. Affected asymptomatic relatives can thus be treated before there is any tissue damage.

Table A. Causes of LBBB

Ischaemic heart disease
Cardiomyopathy
Aortic stenosis
Hypertensive heart disease
Cardiac conduction tissue disease
Following insertion of a pacemaker

Table B. Causes of chondrocalcinosis

Calcium pyrophosphate arthropathy (pseudo gout)
Gout
Hyperparathyroidism
Haemochromatosis
Hypophosphatasia
Hypothyroidism
Wilson's disease
Alkaptonuria
Lead poisoning

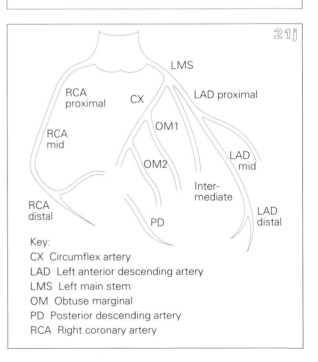

Key:
CX Circumflex artery
LAD Left anterior descending artery
LMS Left main stem
OM Obtuse marginal
PD Posterior descending artery
RCA Right coronary artery

In the absence of alcohol abuse, the combination of a dilated cardiomyopathy with normal coronary arteries, diabetes mellitus, arthropathy, and cirrhosis of the liver in a pigmented individual can all be explained by idiopathic haemochromatosis. Idiopathic haemochromatosis is an autosomal recessive genetic disorder characterized by increased iron absorption from the gastrointestinal tract with subsequent deposition in the skin, liver, heart, pancreas, gonads and the pituitary gland. The genetic defect is a point mutation on the gene HLA FE which is the short arm of chromosome 6. The mutation results in the substitution of the amino acid cysteine by tyrosine at position 282. The actual function of the gene is unknown. There is also an association with HLA-A3, B7 and HLA A3, B14. The most common presentation in homozygotes is with lethargy and malaise, although joint pains, particularly in the knee, symptoms of diabetes mellitus and skin pigmentation may also be the initial presenting complaints. Males are more susceptible than females who are protected by menstruation. Alcohol abuse may cause the same clinical picture in heterozygotes. Cardiac involvement leads to dilated or restrictive cardiomyopathy and an abnormal ECG, but haemochromatosis is a rare cause of cardiomyopathy. Deposition of excess iron in the liver leads to cirrhosis and an increased predisposition to hepatocellular carcinoma.

Chondrocalcinosis is a recognized complication, most commonly affecting the metacarpophalangeal and knee joints. Hypogonadism results from direct infiltration into the gonads and into the pituitary.

The diagnosis can be made genetically, but this is currently expensive and iron studies continue to remain the 'gold standard' test. The serum iron is high, the total iron-binding capacity is low, and the serum ferritin is

> **Table C. Differential diagnosis of conditions causing simultaneous cardiac and liver disease**
>
> | | *Liver* | *Heart* |
> | --- | --- | --- |
> | Alcohol abuse | Cirrhosis | Dilated cardiomyopathy |
> | Haemochromatosis | Cirrhosis | Dilated cardiomyopathy |
> | Pericardial constriction | Cirrhosis | Cardiac failure |
> | Chronic tricuspid regurgitation | Hepatic congestion | Cardiac failure |
> | Carcinoid tumour with hepatic metastases | Metastases | Pulmonary/tricuspid stenosis |
> | Sarcoidosis | Granulomas | Restrictive cardiomyopathy |
> | HIV | Hepatitis | Myopericarditis |
> | Neoplasia | Metastases | Pericardial effusion |
> | Storage disorders | Hepatic dysfunction | Cardiomyopathy |

usually in the thousands. The transferrin saturation or the iron-binding saturation index ([Fe]/[TIBC]) are very sensitive and are typically above 90% in patients with homozygous haemochromatosis. A liver biopsy demonstrates iron overload in the presence or absence of micronodular cirrhosis. There is deposition of iron in the liver parenchyma and the bile duct canaliculi, but the Kupffer cells are spared. A dry iron content of over 180 μg is highly suggestive of the diagnosis.

In some cases, idiopathic haemochromatosis is difficult to differentiate from alcoholic liver disease, which is also associated with raised serum ferritin levels and increased iron deposition in the liver. The liver biopsy is very helpful in this respect because it demonstrates coexisting changes of alcohol-related liver disease such as Mallory's hyaline and, in contrast to idiopathic haemochromatosis, iron deposition occurs in the Kupffer cells.

Question 22

A 55-year-old male was admitted with a three-month history of abdominal pain which was dull in nature and often radiated to his back. The pain was precipitated by meals and started 2 hours after eating. The patient had intermittent diarrhoea productive of foul, bulky stool, and had lost almost half a stone in three months. He was diagnosed as having non-insulin-dependent diabetes mellitus six years ago, and had an inferior myocardial infarction two years later. He smoked 20 cigarettes per day and had never consumed alcohol. There was a strong family of ischaemic heart disease. A barium meal and ultrasound of the hepatobiliary system was normal.

On examination, he was thin. The external appearance of his eyes is shown (**22**). There was no pallor, clubbing or lymphadenopathy. His heart rate was 98 beats/min and blood pressure 140/90 mmHg. The heart sounds were normal and his chest was clear. He had a soft left carotid bruit. On examination of his abdomen he was tender in the epigastrum and umbilical area. There were no abdominal bruits. Neurological examination was normal.

1. What is the diagnosis?
2. How would you confirm the diagnosis?

Answer 22

1. Mesenteric ischaemia. The differential diagnosis includes carcinoma of the pancreas or chronic pancreatitis.
2. Mesenteric angiography.

The patient has chronic abdominal pain after meals, steatorrhoea and weight loss. All three differential diagnoses could account for this picture. He has stigmata of hyperlipidaemia (the eyes reveal xanthelasma and corneal arcus) and peripheral vascular disease (carotid bruit). He is diabetic, and a long-term smoker. All these factors favour atherosclerosis, making the diagnosis of intestinal ischaemia more likely in the examination situation, although there is no reason why an arteriopath should not develop carcinoma of the pancreas or chronic pancreatitis which is idiopathic in almost 50% of cases. Severe atheroma affecting the coeliac axis would account for the symptoms. Increased intestinal motility after a meal exacerbates ischaemia, causing pain. The ischaemic small bowel loses functional capacity and therefore a malabsorption syndrome develops. The combination of fear of pain from eating and malabsorption are responsible for weight loss. Zollinger–Ellison syndrome can present with abdominal pain following meals and steatorrhoea; however, in this case the barium meal is invariably abnormal, revealing multiple gastric, duodenal or jejunal ulcers. The possibility of cholelithiasis is excluded by the normal hepatobiliary ultrasound.

Mesenteric ischaemia is essentially a diagnosis of exclusion. In this situation the patient would have a CT scan of the abdomen and an ERCP to check for carcinoma of the pancreas and chronic pancreatitis. If these tests are negative, mesenteric angiography would help validate the clinical suspicion of mesenteric ischaemia. Some patients can have severe atherosclerosis of the mesenteric arteries and be completely asymptomatic; therefore, this finding does not necessarily diagnose mesenteric ischaemia as the cause of his symptoms unless other potential causes have been excluded.

Question 23

A 34-year-old female was originally presented with a six-week history of epigastric pain that radiated to her back and which was precipitated by meals. There was no accompanying nausea or vomiting. Her general practitioner prescribed ranitidine and antacid solution, which relieved the discomfort to some extent. Just one month previously she had requested a blood sugar check because she had developed nocturia, but the test was normal. According to her husband, she had started to become miserable and spoke very little. She attributed this to fear of having an abdominal malignancy because her maternal aunt had just died from carcinoma of the stomach. The only other family history of significance was that her father had undergone an operation on his neck 20 years ago to treat kidney stones. She did not consume alcohol and was a non-smoker. She worked in a confectioner's shop near the house. She had two daughters, aged eight and six respectively.

On examination, the patient had mild tenderness on palpation of the epigastrum, but all other physical examination was normal.

Investigations are shown (right).

The patient underwent surgery shortly afterwards, which improved all her symptoms, and she remained well for six years; following this, the abdominal pain returned. The pain was associated with dyspepsia. She also complained of intermittent episodes of foul-smelling diarr-

hoea. She was prescribed ranitidine once again; however, on this occasion it proved to be ineffective. She was advised to stay on ranitidine and referred to a gastro-enterologist, who performed upper gastrointestinal endoscopy and demonstrated many small ulcers in the antrum of the stomach and the first and second part of the

FBC	Hb 12 g/dl
	WCC 7×10^9/l
	Platelets 380×10^9/l
	MCV 88 fl
ESR	11 mm/h
Biochemistry	Sodium 135 mmol/l
	Potassium 4 mmol/l
	Urea 7.1 mmol/l
	Creatinine 89 µmol/l
	Chloride 118 mmol/l
Biochemistry	Bicarbonate 19 mmol/l
	Calcium 3.0 mmol/l
	Phosphate 0.7 mmol/l
	Alkaline phosphatase 345 u/l
Blood glucose	4.6 mmol/l
Abdominal X-ray	Fecal loading, but no bowel obstruction
Urinary calcium	20 mmol/l

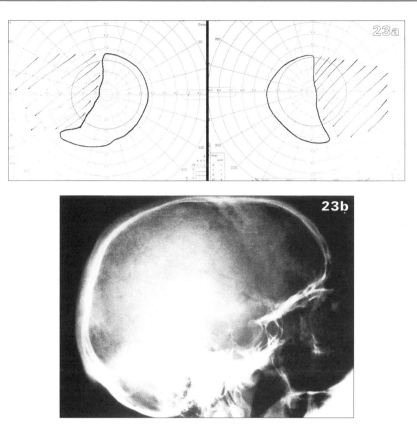

duodenum. A serum gastrin level was also performed which was 500 pg/ml (normal range <100 pg/ml). He commenced the patient on 40 mg of omeprazole, after which her symptoms improved. Her general practitioner had tried to reduce the dose to 20 mg after six weeks, but she started developing abdominal pain and the dose was raised back up to 40 mg.

The patient remained well for a further two years, after which she presented with increasing lethargy and headaches. She had stopped menstruating, and had reduced libido. Her appetite was reduced, but she had not lost any weight.

On examination, she was pale and had very scanty axillary and pubic hair. Her skin was dry. Her pulse was 62 beats/min and blood pressure 105/65 mmHg. Examination of her fundi showed slightly pale discs. Her visual fields are shown (**23a**). Neurological examination of her arms and legs and examination of the other systems was normal.

Investigations are shown (right).

FBC	Hb 10 g/dl
	WCC 6 × 10⁹/l
	Platelets 300 × 10⁹/l
	MCV 81 fl
ESR	25 mm/h
Biochemistry	Sodium 129 mmol/l
	Potassium 4 mmol/l
	Urea 4 mmol/l
	Creatinine 89 µmol/l
	Calcium 2.1 mmol/l
	Phosphate 1.2 mmol/l
	Alkaline phosphatase 92 u/l
Thyroid function	Thyroxine 4 nmol/l
	TSH 0.1 mu/l
FSH	0.3 u/l
LH	0.3 u/l
PRL	4,500 mu/l
Skull X-ray (**23b**)	

1. What was the initial diagnosis?
2. Which surgical procedure had her father undergone?
3. What was the cause of the pain six years later?
4. Which investigation would you have performed to confirm the diagnosis six years later?
5. What is the abnormality on the visual fields?
6. What is demonstrated on the skull X-ray?
7. What was the cause of her headaches?
8. Which single diagnosis accounts for all her presentations?
9. Should anyone else be investigated?

Answer 23

1. Hyperparathyroidism.
2. Parathyroidectomy.
3. Peptic ulceration resulting from a gastrinoma.
4. Assessment of serum gastrin after intravenous secretin or measurement of gastric acid output after the administration of pentagastrin. In normal individuals, secretin causes suppression of serum gastrin levels; however, in patients with gastrinomas, gastrin secretion is not suppressed and may even demonstrate a paradoxical rise. Pentagastrin reduces gastric acid production in normal individuals, but not in patients with gastrinomas.
5. The patient has a bitemporal hemianopia, suggesting a lesion compressing the optic chiasm. This could be a meningioma, an aneurysm, a pituitary tumour or a cerebral metastasis.
6. There is enlargement of the pituitary fossa, a double floor to the sella turcica and erosion of the posterior clinoid process. The findings are consistent with a pituitary tumour.

7. Raised intracranial pressure resulting from a large prolactinoma. A prolactinoma is the most common pituitary tumour associated with multiple endocrine neoplasia (MEN) 1. Prolactinomas are associated with amenorrhoea, galactorrhoea, hirsutism and infertility in females. In males, prolactinomas cause impotence, oligospermia, infertility and galactorrhoea. Note: hyperprolactinaemia does not cause gynaecomastia. There are several causes of raised PRL (*Table*), but a PRL of over 3,000 mu/l is highly suggestive of prolactinoma. Treatment is with bromocriptine for small tumours and surgery for larger ones.
8. Multiple endocrine neoplasia type 1.
9. The condition is autosomal dominant, so there is a 50% chance of her offspring inheriting the condition. Therefore, both daughters should be screened for the condition.

MEN 1 is characterized by tumours of the parathyroid gland (95%), islet cells (50%) and the pituitary gland (33%). Abnormality within a gene termed the menin gene on chromosome 11 is responsible, but the function of the gene is yet to be elucidated. Hypercalcaemia is the first presentation, usually from the third decade onwards. Islet cell tumours (usually gastrinomas or insulinomas) occur in the fourth or fifth decade, and pituitary tumours (usually prolactinomas) occur in the fifth or sixth decade.

Screening is with yearly calcium/PTH and PRL, and a two-yearly pituitary MRI. Patients are made aware of symptoms of islet cell tumours so that they present early.

Causes of hyperprolactinaemia

Prolactinoma
Hypothalamic or pituitary stalk lesions
Hypothyroidism
Coitus
Pregnancy
Nipple suckling
Stress
Oral contraceptive pill
Dopamine antagonist drugs, e.g. phenothiazines
PCOS
Chronic renal failure
Chest wall damage/trauma

Question 24

A 48-year-old male with rheumatoid arthritis presented with a cough, high fever and painless jaundice. He had a seven-year history of rheumatoid arthritis affecting his shoulders, elbows, wrists, hands and feet, and which was refractory to therapy with NSAID. Over the past 16 months, his symptoms had progressed, and he had been switched to immunosuppressant drugs which had controlled his symptoms. He was a non-smoker and consumed less than 2 units of alcohol per week.

On examination, he was unwell, jaundiced and had a temperature of 39°C (102.2°F). Examination of the oral cavity revealed candidal infection and palatal petechiae. On auscultation of the lung fields there were coarse crackles at the right lung base. On abdominal examination, there was evidence of a palpable spleen 3 cm below the costal margin.

Investigations are shown.

FBC	Hb 7.1 g/dl
	WCC $1.4 \times 10^9/l$
	Platelets $33 \times 10^9/l$
	MCV 103 fl
	Reticulocyte count <1%
INR	1.9
ESR	70 mm/h
CRP	190 g/l
Biochemistry	Sodium 136 mmol/l
	Potassium 4 mmol/l
	Urea 6 mmol/l
	Creatinine 110 µmol/l
	Bilirubin 180 µmol/l
	AST 180 u/l
	Alkaline phosphatase 450 u/l
	Albumin 29 g/l

1. Give three possible causes for this patient's presentation.
2. Which six investigations would you perform on admission?
3. Give three explanations for the raised MCV.
4. List two immediate management steps.

Question 25

The following cardiac catheter data is from a 10-year-old male after a murmur was heard during a school medical.

1. What are the two main abnormalities?
2. What is the diagnosis?

Chamber	Pressure (mmHg)	Oxygen saturation (%)
Right atrium	5	74
Right ventricle	20/6	74
Pulmonary artery	32/12	92
PCWP	3	
Left ventricle	100/8	96
Aorta	90/65	96

Answer 24

1. i. Septicaemia secondary to respiratory infection precipitated by methotrexate-induced neutropenia.
ii. Septicaemia secondary to respiratory infection precipitated by azathioprine-induced neutropenia.
iii. Septicaemia secondary to respiratory tract infection due to Felty's syndrome.
2. i. Chest X-ray.
ii. Oxygen saturation.
iii. Blood cultures.
iv. Urine culture.
v. Throat swab for culture.
vi. Hepatobiliary ultrasound.
3. i. Megaloblastic anaemia due to methotrexate or azathioprine.
ii. Megaloblastic anaemia due to folate deficiency (methotrexate inhibits dihydrofolate reductase).
iii. Liver cirrhosis.
4. i. Stop immunosuppressant drug.
ii. Broad-spectrum intravenous antibiotics following a septic screen. Usually the combination of a penicillin and aminoglycoside or a third line cephalosporin is used.

This patient with rheumatoid arthritis presents with a respiratory tract infection and high fever. The blood tests reveal a profound neutropenia which has almost certainly predisposed him to the respiratory and oral *Candida* infection. In the context of rheumatoid arthritis, the neutropenia is either drug-induced or secondary to hypersplenism (part of Felty's syndrome). Felty's syndrome alone cannot explain the abnormal bilirubin and alkaline phosphatase which, in the absence of abdominal pain, suggests either a cholestatic hepatitis or cirrhosis of the liver. Both methotrexate and azathioprine, which are sometimes used as immunosuppressants in rheumatoid arthritis, may also cause hepatitis and cirrhosis. The mode of action of these drugs is to interfere with purine nucleotide synthesis required for nucleic acid generation. All cells in the body with a rapid turnover time are affected, particularly the cells in the marrow – hence the pancytopenia. The raised MCV is due to a megaloblastic anaemia, but may be due to chronic liver disease.

Methotrexate-induced liver cirrhosis only complicates 1% of all patients taking the drug. Liver disease is more common in patients consuming over 10 units of alcohol per week, patients with diabetes and patients taking the drug frequently. In the early stages, the symptoms are non-specific and comprise anorexia and nausea; however, late disease presents with portal hypertension, varices or hepatocellular failure. Azathioprine-induced hepatitis is rare but may occur early in patients taking allopurinol, as the latter drug potentiates the effects of azathioprine.

The immediate management of this patient is a septic screen (blood cultures, urine culture, throat and nasal swabs) followed by broad-spectrum antibiotics. Be careful when performing blood gases in a patient with low platelets and abnormal clotting. Oxygen saturation using a pulse oximeter is the safest method of determining arterial oxygenation in this case. An ultrasound of the biliary system should be requested to exclude biliary obstruction.

Answer 25

1. i. Elevated pulmonary artery pressure.
ii. Step up in oxygen saturation in the pulmonary artery.
2. The findings are consistent with a patent ductus arteriosus with a left-to-right shunt.

Question 26

A 25-year-old male presented to the accident and emergency department with a three-day history of pleuritic, left-sided chest pain and increasing breathlessness. The symptoms started suddenly while he was playing football. He denied any chest trauma. Until then he had been fit and well, and there was no past medical history of note. His father died suddenly at the age of 32 years.

On examination, he was thin and tall and distressed with pain. There was no pallor or cyanosis. He had a wide arm span. The heart rate was 100 beats/min and blood pressure 150/80 mmHg. The respiratory rate was 32/min. The trachea was deviated to the right. Percussion appeared to be reduced on the right side and was loud on the left side. The left lung base was dull to percussion. On auscultation of the lung fields breath sounds were absent on the left side and normal on the right side. Auscultation of the precordium demonstrated quiet heart sounds and a soft mid-systolic murmur. The femoral pulses were easily palpable. The left calf was bruised and slightly tender. He attributed this to an injury sustained during the football match.

The ECG revealed normal sinus rhythm. The ECG complexes were small, but there were no other abnormalities.

1. Which test would you perform to reach a diagnosis?
2. What is the cause of his respiratory symptoms?
3. What is the management?
4. What is the unifying diagnosis?

Question 27

A 66-year-old female was investigated for a six-month history of increasing breathlessness and palpitation. She had a long history of hypertension. A chest X-ray (27a), ECG (27b), M-mode and 2-D echocardiograms (27c, 27d, respectively) are shown.

1. What does the chest X-ray reveal?
2. What is the abnormality on the ECG?
3. List two abnormalities on the 2-D echocardiogram.
4. List four abnormalities on the M-mode echocardiogram.
5. Which three pharmacological agents would you prescribe for this patient?

Answer 26

1. Chest radiography.
2. A large, left-sided pneumothorax.
3. Insertion of a chest drain.
4. Marfan's syndrome

A large pneumothorax in a symptomatic patient receives relief with chest drain insertion rather than simple needle aspiration.

Pleuritic chest pain and increasing breathlessness occur in pleurisy with or without pleural effusion, pneumonia, pulmonary embolism and lung malignancy. The physical signs are suggestive of a large left pleural effusion. The trachea is deviated to the right, and there are no breath sounds on auscultating the left lung. The right lung sounds comparatively dull to percussion when compared with the left lung, which is hyper-resonant. There also appears to be a small effusion at the left lung base which is not uncommon with pneumothoraces and represents either blood or an inflammatory exudate.

Causes of pneumothorax include asthma, emphysema, stab wound to the lung or following a fractured rib, fibrotic lung disease, suppurative lung disease (rupture of a lung abscess into a bronchus, staphylococcal pneu-monia), pneumoconiosis, neurofibromatosis, tuberose sclerosis, Marfan's syndrome, Ehlers–Danlos syndrome, and lymphangioleiomyomatosis. Most cases are idiopathic and occur in tall, thin men. A rare form, usually left-sided, occurs in women during menstruation (cata-menial pneumothorax). It is possibly due to pulmonary endometriosis.

The underlying diagnosis and the cause of the pnemo-thorax in this case is Marfan's syndrome. This is suggested by his tall height, cardiac mumur consistent with mitral valve prolapse and a possible family history of the condition, i.e. his father died premaurely. The syndrome is caused by a mutation in the gene encoding the connective tissue protein fibrillin on chromosome 15. The condition is inherited as an autosomal dominant trait. Affected individuals are tall, have a wide arm span, arachnodactyly and skeletal deformities which include kyphoscoliosis, high arched palate, and pectus excavatum. The joints are hyperextensile. Other associations include lens dislocation and retinal detachment. Mitral valve prolapse and aortic dilatation are recognised cardiac manifestations. Aortic dissection or rupture are the commonest cause of death. Patients with Marfan's syndrome have a higher incidence of pneumothorax than the general population.

Answer 27

1. An enlarged cardiothoracic ratio and evidence of an enlarged left atrium.
Features of an enlarged left atrium include a prominent left heart border, a double shadow at the front of the heart, splaying of the carinii, and sometimes elevation of the left hilum.
2. Atrial fibrillation (for causes, see *Table*, Answer **35**, page 54). There is a complete absence of P-waves and a beat-to-beat variation of the RR-interval. This patient also has voltage criteria for left ventricular hypertrophy, presumably secondary to the hypertension or coexisting mitral regurgitation.
3. i. Enlarged left atrium.
ii. A thickened dome-shaped appearance of the mitral valve in diastole which is consistent with mitral stenosis.
4. i. Thickening of the anterior mitral valve leaflet which is characterized by loss of its normal 'M'-shape in diastole.
ii. Multiple echoes on the anterior mitral valve leaflet which suggest fibrosis.
iii. Reduced mitral valve excursion.
iv. Anterior movement of the posterior leaflet in diastole (in normal individuals the posterior leaflet moves backwards in diastole). (See Echocardiography, page 223.)
5. i. Digoxin to control ventricular rate.
ii. Frusemide to help improve breathlessness from pulmonary congestion.
iii. Warfarin as a prophylaxis to thromboembolism.
Patients with mitral stenosis and atrial fibrillation have a 35% chance of having an embolic CVA per annum.

Question 28

A 47-year-old business male was referred to dermatology clinic with a rash over his hands, scalp and face. He had been generally well. He smoked 20 cigarettes per day and drank 8–10 units of alcohol on a daily basis. There was no other significant medical history of note. The patient had not taken any medication, with the exception of occasional chlorpheniramine to help relieve his symptoms.

On examination, he had vesicular lesions affecting his face, forearms, hands (28) and scalp. All other physical examination was essentially normal.

Investigations are shown.

FBC	Hb 18.5 g/dl
	WCC 7 × 10⁹/l
	Platelets 149 × 10⁹/l
	MCV 101 fl
Biochemistry	Sodium 135 mmol/l
	Potassium 3.9 mmol/l
	Urea 4 mmol/l
	Creatinine 80 µmol/l
	Blood glucose 10 mmol/l
Bilirubin	25 µmol/l
AST	52 u/l
Alkaline phosphatase	450 u/l
Albumin	37 g/l
Globulins	30 g/l
Gamma GT	52 u/l
Serum ferritin	550 µg/l
Skin biopsy	Subepidermal blisters with perivascular deposition of PAS-staining material

1. What is the most probable diagnosis?
2. State two tests to confirm the diagnosis.
3. What two factors should this patient avoid?
4. Apart from avoidance, give two other therapeutic measures.

Question 29

A 13-year-old female is admitted under the surgeons with acute abdominal pain. The blood pressure was 100/60 mmHg.

Investigations are shown.

1. What is the acid–base disturbance?
2. What is the most likely cause for the abnormality?
3. List three therapeutic management steps.

Biochemistry	Sodium 131 mmol/l
	Potassium 7.2 mmol/l
	Urea 13 mmol/l
	Creatinine 121 µmol/l
Biochemistry	Bicarbonate 8 mmol/l
	Chloride 96 mmol/l
Abdominal X-ray	Normal
Urinalysis	Glucose +++

Answer 28

1. PCT.
2. i. Urinary uroporphyrin level.
ii. Uroporphyrin decarboxylase assay on red blood cells.
3. i. Sunlight.
ii. Alcohol.
4. i. Venesection.
ii. Chloroquine.

The blistering skin rash in a patient with a history of excess alcohol consumption and biochemical evidence of liver disease is suggestive of the diagnosis of PCT.

PCT is a rare disorder of haem synthesis which is inherited as an autosomal dominant trait. It is one of the most commonly tested porphyrias in higher medical examinations, and is caused by a reduced activity or complete absence of the enzyme, uroporphyrin decarboxylase, which catalyses the conversion of uroporphyrin to coproporphyrin. This leads to an excess of uroporphyrins in the blood and urine. The result is a pruritic photosensitive blistering rash which affects areas exposed to the sunlight, and cirrhosis of the liver. Blisters on the skin lesion contain PAS-positive material. The clinical effect of this deficiency becomes most apparent in genetically predisposed patients who consume excess alcohol or other drugs which are enzyme inducers for haem synthesis (most commonly anticonvulsants and oestrogens). Hepatic involvement is common and is predominantly due to the effects of excess alcohol. The liver biopsy demonstrates macronodular cirrhosis and Mallory's hyaline. A proportion of patients with liver disease also have evidence of iron overload in the blood and liver resulting in a raised serum ferritin and a positive Perl's stain on liver biopsy, respectively; in addition, approximately 20% develop diabetes mellitus. The condition may be confused with haemochromatosis (iron overload, cirrhosis and diabetes); however, haemochromatosis is not associated with a blistering rash. A secondary polycythaemia may also occur and appears to compound the condition.

Treatment is by abstaining from alcohol and avoiding sunlight. In patients with a high Hb, weekly venesection (not more than 1 unit) until the Hb is less than 12 g/dl helps to alleviate the skin manifestations. Chloroquine is commonly used in the management of PCT. It binds uroporphyrin and helps urinary clearance.

Answer 29

1. Metabolic acidosis with a high anion gap.
2. Diabetic ketoacidosis.
3. i. Intravenous calcium gluconate to prevent hyperkalaemic cardiac arrest.
ii. Intravenous insulin infusion to halt further ketoacidosis.
iii. Intravenous saline to rehydrate patient and correct acidosis.

The patient has a very low serum bicarbonate, which is indicative of a metabolic acidosis. The heavy glycosuria is the clue to the cause of the acidosis. Diabetic ketoacidosis is the result of insulin deficiency. It may occur in previously undiagnosed insulin-dependent diabetes mellitus, established insulin-dependent diabetics who are on suboptimal insulin doses or who have interrupted insulin therapy, and insulin-dependent diabetics who have intercurrent illness resulting in increases in hormones which antagonize the effects of insulin. In the absence of insulin, hepatic gluconeogenesis is increased, but peripheral glucose uptake is decreased; the result is an osmotic diuresis and dehydration. Peripheral oxidation of free fatty acids is increased, which results in an increase in ketones, leading to a metabolic acidosis. Both the acidosis and hypoperfusion of the kidneys due to hypovolaemia contribute to the hyperkalaemia (reduced potassium excretion). Treatment involves rehydration and insulin replacement. If the serum potassium is above 6.8 mmol/l, calcium gluconate is advised to prevent hyperkalaemia-induced cardiac arrest. Intravenous bicarbonate should only be given if the arterial pH is less than 7. (See Acid–base Disturbance, page 228.)

Question 30

A 14-year-old male was admitted with a headache and drowsiness. Three days previously he had complained of a sore throat.

Investigations are shown.

CT scan of brain	Normal
CSF	Opening pressure
	160 cm H_2O
Cells	200 neutrophils/mm^3
	20 red cells/mm^3
	Protein 1.2 g/l
	Glucose 2.4 mmol/l
Gram stain (**30a**)	

1. What is the diagnosis?
2. What is the management?

Question 31

A 64-year-old West Indian male was admitted after his daughter noted that he had become increasingly drowsy over the past 48 hours. He had a 10-year history of diabetes mellitus for which he was taking chlorpropamide. Before the deterioration, he had complained of increasing urinary frequency and excessive thirst. He recently saw his general practitioner, and was noted to have a blood pressure of 170/100 mmHg for which he had been commenced on a thiazide diuretic.

On examination, he was drowsy and apyrexial, but answered questions appropriately. There was reduced skin turgor. The heart rate was 110 beats/min and regular, and the blood pressure was 115/60 mmHg. The heart sounds were normal, and the chest was clear. Examination of the abdomen did not reveal any abnormality, and there was no focal neurological deficit.

Investigations are shown.

FBC	Hb 15 g/dl
	WCC 13 × 10^9/l
	Platelets 179 × 10^9/l
Biochemistry	Sodium 151 mmol/l
	Potassium 5 mmol/
Biochemistry	Urea 17 mmol/l
	Creatinine 140 µmol/l.
Urinalysis	Glucose +++
	Protein +

1. What is the diagnosis?
2. List six investigations which should be performed on this patient.
3. List four steps in your management.

Answer 30

1. Streptococcal meningitis.
2. Intravenous cefotaxime on admission. The antibiotic can be switched to benzylpenicillin if the organism is sensitive to penicillin.

The CSF neutrophil count is consistent with a bacterial meningitis (see Answer **106**, page 138). The three commonest bacterial meningitides worldwide include those due to *Streptococcus pnemoniae*, *Neisseria menigitidis*, and *Haemophilus influenzae*. The Gram stain reveals Gram-positive (stain blue-purple) cocci, therefore the most likely diagnosis is *S. pnuemoniae*.

N. menigitidis is a Gram-negative (stains pink) diploccocus (**30b**). *H. influenzae* is a Gram-negative bacillus (pink rods in **30c**).

All three present with fever, headache, neck stiffness and photophobia. A necrotic purpuric rash is characteristic of menigitis due to *N. meningitids*, but may occur with all three types.

Answer 31

1. Hyperosmolar non-ketotic diabetic coma (HONK).
2. i. Plasma osmolality.
ii. Blood glucose.
iii. Blood cultures.
iv. Urine culture.
v. Chest X-ray.
vi. ECG.
3. i. Rehydration with 0.45% saline.
ii. Insulin infusion of 1–3 units/hour.
iii. Anticoagulation.
iv. Treat underlying cause.

Hyperosmolar non ketotic diabetic coma usually complicates middle-aged or elderly patients with non-insulin-dependent diabetes mellitus and is characterized by a marked increase in blood glucose (usually higher than 50 mmol/l) and a consequent increase in plasma osmolality. Ketonuria is absent and acidosis is mild or absent. The actual pathogenesis of the condition is unclear, but possible triggers include consumption of large amounts of sugary drinks, infection, recent prescription of thiazide diuretics or steroids, and myocardial infarction. Patients present with thirst, polyuria, impaired level of conscious-ness and sometimes evidence of the precipitating disorder.

Investigations reveal a high blood glucose and plasma osmolality. The plasma sodium is usually elevated due to pure water loss from osmotic diuresis; however, it may be falsely low (pseudohyponatraemia) due to the presence of excess lipids. The serum pH is usually normal, but the patient may have a mild acidosis. Other investigations which should be performed are an infection screen and an ECG (beware of silent myocardial infarction in a diabetic patient!).

Management includes rehydration with saline. In cases of severe hypernatraemia (sodium >150 mmol/l), half-strength saline is used. Insulin is infused carefully as HONK is more sensitive to insulin than diabetic ketoacidosis. The patient is given 4 units immediately followed by an infusion of 1–3 units per hour. The aim is to reduce the plasma osmolality by approximately 3 mOsm per hour. A rapid reduction in plasma osmolality is dangerous because it may precipitate cerebral oedema. Bicarbonate infusion is not required. Prophylactic anticoagulation with heparin is recommended because the high glucose concentration and dehydration results in hyperviscosity. After treatment of the acute state the patient should be recommenced on an oral hypoglycaemic agent.

Question 32

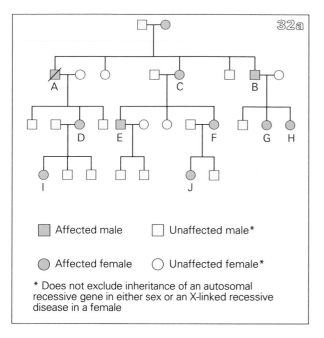

Affected male □ **Unaffected male***

Affected female ○ **Unaffected female***

* Does not exclude inheritance of an autosomal recessive gene in either sex or an X-linked recessive disease in a female

The chart above (**32a**) is the pedigree of a family with a rare condition. All members are affected by the same condition. Patient A is dead, but he had a history of progressive renal failure, and had a renal transplant which was affected by a separate renal disease causing haematuria and rapid deterioration of renal function. An audiogram and a picture of his fundus have been removed from his case notes and are shown (**32b, c**). His sister (patient C), aged 70 years, was deaf and had intermittent haematuria, but her creatinine was 89 μmol/l. His brother (patient B), aged 65 years, had a renal transplant 14 years previously and was also deaf. Patients D, F, G, H, I and J all had a history of intermittent haematuria, but serum creatinine was within the normal range in each case. Patients D and H had premature cataracts, and patient J was blind, but did not have cataracts. Patient E was aged 38 and was on the transplant list for renal failure. He had been fitted with a hearing aid aged 26 years, and had had intermittent haematuria since he was aged 7 years.

1. What is the mode of transmission of the disorder?
2. What is shown on the audiogram?
3. Why may patient J have been blind?

4. What is the underlying condition in the affected members of this family?
5. Which renal disease did patient A develop in his transplanted kidney?

Question 33

A 45-year-old male attended to become a blood donor. Blood results were as follows (0 = no agglutination, + = agglutination):

1. What is the patient's blood group?
2. Give at least two possible underlying diagnoses.

Patient's cells against anti-A = 0
Patient's cells against anti-B = 0
Patient's cells against anti-A and anti-B = 0
Patient's serum against red cells with antigen A = 0
Patient's serum against red cells with antigen B = 0
Patient's cells against anti-D = +
Immunoglobulins: IgM 0.2 g/l; IgG 1.5 g/l; IgA 0.1 g/l

Answer 32

1. The mode of inheritance is X-linked dominant.
2. There is progressive and severe hearing loss at higher frequencies which is typical of sensorineuronal deafness. (See also Audiograms, page 218.)
3. It is possible that she had retinitis pigmentosa just like her great uncle (patient A).
4. The condition is Alport's syndrome.
5. Anti-GBM disease.

There is no male-to-male transmission which is characteristic of X-linked conditions. Affected males transmit the disease to all female offspring in conditions inherited by an X-linked dominant trait, whereas affected females pass the disease to 50% of all their offspring.

Alports's syndrome is an X-linked hereditary nephritis characterized by progressive glomerular disease, ocular and auditory abnormalities. The renal manifestations begin early in childhood, comprising asymptomatic haematuria and proteinuria. Progressive renal deterioration has a bimodal age distribution, presenting between 16–35 years and 45–60 years. Only males develop progressive renal failure. Affected females develop asymptomatic haematuria, but progression to renal failure does not occur. Sensorineuronal loss occurs in 30–50% of patients, and many patients have ocular abnormalities which include myopia, retinitis pigmentosa (**32c**) and cataracts. Renal biopsy reveals thinning of the GBM, but as the disease progresses the membranes become thin and start to split. The genetic defect is in the α-5 chain of type IV collagen which is located on the X chromosome, but collagen defects in the α-3 and α-4 chains of type IV collagen on chromosome 2 have also been described in some families. All three types of α chains combine to form the collagen network in the GBM. Some patients with Alport's syndrome develop anti-GBM antibodies after renal transplantation. The risk is greatest in patients with a large deletion in the gene encoding the α-3 chain of type IV collagen, in which case the Goodpasture antigen is not expressed and therefore the Goodpasture antigen in the transplanted organ is recognized as foreign. Some 5% of patients with transplants for Alport's syndrome will develop anti-GBM disease.

Answer 33

1. Blood group O rhesus-positive (absent anti-A and anti-B).
2. Hypogammaglobulinaemia due to:
i. Thymoma.
ii. Chronic lymphatic leukaemia.
iii. Myeloma.
iv. Lymphoma.
v. Drugs.
vi. Common variable hypogammaglobulinaemia.
vii. HIV infection.

The patient's red cells fail to agglutinate with sera containing anti-A and anti-B, suggesting that the patient is blood group O, i.e. the cells do not express the antigens A or B on the cell surface. His cells agglutinate with serum containing anti-D, indicating that his cells express the rhesus D antigen. Patients with blood group O have anti-A and anti-B antibodies which are of the IgG, IgM and the IgA class. The serum from an O-positive individual should normally agglutinate blood cells expressing antigens A and B, unless the antibodies are present in very low titre. Failure of the appropriate agglutination may arise in conditions predisposing to hypogammaglobulinaemia and with paraproteinaemias. In generalized hypogammaglobulinaemia the low levels of IgG, IgM and IgA are responsible for the poor response. With paraproteinaemias, one of the immunoglobulin subset levels may be elevated (usually IgG) due to autonomous production. These antibodies are monoclonal and are not directed towards any specific antigen. They are generally ineffective. Autonomous production of a monoclonal antibody also leads to paraparesis of the other immunoglobulin subtypes, causing further immunosuppression.

This man has evidence of hypogammaglobulinaemia. He is 40 years of age and is unlikely to have an inherited hypogammaglobulinaemia because one would associate this with a previous history of infections. An acquired hypogammaglobulinaemia is more likely, and examples include chronic lymphatic leukaemia, lymphoma, myeloma and thymoma.

Question 34

A 5-year-old male was admitted for investigation of ankle swelling and abdominal distension which had occurred over three months. His appetite was satisfactory, and there was no history of diarrhoea, breathlessness, arthralgia or syncope. He was born by a normal vaginal delivery and weighed 3.6 kg at birth. He was well as a neonate and had achieved his milestones normally thus far. Apart from having mild eczema there was no past medical history of note. His father was a solicitor, and his mother had just returned to full-time teaching after giving birth to his 16-month-old brother, who was the only other sibling. There was no history of travel abroad or any drug history.

On examination, he had facial swelling. There was no pallor or cyanosis. The most striking feature was pitting oedema of the lower limbs from the ankles to the thighs. The heart rate was 100 beats/min and regular. The blood pressure was 95/55 mmHg. The JVP was not raised. Palpation of the precordium was normal. On auscultation, heart sounds I and II were normal, but there was an additional third heart sound. Examination of the respiratory system revealed dullness to percussion at the right lung base and reduced air entry on auscultation. Abdominal examination demonstrated a non-tender, distended abdomen with shifting dullness. There was no palpable organomegaly.

Investigations are shown (first panel).

The patient was treated with 60 mg prednisolone and 40 mg frusemide. The oedema started improving after one week, and renal function remained normal. After two weeks he was discharged and seen at weekly intervals. In the sixth week the oedema had completely subsided, and his abdomen was soft and non-distended. A 24-hour urinary protein estimation was 0.7 g. The frusemide was stopped and plans were made to re-review the patient in two weeks, but three days later he was admitted with right upper quadrant pain and abdominal distension. On examination, the JVP was not raised. There was palpable tender hepatomegaly and shifting dullness. There was no lower-limb oedema.

Further investigations are shown (second panel).

FBC	Hb 10 g/dl
	WCC 5 × 10⁹/l
	Platelets 166 × 10⁹/l
	MCV 80 fl
Urinalysis	Microscopy revealed occasional transitional cells
	24-hour urinary protein 5.2 g
	Selective protein clearance ratio was low
Ascitic fluid	Protein 8 g/l
Chest X-ray	Normal
Biochemistry	Sodium 135 mmol/l
	Potassium 3.7 mmol/l
	Urea 2.1 mmol/l
	Creatinine 65 µmol/l
	Bilirubin 10 µmol/l
	AST 19 u/l
	Alkaline phosphatase 80 u/l
	Total protein 36 g/l
	Albumin 13 g/l
	Glucose 4 mmol/l

Biochemistry	Bilirubin 15 µmol/l
	AST 90 u/l
	Alkaline phosphatase 89 u/l
	Albumin 35 g/l

1. What was the original cause of oedema?
2. What was the subsequent cause of abdominal pain and distension?
3. List two tests which will help confirm the cause of abdominal pain.
4. In one step, what is the management?

Question 35

1. What is the rhythm disturbance in this rhythm strip (35)?

Answer 34

1. Nephrotic syndrome.
2. Hepatic vein thrombosis.
3. i. Ultrasound or CT scan of the liver looking particularly at the hepatic and portal veins.
ii. Liver biopsy.
4. Thrombolysis to prevent severe hepatic congestion.

The combination of hypoalbuminaemia, heavy proteinuria and oedema is strongly suggestive of the diagnosis of nephrotic syndrome, which, in young children is most often due to minimal change glomerulonephritis. Minimal change glomerulonephritis is thought to be an autoimmune disorder, and usually responds extremely well to steroids and other immunosupressants such as cyclophosphamide and chlorambucil. There is a well-recognized association of the disorder with Hodgkin's lymphoma, bee stings, cow's milk allergy and ingestion of NSAID. Minimal change nephropathy is found in 80% of children with nephrotic syndrome. Treatment is with high-dose steroids, and diuretics are often necessary to treat the oedema. Relapses are common and are treated with steroids until the urine is completely free of protein for three days. Steroids are prescribed for a maximum of four weeks. Recurrent relapses are managed with cyclo-

phosphamide or chlorambucil. Complications of nephrotic syndrome include susceptibility to infection due to loss of immunoglobulins in the urine, protein malnutrition, hyperlipidaemia, arterial and venous thromboses and acute renal failure.

Thrombosis is a frequent and serious complication. Corticosteroids and diuretic therapy contribute to thrombosis. Whole blood viscosity is increased, and there is alteration in the concentration of clotting factors in the blood. The levels of anti-thrombin III and plasminogen are reduced, increasing the tendency to thrombosis. In this case the onset of abdominal pain, tender right upper quadrant, ascites and abnormal LFT reflect hepatic vein or portal vein thrombosis. Patients may present rapidly with fulminant hepatic failure or with gradual-onset ascites and jaundice. Early revascularization with a thrombolytic agent is important to prevent hepatic infarction and fibrosis leading to chronic portal hypertension. In patients where thrombolysis is contraindicated, a shunt procedure is necessary.

The diagnosis can be confirmed by ultrasonography and Doppler. The hepatic veins, portal vein and inferior vena cava should be examined by venography. Liver biopsy helps make the diagnosis, and is also important to assess hepatic necrosis and fibrosis.

Answer 35

1. Atrial flutter with 2:1/3:1 atrioventricular block.

There is an irregular narrow complex tachycardia and the differential diagnosis is between atrial fibrillation, atrial flutter with varying atrioventricular block, and an atrial tachycardia with varying atrioventricular block. The clue is in the rhythm strip which reveals a 'saw-tooth' pattern to the ECG complexes, indicating flutter. The RR-interval is not constant; therefore there is flutter with varying block. In this case there are between two and three flutter waves between each RR-interval, and hence the diagnosis is atrial flutter with 2:1/3:1 atrioventricular block. The causes of atrial flutter are the same as those for atrial fibrillation. The most effective treatment for atrial flutter is DC cardioversion delivering small energy shocks between 50 and 100 J. Chemical cardioversion is difficult, but the most effective drugs for this purpose are flecainide and amiodarone. Like atrial fibrillation, patients with atrial flutter should be anticoagulated to prevent the risk of thromboembolism.

Causes of atrial flutter/fibrillation
Ischaemic heart disease
Hypertension
Mitral stenosis
Thyrotoxicosis
Myocarditis
Cardiomyopathy
Pericarditis
Bronchial carcinoma
Severe pneumonia
Chronic lung disease
Pulmonary emboli
Wolff–Parkinson–White syndrome
Alcohol abuse
Cocaine abuse

Question 36

A 66-year-old retired school teacher presented with a six-month history of progressive weakness, fatigue and breathlessness which was accompanied by weight loss of 5 kg. He had difficulty climbing stairs because his 'legs would not carry him', and had noticed that he had difficulty holding light objects with his left hand without dropping them. Over the past week his wife had noticed that his speech appeared slurred and nasal, and he was having difficulty swallowing his meals. He had a past history of pernicious anaemia for which he was taking regular intramuscular B_{12} injections. On examination, he was thin. There was no evidence of pallor or clubbing. The patient had dysarthria. Examination of the cranial nerves revealed normal eye movements, but tongue movement was sluggish and there was reduced palatal movement. The jaw jerk was brisk. On examination of his limbs there was wasting and fasciculation of the small muscles of the left hand. The tone and power in the left upper limb was generally reduced. The upper-limb reflexes were brisk. There was wasting and fasciculation in both thigh muscles. The tone was increased and the power was reduced. The ankle and knee jerks were brisk,

FBC	Hb 12 g/dl
	WCC 5 × 10⁹/l
	Platelets 180 × 10⁹/l
	MCV 86 fl
Biochemistry	Sodium 137 mmol/l
	Potassium 4.1 mmol/l
	Urea 6 mmol/l
	Creatinine 110 µmol/l
Chest X-ray	Normal

and there was obvious clonus at the ankle joint. Sensation was normal and Romberg's test was negative. Examination of the fundi revealed bitemporal pallor.

Investigations are shown.

1. What is the diagnosis?
2. Which two investigations could be performed to confirm your suspicion?

Question 37

An 86-year-old male was found collapsed in his home by his neighbour after his son raised concern about not being able to contact him by telephone. There was no significant past medical history. He was independent. He was last seen two days earlier when he joined his neighbour for Christmas dinner.

On examination, he was unconscious and had a Glasgow coma scale of 5 out of 15. There was no nuchal rigidity. Pupillary reflexes were sluggish, but examination of the fundi was normal. Tone was slightly increased in all the limbs. The peripheral reflexes were present and both plantar reflexes were flexor. The heart rate was 40 beats/min, and blood pressure was 80/40 mmHg. Heart sounds were normal, and the chest was clear.

An ECG was performed in the accident and emergency department (**37**).

1. List four abnormalities on the ECG.
2. Which single investigation should the medical officer have performed?
3. In one sentence, what is the management of this case?

Answer 36

1. Motor neurone disease.
2. i. Electromyography.
ii. Nerve conduction studies.

There is evidence of combined lower motor neurone and upper motor neurone lesions and a pseudobulbar palsy. There is no sensory abnormality, and ocular movements are normal. These findings are characteristic of motor neurone disease, which is characterized by a progressive degeneration of the motor neurones in the cortex, spinal cord and motor nuclei of the cranial nerves. The breathlessness is probably due to involvement of the respiratory muscles. The bitemporal pallor is a 'red herring', and although it may have led some readers to diagnose multiple sclerosis, it is important to note that bitemporal pallor is a normal finding in some individuals. Moreover, wasting and fasciculation are not features of multiple sclerosis because it does not affect lower motor neurones. Although the patient has a history of pernicious anaemia, his blood count does not suggest B_{12} deficiency and therefore subacute degeneration of the spinal cord is unlikely. The absence of a sensory neuropathy is also against the diagnosis.

The cause of motor neurone disease is unknown. In approximately 15% of cases the disease is familial and is due to mutations in the copper/zinc superoxide dismutase gene on chromosome 21. The incidence is 1/50,000, and the male-to-female ratio is 1.5:1. There are three distinct patterns known as progressive muscular atrophy, amyotrophic lateral sclerosis and progressive bulbar palsy which are characterized by predominantly lower motor lesions, predominantly upper motor neurone lesions, and bulbar and pseudobulbar palsy, respectively. Usually, a combination of all three is present. Female sex, bulbar onset and old age are poor prognostic markers. The disease usually progresses inexorably and death is usually from bronchopneumonia within five years of onset of symptoms.

The diagnosis is clinical, but electromyography characteristically reveals a reduced number of action potentials in the muscles which have an increased amplitude and duration. Nerve conduction studies reveal normal motor conduction and exclude an underlying neuropathy, particularly in patients with the progressive muscular atrophy variety of the disorder.

There are no curative therapies, but glutamate antagonists such as riluzole appear promising, as does ciliary neurotrophic factor, which has been shown to promote survival of cultured rat and human motor neurones. Both agents are currently being tested on affected humans.

Answer 37

1. i. Bradycardia.
ii. Tremor artefact.
iii. J-waves.
iv. Prolonged QT-interval.
2. Rectal (core) temperature with a low-reading thermometer.
3. Gradual rewarming using space blankets and possibly warmed intravenous fluids, depending on the severity of hypothermia.

Hypothermia is common among the elderly. It is usually attributable to cold environment (no heating at home), inadequate clothing, poor nutrition, neuroleptic drugs, alcohol and hypothyroidism. Hypothermia is defined as a fall in the core temperature to below 35°C (95°F). Severe hypothermia causes impaired consciousness and cardiac embarrassment. Bradycardia, hypotension, hypopnoea, sluggish pupillary and peripheral reflexes, muscle rigidity and coma are recognized features of severe hypothermia. Ventricular fibrillation and asystole are the usual causes of death.

ECG abnormalities include bradycardia, atrial fibrillation with a slow ventricular rate, prolonged PR- and QT-intervals and J-waves. A baseline artefact due to muscle tremor may also be seen, and should help make the diagnosis in the examination situation.

Gentle rewarming is indicated. If the temperature is above 32°C (89.6°F), space blankets and warm oral fluids are usually sufficient. If the temperature is lower than this, and the patient is unconscious, then warmed intravenous fluids should be given. In this situation there is a danger of severe metabolic acidosis due to sluggish circulation, which should be corrected promptly. The aim is to increase the temperature by 1°C (1.8°F) per hour.

Question 38

38a

A 21-year-old chef presented with a two-week history of general malaise, cough and headaches. He had just returned from a ten-day holiday in a hotel resort in Spain. He consulted his general practitioner on arrival, who diagnosed a respiratory tract infection and prescribed erythromycin. Despite this, the patient's symptoms continued to persist. He had now developed a foul-smelling, blood-stained nasal discharge and was deaf in his left ear. His cough was worse, but was non-productive. He felt 'hot and cold' and had a reduced appetite due to nausea. He was a non-smoker and consumed 20 units of alcohol per week.

On examination, he appeared relatively well. There was no skin rash, pallor, cyanosis, clubbing, lymphadenopathy or ankle oedema. He was tender over his frontal sinuses, and had crusting around the nasal septum on the right side. Inspection of the outer ears and tympanic membranes was normal. The Rinne's test revealed reduced air and bone conduction on the left side. Weber's test lateralized to the right side. Apart from the abnormal hearing tests, all other neurological examination was normal. The heart rate was 96 beats/min and blood pressure 140/90 mmHg. The patient was tachypnoeic on mild exertion, and had a respiratory rate of 20/min. Chest expansion was moderate. The trachea was central. On auscultation of the lung fields there was evidence of bronchial breathing at the left lung base and a few inspiratory crackles at the right lung base. Examination of the heart and abdomen was normal.

Investigations are shown.

FBC	Hb 11 g/dl
	WCC 14 × 10⁹/l
	(neutrophil leucocytosis)
	Platelets 480 × 10⁹/l
ESR	110 mm/h
CRP	209 g/l
Biochemistry	Sodium 134 mmol/l
	Potassium 4.1 mmol/l
	Urea 6 mmol/l
	Creatinine 89 µmol/l
Urinalysis	Protein +1
	Blood not detected
Chest X-ray (38a)	

1. Describe the abnormalities on the chest X-ray.
2. How would you interpret the findings from the Rinne's and Weber's tests?
3. Which two tests could you perform to help achieve the diagnosis?
4. What is the underlying diagnosis?

Answer 38

1. The chest X-ray demonstrates alveolar shadowing affecting the right middle and lower lobes and in the left lower lobe. In addition, there is a round cavitating lesion in the left lower lobe. The findings are consistent with either a purulent pneumonia with left lower lobe abscess formation, or pulmonary haemorrhage and a cavitating granuloma due to Wegener's granulomatosis.

2. The Rinne's test revealed reduced bone and air hearing conduction, suggesting sensorineuronal deafness on the left side. The Weber's test does not normally lateralize to either ear, but in this case it lateralized to the right. This is in keeping with sensorineuronal hearing loss in the left ear. Because both air and bone conduction are impaired in sensorineuronal deafness, the sound from the tuning fork (which is conducted via bone in the Weber's test) is heard loudest in the ear which is not affected. In the case of pure conduction deafness, the Weber's test lateralizes to the affected ear. Wegener's granulomatosis can produce conduction and sensorineuronal deafness by blockage of the Eustachian tube when it involves the upper respiratory tract and 8th cranial nerve, respectively.

3. i. Nasal or transbronchial lung biopsy.
ii. c-ANCA (anti proteinase 3).
4. Wegener's granulomatosis.

Wegener's granulomatosis is a necrotizing granulomatous vasculitis affecting the upper and lower respiratory tract and the kidneys, although several other organs can be affected. Granulomas occur in small arterioles. The diagnosis should be suspected when two of these systems are involved in the presence of systemic features such as malaise, night sweats, fever and weight loss. This patient has features of upper and lower respiratory tract involvement which include frontal sinusitis, purulent nasal discharge and nasal septal crusting, dry cough and evidence of gross respiratory involvement on the chest X-ray. The deafness in the left ear is indicative of 8th nerve involve-

ment. The kidneys do not appear to be significantly affected. The trace of protein may be a response to a febrile illness. Upper respiratory involvement can also lead to hoarseness and stridor due to vocal cord and tracheal involvement respectively, and lower respiratory involvement may present with pleurisy and haemoptysis. Renal involvement can vary from asymptomatic proteinuria and haematuria to fulminant renal failure due to crescentic glomerulonephritis. Other organs affected include the eye, cardiovascular system, central nervous system and the skin. In the eye, the disease can present with scleritis, uveitis and pseudotumour due to retro-orbital granuloma formation. Cardiovascular involvement is rare. The most common manifestation is pericarditis, but conduction tissue involvement produces tachy- and bradyarrhythmias. Involvement of the central nervous system is also rare and comprises a mononeuritis multiplex, isolated cranial nerve palsies, and meningeal involvement.

The diagnosis is based on demonstrating a necrotizing granulomatous vasculitis biopsy of the affected tissue. The best yield of a positive biopsy comes from the kidney or the lungs when they are involved. ANCA are present in over 80% of untreated cases. Immunofluorescence studies have revealed two main types of ANCA which are determined by the pattern of cytoplasmic staining. c-ANCA stains the outer cytoplasm, whereas p-ANCA stains the perinuclear cytoplasm. It is now clear that c-ANCA binds the enzyme proteinase 3 (PF3) and is specific for Wegener's granulomatosis, although it may be positive in some cases of polyarteritis nodosa. p-ANCA is heterogeneous. One subset binds the cytoplasmic enzyme MPO which is positive in microscopic polyangiitis and idiopathic crescentic glomerulonephritis. Other subsets of p-ANCA bind elastase, lactoferrin, lysozyme and cathepsin G and are present in a variety of autoimmune conditions including CAH, sclerosing cholangitis, ulcerative colitis and SLE (**38b**).

The management of Wegener's granulomatosis is with steroids and other immunosupressants such as cyclophosphamide. Disease progress is monitored by estimating ANCA titres. There is good correlation between ANCA titres and underlying inflammatory activity in most patients.

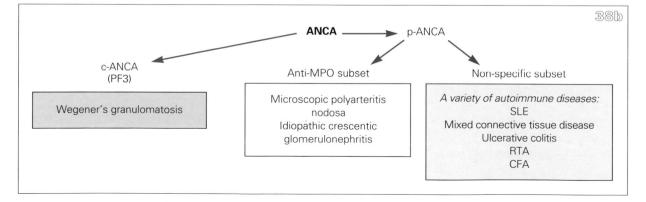

Question 39

A 28-year-old male presented with a three-day history of rigors and pleuritic pain affecting the left lung. There were signs of consolidation in the left lung. There was no evidence of lymphadenopathy or hepatosplenomegaly.

Investigations are shown.

1. What is the characteristic term given to this blood picture?
2. Which two features on the blood film would confirm your suspicions?

FBC	Hb 12 g/dl
	WCC $24 \times 10^9/l$
	Platelets $149 \times 10^9/l$
Blood film	Neutrophils 85%
	Normoblasts 7%
	Myeloblasts 3%
	Myelocytes 2%
	Lymphocytes 3%

Question 40

The following are serial LFT on a 51-year-old married school teacher who had a partial gastrectomy for a perforated peptic ulcer 10 years previously. He was asymptomatic. He was currently taking ranitidine. He consumed approximately 4 units of alcohol per week. Apart from very slight jaundice, the physical examination was normal.

LFT	1987	1988	1990	1992	1993
Alanine aminotransferase (normal 5–30 u/l)	30	36	40	44	49
Aspartate aminotransferase (normal 10–40 u/l)	42	65	69	73	78
Alkaline phosphatase (normal 25–115 u/l)	100	112	118	125	135
Bilirubin (normal <17 µmol/l)	17	20	24	29	36

1. What is the most likely cause for the abnormality of the LFT?
2. Which two investigations would you perform?
3. What treatment should be considered?

Question 41

The following are cardiac catheter data on a 4-year-old male with cyanosis and failure to thrive:

Chamber	Pressure (mmHg)	Oxygen saturation (%) (on air)	Oxygen saturation (%) (on 28% oxygen)
Right atrium	8	52	52
Right ventricle	90/30	53	54
Pulmonary artery	22/12	53	54
PCWP	4		
Left ventricle	80/20	82	81
Aorta	77/50	66	66

1. List four abnormalities.
2. What is the underlying diagnosis?
3. Explain the lack of rise in oxygen tension after inspiring 28% oxygen.

Answer 39

1. 'Leukaemoid reaction'.
2. i. The presence of toxic granulations or Dohle bodies in the white cells.
ii. Neutrophils exhibiting a toxic shift to the left, i.e. three or less segments of the nucleus.

A leukaemoid reaction is a descriptive term given to a leucoerythroblastic blood picture which follows sepsis. In some cases of overwhelming infection, the 'sick' marrow releases immature cells into the blood stream; thus, there is an abundance of myelocytes and normoblasts. In contrast to a true leucoerythroblastic anaemia where the marrow is characteristically replaced by neoplastic cells, there is no lymphadenopathy or hepatosplenomegaly.

Answer 40

1. Chronic active hepatitis due to hepatitis B or hepatitis C.
2. i. Hepatitis B and C serology.
ii. Liver biopsy.
3. Interferon therapy.

The patient has had major surgery in the past that almost certainly required blood transfusion. Both hepatitis B and C are readily contracted from blood transfusions. Since screening donated blood for hepatitis B was initiated in the 1980s, hepatitis C has become the most common cause of post-transfusion hepatitis in the Western world.

Almost 20% of patients with hepatitis B infection will develop CAH. The cause is unknown, but is thought to be a defective T-cell immune response. Most patients affected are male. The condition is usually asymptomatic, or may present as very slowly progressive hepatitis. About 50% of those affected present with established chronic liver disease.

CAH may also occur following hepatitis C infection. The acute hepatitic event is usually very mild, and often goes unnoticed. The sequelae are similar to those of hepatitis B infection; however the incidence of CAH is almost 50%. Other causes of CAH are given (*Table*). There is nothing in the patient's history to suggest any of these other causes.

The aminotransferases and bilirubin are usually modestly raised and the alkaline phosphatase is very slightly raised. The blood transaminase level bears no correlation with the severity of the hepatic damage. In hepatitis B-related CAH, the hepatitis B surface antigen and the e antigen is present. In hepatitis C-related CAH, anti-hepatitis C antibodies are present. The histological landmark of CAH is piecemeal necrosis. There is destruction of the liver cells between the interface of the hepatic parenchyma and the connective tissue. In hepatitis B-related CAH, the presence of hepatitis B surface antigen in the hepatocytes produces a ground-glass appearance on haematoxylin and eosin staining.

Patients with evidence of CAH should be treated with intravenous interferon for several months to prevent viral replication and allow seroconversion. The success rate is below 30%, and relapse often occurs soon after cessation of therapy.

Other causes of CAH

Autoimmune
Lupoid hepatitis
Anti-LKM antibody-associated CAH

Drugs
Methyl dopa
Isoniazid

α-1 antitrypsin deficiency

Wilson's disease

Inflammatory bowel disease (usually ulcerative colitis)

Answer 41

1. i. Elevated right ventricular pressure.
ii. Pressure drop across the pulmonary valve, suggesting pulmonary stenosis.
iii. Low oxygen saturation in the left ventricle, suggestive of a VSD with a right-to-left shunt.
iv. Saturation in the ascending aorta much lower than the left ventricle, indicating an overriding aorta.
2. Fallot's tetralogy.
3. The right-to-left shunt means that the majority of the blood does not pass through the lungs to be oxygenated.

(See Guidelines for the Interpretation of Cardiac Catheter Data, page 220.)

Question 42

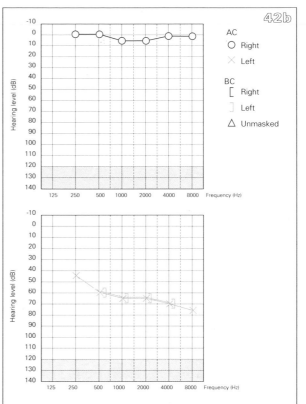

A 30-year-old male presented with vertigo and deafness in the left ear. His trunk was examined (**42a**), and he had an audiogram as part of the investigation for his symptoms (**42b**). There was no air–bone gap.

1. What is the audiographic abnormality?
2. What is the unifying diagnosis?
3. What other abnormalities would you expect to find on neurological examination?

Question 43

A 17-year-old male was referred with poorly developed secondary sexual characteristics. He was a slow developer, and had been to a special school for his entire education. He had a brother who was severely handicapped and wheelchair-bound who had died at the age of 17 years.

On examination, there was absence of axillary and pubic hair. His penis and testicles were small. There was bilateral gynaecomastia. Neurological examination was normal.

Investigations are shown.

1. What is the endocrine abnormality?
2. What is the most probable diagnosis?
3. How would you confirm the diagnosis?
4. How would you explain the abnormal creatinine kinase level?

FBC	Hb 12 g/dl
	WCC 5×10^9/l
	Platelets 190×10^9/l
Biochemistry	Sodium 137 mmol/l
	Potassium 3.7 mmol/l
	Urea 5 mmol/l
Biochemistry	Creatinine kinase 350 u/l
Testosterone	4 nmol/l
LH	35 u/l (normal range 1–10 u/l)
FSH	30 u/l (normal range 1–7 u/l)

Answer 42

1. There is severe hearing loss at progressively higher frequencies in the left ear.
2. The trunk demonstrates café au lait spots, a feature of neurofibromatosis. An important association of neurofibromatosis is acoustic neuroma, which is a recognized cause of sensorineuronal deafness (*Table A*).
3. On neurological examination, the patient may also have an absent ipsilateral corneal reflex and ipsilateral cerebellar signs. In a minority of cases acoustic neuromas may be bilateral.

Neurofibromatosis is inherited as an autosomal dominant condition. Abnormalities on two chromosomes may cause disease with either a predominantly peripheral or central manifestation (*Table B*). Regular audiometry is mandatory to detect acoustic neuroma early. MRI of the brain revealed an acoustic neuroma (**42c**)

(See Audiograms, page 218.)

Table A. Causes of sensorineuronal deafness

Unilateral (lesion in the cerebellopontine angle)
Meningioma
Acoustic neuroma
Granuloma
Metastasis

Bilateral
Degenerative (presbycusis)
Aminoglycosides
Amphotericin
High-dose loop diuretics
Mumps
Rubella

Table B. Other associations of neurofibromatosis

Chromosome 17 (peripheral abnormalities)
Renal artery stenosis
Pulmonary fibrosis
Cardiomyopathy (hypertrophic, restrictive and dilated)
Fibrous dysplasia of bone
Phaeochromocytoma

Chromosome 22 (central abnormalities)
Acoustic neuroma
Meningioma
Optic glioma
Ependymoma

Answer 43

1. Primary hypogonadism (hypergonadotrophic hypogonadism).
2. Kleinfelter's syndrome.
3. Demonstration of Barr body on buccal smear or karyotyping.
4. Carrier for Duchenne muscular dystrophy.

The most common cause of primary hypogonadism is Kleinfelter's syndrome, which has an incidence of 1/1,000 births. Patients are tall, lack secondary sexual characteristics, have gynaecomastia, and are often mentally subnormal. The condition is characterized by failure of development of Leydig cells and seminiferous tubules. Other causes of primary hypogonadism include Prader–Willi syndrome, Lawrence–Moon–Biedel syndrome, Leydig cell agenesis (Castelli's syndrome), 5α-reductase deficiency, mumps orchitis, renal failure, sickle cell disease, alcohol excess, chemotherapy and radiotherapy (see *Table* in Answer 99, page 128).

Patients have XXY karyotype due to non-dysjunction and have the potential of being carriers for X-linked recessive conditions (as with females) such as Duchenne muscular dystrophy, glucose-6-phosphate dehydrogenase deficiency, and haemophilia A. Kleinfelter patients are infertile. They are capable of having erections and ejaculation, but the semen does not contain spermatozoa.

Kleinfelter's syndrome is associated with a higher incidence of carcinoma of the breast, hypothyroidism, diabetes mellitus and chronic respiratory disease than the general male population.

Question 44

A 17-year-old female was admitted with a seven-hour history of severe central abdominal pain radiating to her back, which was accompanied by bilious vomiting. She had been constipated for 72 hours. There was no significant past medical history; in particular, there was no history of abdominal surgery. She was a non-smoker and had a very occasional glass of wine. She was an only child. Her father died when she was aged two. She was not certain about the cause of death, but mentioned that he had a history of psychosis and epilepsy. Her mother had gall stones, but was otherwise well. She took paracetamol for infrequent 'period pains'. The only other drug history was that of the contraceptive pill which had been commenced 10 days previously.

On examination, she was unwell and distressed with pain. She was sweating profusely. Her heart rate was 130 beats/min and blood pressure 190/110 mmHg. Examination of the precordium revealed normal heart sounds. Peripheral pulses were easily palpable. The chest was clear. The abdomen was generally very tender, with guarding around the umbilical area. The hernial orifice was normal. There was a positive succussion splash and the bowel sounds were present. Rectal examination revealed an empty rectum. Neurological examination was normal.

The patient was prescribed pethidine for her pain and metoclopramide for the vomiting. She received intravenous saline. A few hours later she complained of weakness affecting her left shoulder. She was unable to abduct or adduct the shoulder. Shortly afterwards she developed weakness in both her legs, in addition to urinary retention. She was due to be catheterized when she had a grand mal epileptic seizure.

Investigations are shown.

FBC	Hb 13 g/dl
	WCC 19×10^9/l
	Platelets 400×10^9/l
ESR	12 mm/h
Biochemistry	Sodium 121 mmol/l
	Potassium 3 mmol/l
	Urea 5 mmol/l
	Calcium 2.5 mmol/l
	Albumin 44 g/l
	Bilirubin 15 µmol/l
	AST 44 u/l
Blood glucose	4 mmol/l
Abdominal X-ray	Normal
Chest X-ray	Normal
CT scan brain	Normal
Lumbar puncture	1 lymphocyte/mm^3
	No red cells
	Protein 0.3 g/l
	Glucose 3.3 mmol/l

1. What is the diagnosis?
2. Which two investigations would you perform to confirm the diagnosis?
3. What is the precipitating factor?
4. List four management steps which you would take in this patient.
5. How will you manage her epileptic seizures?

Question 45

A 68-year-old male presented with a 48-hour history of right upper quadrant pain, dark urine and pale stools. Shortly after admission he had an investigation (**45**).

1. What investigation has been performed?
2. What does it reveal?
3. What is the diagnosis?

Answer 44

1. Acute intermittent porphyria (AIP). The combination of abdominal pain, neurological features, hypertension and tachycardia in a young person should raise the suspicion of AIP.
2. i. Urinary PGB.
ii. Assay red cells for the enzyme PBG deaminase.
3. The oral contraceptive pill.
4. i. Stop oral contraceptive pill.
ii. High calorie intake with intravenous infusion 500 ml of 50% dextrose per 24 hours via a large central vein in this case. The normal regime is 2 litres of 20% dextrose per 24 hours; however, in the case of syndrome of inappropriate ADH secretion, fluid restriction demands the use of smaller volumes of high-concentration dextrose.
iii. Start intravenous haematin.
iv. Intravenous beta-blocker to control tachycardia and hypertension.
5. Intravenous diazepam or chlormethiazole.

Acute intermittent porphyria is the most common type of acute porphyria. It is a rare condition caused by a genetic mutation in the gene encoding the enzyme PBG deaminase on chromosome 11, and is inherited as an autosomal dominant trait. A family history is usually present, but in up to one-third of cases this may be absent, either because the condition has not been diagnosed in first-degree relatives, or because the condition is running a latent course. It is five times more common in females than males, and usually presents between the ages of 14 and 30 years. The absence of PBG deaminase leads to elevated δ-ALA and PBG in the blood stream (**44**), both of which are responsible for the clinical manifestations of the condition. AIP is characterized mainly by gastrointestinal and neurological symptoms. Unlike the chronic porphyrias, skin photosensitivity is extremely unusual in AIP. Attacks are usually precipitated by drugs, alcohol, fasting and sepsis. Several drugs, particularly barbiturates and other anticonvulsants, have been implicated. The oral contraceptive pill has also been associated with acute attacks of porphyria and is the most likely precipitating factor in this case. The most common symptoms are acute abdominal pain which can simulate a surgical emergency, nausea, vomiting and constipation. Abdominal guarding may be present, but bowel sounds are usually present. There is often evidence of delayed gastric emptying, and it is not unusual to elicit a succussion splash due to a stomach full of gastric contents. The abdominal X-ray is normal. Neurological manifestations of the disease include a peripheral and autonomic neuropathy. Autonomic neuropathy most commonly manifests as tachycardia which is out of proportion to the extent of abdominal pain, hypertension and excess sweating. In approximately 50% of cases there is evidence of a motor neuropathy which often affects the proximal muscles. Both bulbar palsy and

quadriplegia are recognized manifestations. Respiratory muscle paralysis is life-threatening, and requires assisted ventilation. In this case there was involvement of the left shoulder girdle and then a paraparesis. Epilepsy occurs when the disease is in its most aggressive phase. It often heralds the onset of hyponatraemia due to SIADH.

The management is by withdrawing the offending drug, if this is applicable. A high calorie intake reduces precursors of haem synthesis in the blood by reducing the activity of the rate-limiting enzyme ALA synthetase. Intravenous haematin is used in the acute situation and also acts by inhibiting the action of ALA synthetase. The control of abdominal pain requires narcotic analgesia. Vomiting can be prevented by insertion of a nasogastric tube to empty the stomach contents.

Metoclopramide is another drug which can precipitate acute porphyria, and should be avoided. Beta-blockers are used to manage the tachycardia and hypertension.

The management of epilepsy is by trying to abate the condition with a high calorie intake and by fluid restriction to prevent further hyponatraemia from SIADH. Epilepsy in the acute situation is managed with chlormethiazole, which is one of the very few anticonvulsant agents not known to cause acute porphyria. Prevention of the condition is mainly based on avoiding precipitating drugs and recognizing warning symptoms early.

The diagnosis is made by demonstrating high levels of δ-ALA and PBG in the urine. The addition of Ehrlich's dye to the urine will cause a red discoloration in the presence of PBG; however, this phenomenon is also observed in the

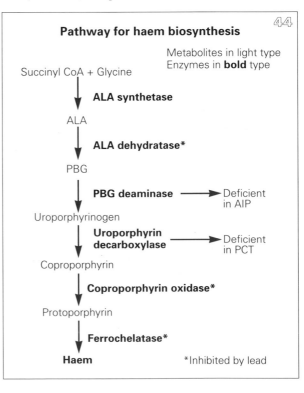

Pathway for haem biosynthesis   44

Metabolites in light type
Enzymes in **bold** type

Succinyl CoA + Glycine

↓ **ALA synthetase**

ALA

↓ **ALA dehydratase***

PBG

↓ **PBG deaminase** ──→ Deficient in AIP

Uroporphyrinogen

↓ **Uroporphyrin decarboxylase** ──→ Deficient in PCT

Coproporphyrin

↓ **Coproporphyrin oxidase***

Protoporphyrin

↓ **Ferrochelatase***

Haem   *Inhibited by lead

presence of urobilinogen in the urine. Differentiation of urobilinogen from PBG involves the addition of chloroform, which will cause PBG to separate out in the aqueous layer as a purple sediment, whereas the urobilinogen is soluble and becomes colourless. This is the basis of the Watson–Schwartz test. The urinary levels of ALA and PBG are always elevated during an attack, though they may be normal when the patient is well. The red cells can also be assayed for the enzyme PBG deaminase, which is very low in AIP. The enzyme ALA dehydratase is elevated. See also Answer **161** (page 212).

Answer 45

1. The investigation is a percutaneous transhepatic cholangiogram.
2. Both the common bile duct and the internal hepatic ducts are dilated. There is a large filling defect at the distal end of the common bile duct.
3. A gall stone in the common bile duct causing obstructive jaundice.

Question 46

A 25-year-old female presented to her general practitioner after noticing asymmetry of her face (**46a**). For the past two days she had also experienced dizziness and lethargy, particularly on exertion. She had no past medical history. Six weeks previously she had been to visit friends in North America. While on holiday, she developed a painful rash on her left arm which she described as a small red nodule which gradually expanded over the next few days before subsiding. A friend had taken a photograph of the rash (**46b**).

On examination, she had a temperature of 37°C (98.6°F) and a slow pulse. Examination of the ears was normal. The doctor was concerned and performed an ECG (**46c**).

1. What is the cause of the abnormality on her face?
2. What is the characteristic name given to the rash?
3. Give two other dermatological manifestations of this disorder.

4. What is the ECG diagnosis?
5. What is the overall diagnosis?
6. List two therapeutic steps in the management of this patient.

Answer 46

1. Left facial nerve palsy.
2. Erythema chronicum migrans.
3. i. *Borrelia* lymphocytoma.
ii. Acrodermatitis chronica atrophicans.
4. Complete heart block. (Third-degree atrioventricular block.)
5. Lyme disease.
6. i. Therapy with doxycycline, benzyl penicillin, azithromycin, or cefotaxime.
ii. Temporary cardiac pacing.

The patient presented with a facial palsy and has ECG evidence of third-degree atrioventricular block. In addition, she had a macular rash which appears to be fading in the centre (**46b**) and is characteristic of erythema chronicum migrans. While there are several medical conditions which may involve the cardiovascular and central nervous system simultaneously (*Table*), the rash makes Lyme disease the most likely diagnosis.

Lyme disease is caused by the spirochaete, *Borrelia burgdorferi*. It is transmitted by hard-bodied ticks (*Ixodes* species). The disease has a wide clinical spectrum, ranging from asymptomatic infection to multisystem involvement. The first presentation is a characteristic skin lesion at the site of the tick bite, which begins as a macule between 2–40 days after exposure, and expands with central clearing. This is termed erythema chronicum migrans and may be associated with fever and regional lympha-denopathy. Early localized infection may present as *Borrelia* lymphocytoma, which is a bluish-red nodule on the ear lobe or nose. The second stage of the disease occurs several weeks or months after exposure, and is due to spread of the organism via the blood or the lymphatics. At this stage there may be fever and flu-like symptoms, several skin lesions similar to erythema chronicum migrans, and cardiac and neurological involvement. Cardiac disease occurs in 5% of affected individuals and is characterized by varying degrees of heart block and myopericarditis. It is usually brief and seldom lasts more than one week. Temporary pacing is only indicated in patients who are symptomatic from heart block, as in this case. Neurological disease comprises a mild meningoencephalitis, peripheral neuritis, cranial nerve involvement, particularly the facial nerve, and Bannworth's syndrome (lymphocytic meningoradiculitis).

Chronic Lyme disease may manifest years later as an erosive oligoarthritis or as acrodermatitis chronica atrophicans, which is characterized by atrophy of the skin on the lower limbs.

The diagnosis is clinical and confirmed by serological testing. Serology may be negative during the early erythema chronicum migrans stage. All stages of the disease are amenable to therapy with antibiotics, and the clinical response is usually good. The antibiotics used with success include doxycycline, benzyl penicillin, cefotaxime, amoxycillin and azithromycin.

Conditions simultaneously affecting the cardiovascular and central nervous system

Infections
TB
HIV
Syphilis
Lyme disease
Rheumatic fever
Infective endocarditis

Multisystem conditions
Connective tissue diseases
Vasculitides
Sarcoidosis

Toxins
Alcohol

Drugs
Amphetamines
Tricyclic antidepressant drugs
Lithium

Neuroectodermal syndromes
Neurofibromatosis
Tuberose sclerosis

Hereditary neuropathies
Friedreich's ataxia
Dystrophia myotonica
Duchenne muscular dystrophy

Miscellaneous
AIP
Guillain–Barré syndrome

Question 47

A 69-year-old male was admitted to the Coronary Care Unit after presenting with a three-hour history of chest pain, palpitations and breathlessness. He had a past history of hypertension and three myocardial infarctions. His regular medication comprised aspirin 150 mg once daily, captopril 50 mg three times daily, frusemide 40 mg once daily, and simvastatin 10 mg once daily. An ECG performed on admission is shown in **47a**. (Do not answer **4** until you have finished answering **1–3**.)

1. What is the ECG diagnosis?
2. Give four reasons in favour of your diagnosis.
3. What is the drug of choice?
4. Shortly after administering the drug, the patient becomes very clammy and cyanosed. His conscious level deteriorates and his blood pressure recording is 70/40 mmHg. What is the next step in his management?

Question 48

A deaf couple both have a hereditary form of deafness. They have recently married, and want advice on the chances of their children being affected. The family tree of both parents is shown (**48**).

1. What is the pattern of inheritance for family A?
2. What is the inheritance for family B?
3. Assuming that both families have the same mutation causing deafness, what is the chance of their children being affected?

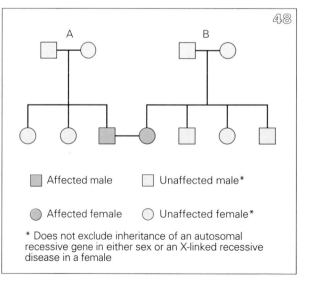

Affected male   Unaffected male*

Affected female   Unaffected female*

* Does not exclude inheritance of an autosomal recessive gene in either sex or an X-linked recessive disease in a female

Answer 47

1. Ventricular tachycardia (VT).
2. i. Broad complex tachycardia.
ii. Extreme axis deviation.
iii. Concordance in the precordial leads.
iv. Dissociated P waves (**47b**).
3. Intravenous lignocaine.
4. DC cardioversion.

Factors favouring VT rather than supraventricular tachycardia (SVT) include all of the above. The diagnosis of VT rather than SVT in a patient with a broad complex tachycardia is also more likely when there is a history of ischaemic heart disease or cardiomyopathy.

Most VT has a RBBB morphology because it arises from the left ventricle; however, VT from the right ventricle is also recognized, in which case it has a LBBB morphology. Examples of right ventricular VT include right ventricular outflow tachycardia, congenital heart disease with right-to-left shunts, and arrhythmogenic right VT.

The management of sustained VT is dependent on haemodynamic status. Patients who are haemodynamically stable (not hypotensive or clammy) should be treated with a class Ia anti-arrhythmic agent. The drug of choice is lignocaine. There is a potential for all class Ia agents to precipitate cardiogenic shock in a patient with poor myocardial function because of their negative inotropic effect. Patients with haemodynamic collapse should be cardioverted immediately.

Features of ventricular tachycardia

Broad complex (QRS usually >140 ms)
Extreme axis deviation
Positive or negative concordance in the precordial leads
RSr pattern in V1
Deep S-wave in V6
Fusion and capture beats
Dissociated P-waves

Answer 48

1. Family A autosomal recessive.
2. Family B autosomal recessive.
3. 100%.

In both families, neither parent is affected, which excludes an autosomal dominant or an X-linked dominant condition in any of the parents and an X-linked recessive condition in both fathers (the presence of a defective X-linked gene in the fathers would manifest as abnormal phenotype). This leaves the possibility of an autosomal recessive condition, or that the mothers are carriers of an X-linked condition. However, an X-linked recessive mode of inheritance is excluded by the fact that there are affected daughters in both families. If a mother is a carrier for an X-linked recessive condition there is a 50% chance that her daughters will be carriers, but none will have the disease, and there is a 50% chance that her sons will be affected. If both parents are carriers of autosomal recessive genes for deafness, then there is a 25% chance that their children will be affected, irrespective of their sex.

Both the couple in question are affected, which implies that both carry two autosomal recessive genes for deafness. The chance of their children being affected is 100%, because they will inherit one autosomal recessive gene for deafness from each parent.

Question 49

A 5-year-old male was admitted with a two-day history of blood-stained diarrhoea. Three days after, he felt nauseous and generally unwell. On examination he had periorbital oedema and a blood pressure of 150/95 mmHg.

Investigations are shown.

FBC	Hb 8 g/dl
	WCC 13×10^9/l
	Platelets 36×10^9/l
Clotting	PT 13 s (control 13 s)
	APTT 34 s (control 36 s)
Blood film (**49**)	
Biochemistry	Sodium 138 mmol/l
	Potassium 5.9 mmol/l
	Creatinine 130 µmol/l
	Urea 11 mmol/l

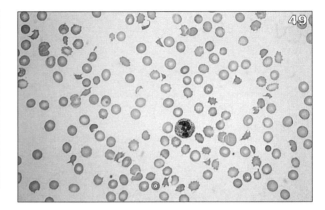

1. What is the diagnosis?
2. What investigation would you request to confirm your suspicion?

Question 50

A 67-year-old patient with diet-controlled diabetes was found collapsed at the bottom of the stairs in his home by his daughter. The only other medical history available was that he had a history of hypertension for which he was taking bendrofluazide. On examination, he was drowsy. His heart rate was 41 beats/min, and blood pressure 140/90 mmHg. The temperature was 36.8°C (98.2°F). The JVP was not raised. The heart sounds were normal, and his chest was clear. Abdominal examination was normal. His left lower limb was externally rotated and painful to move, and there was extensive bruising of the buttock and left thigh.

Investigations are shown.

1. What is the diagnosis?
2. List two investigations you would perform to confirm the cause of the metabolic abnormality .

FBC	Hb 9.8 g/dl
	WCC 14×10^9/l
	Platelets 350×10^9/l
	MCV 84 fl
Clotting	Normal
Biochemistry	Sodium 135 mmol/l
	Potassium 6.8 mmol/l
	Urea 16 mmol/l
	Creatinine 670 µmmol/l
	Bicarbonate 15 mmol/l
	Calcium 2.0 mmol/l
	Phosphate 2.8 mmol/l
	Bilirubin 14 µmol/l
	AST 26 u/l
	Alkaline phosphatase 100 u/l
	Albumin 40 g/l
	Glucose 9 mmol/l
Urinalysis	Blood +++
	Protein +
Chest X-ray	Normal
X-ray of left hip	Fracture and dislocation of the neck of femur
ECG	Minor T-wave abnormalities in the lateral leads

Answer 49

1. Haemolytic uraemic syndrome (HUS).
2. Stool inspection for *Escherichia coli* 0157:H7.

E. coli 0157:H7 is most commonly transmitted by eating under-cooked beef. The bacterium produces a toxin which is responsible for the gastrointestinal effects, which include colicky pain and diarrhoea which may be blood-stained. Fever is very mild or completely absent. Symptoms of infection usually subside after about a week; however, the HUS develops in approximately 6% of patients. This is characterized by a MAHA which is a result of endothelial damage by the toxin, leading to adherence of fibrin strands which trap and fragment red cells and platelets. This produces a characteristic blood picture of anaemia, red cell fragments, thrombocytopenia and increased reticulocytes. Small vessel fibrin deposition and thrombosis resulting from MAHA lead to renal damage and oliguric renal failure. Bleeding and bruising are common. In pure MAHA clotting is usually normal; however, MAHA often coexists with disseminated intravascular coagulation, where clotting is impaired and the serum fibrinogen degradation product level is elevated. Treatment of HUS complicated by MAHA and renal failure is supportive. Blood transfusions are often necessary. Some 50% of patients require dialysis. The mortality rate is 3–5%. A variant of HUS occurring in the same circumstances and characterized by neurological involvement is known as thrombotic thrombocytopenic purpura. This is caused by a circulating inhibitor for the Von Willebrand Factor protease enzyme. This results in uncontrolled thrombotic tendencies in small vessels.

The combination of MAHA and DIC occurs in sepsis, malignancy and obstetric emergencies such as septic abortion, abruptio placentae, and amniotic fluid embolism.

Causes of MAHA

HUS
Thrombotic thrombocytopenic purpura
Accelerated hypertension
Septicaemia
Vasculitides
Connective tissue diseases
Mucinous adenocarcinoma
Burns
Prosthetic valve-induced haemolysis
Drugs (cyclosporin, mitomycin)

Answer 50

1. Rhabdomyolysis.
2. i. Measuring creatinine kinase levels, which are elevated due to skeletal muscle damage
ii. Detection of myoglobin in the urine.

There are two important clues for diagnosing rhabdomyolysis. Firstly, the patient has had a fall. Secondly, there is renal failure with a disproportionately raised creatinine level. Other causes of rhabdomyolysis are tabulated below (*Table A*). The common pathology is myositis, skeletal muscle trauma or infarction leading to raised myoglobin levels in the blood. Myoglobin is toxic to the renal tubules and precipitates renal failure. In rhabdomyolysis, the serum calcium is low because free calcium becomes bound by myoglobin. The serum potassium and phosphate are high because large amounts of these electrolytes are released from damaged muscle cells. (*Table B.*)

The management involves adequate hydration and alkalinization of the urine to reduce precipitation of myoglobin in the renal tubules. Loop diuretics should be avoided as they result in an acidic urinary pH.

Table A. Causes of rhabdomyolysis

Muscle trauma/infarction
Electrocution
Hypothermia
Status epilepticus
Neuroleptic malignant syndrome
Ecstasy/amphetamine abuse
Burns
Septicaemia
Therapy with statins
Very strenuous exercise (e.g. marathon running)

Table B. Causes of low calcium and high phosphate

Chronic renal failure
Hypoparathyroidism
Pseudohypoparathyroidism
Magnesium deficiency*
Rhabdomyolysis

* Due to end-organ resistance to the effects of PTH

Question 51

A 16-year-old male presented with a four-day history of a dry cough, right-sided pleuritic chest pain and increasing breathlessness. On examination, he had a temperature of 38°C (100.4°F). He had a widespread rash affecting his arms and legs and his face (51).

Investigations are shown.

FBC	Hb 9 g/dl
	WCC 5×10^9/l
	Platelets 150×10^9/l
Blood film	Red cell agglutination
Biochemistry	Sodium 131 mmol/l
	Potassium 4.0 mmol/l
	Urea 4.0 mmol/l
	Creatinine 70 μmol/l
	Bilirubin 26 μmol/l
	AST 60 u/l
	ALT 83 u/l
	Alkaline phosphatase 110 u/l
	Albumin 36 g/l
Chest X-ray	Right middle lobe consolidation

1. What is the rash?
2. What is the cause of the low sodium?
3. What is the cause of his anaemia?
4. Which single investigation would you perform to confirm the cause of the anaemia?
5. What is the cause of his chest X-ray findings?
6. Which two tests would you perform to confirm the diagnosis?

Question 52

A 14-year-old female was admitted for investigation of intermittent colicky abdominal pain associated with vomiting. She had experienced several episodes in the past six months requiring hospital admissions. Physical examination during these episodes revealed a distended abdomen which was tympanic to percussion. Bowel sounds were tinkling. Hernial orifice examination was normal. The patient usually developed two painful 4 cm macular lesions on her left hand and forearm respectively which were only present while she was symptomatic. She was never in hospital for more than 48 hours, during which time she was managed with intravenous fluids and resting the bowel. She always made a spontaneous recovery. In between episodes of abdominal pain she was perfectly well. She had a five-year-old cousin who had also recently been admitted to hospital on three occasions with the same symptoms.

These investigations were performed while the patient was symptomatic:

The patient had a small bowel meal when her symptoms had recovered, which was also normal.

FBC	Hb 12 g/dl
	WCC 6×10^9/l
	Platelets 390×10^9/l
U&E	Normal
LFT	Normal
Thyroid function tests	Normal
Bone biochemistry	Normal
Blood glucose	5 mmol/l
Serum amylase	Normal
Serum lead	Undetectable
Urinary δ-ALA	Undetectable
Urinary PGB	Undetectable
Serum immunoglobulins	Normal

1. What is the cause of the abdominal pain?
2. How would you manage her symptoms if she remained symptomatic for several days, or if her symptoms deteriorated?

Answer 51

1. Erythema multiforme.
2. Syndrome of inappropriate ADH secretion (SIADH).
3. Autoimmune haemolytic anaemia.
4. Direct Coomb's test at 4°C (39.2°F).
5. *Mycoplasma* pneumonia.
6. i. *Mycoplasma* serology.
ii. Cold agglutinin estimation.

The patient has a right middle lobe pneumonia and a rash which is characterized by blistering target lesions (erythema multiforme). The patient has an anaemia, and the agglutination on the blood film points to an immune haemolytic anaemia. *Mycoplasma* pneumonia is associated with both erythema multiforme and a cold autoimmune haemolytic anaemia. Other causes of erythema multiforme and complications of *Mycoplasma* pneumonia are listed in *Tables A* and *B*. The low sodium is a consequence of SIADH complicating pneumonia. The causes of SIADH are discussed in Examination Answer **13**, page 248.

Table A. Causes of erythema multiforme

Infections
Mycoplasma pneumonias
Herpes simplex virus
Orf
TB

Drugs
Penicillins
Sulphonamides
Barbiturates
NSAID

Miscellaneous
Connective tissue diseases
Vasculitides
Internal malignancy

Table B. Complications of *Mycoplasma* pneumonia

Neurological	Aseptic meningitis
	Encephalitis
	Transverse myelitis
	Guillain–Barré syndrome
	Peripheral neuropathy
Cardiac	Myocarditis
	Pericarditis
Haematological	Thrombocytopenia
	Cold autoimmune haemolytic anaemia
Locomotor	Myositis
	Arthritis
Skin	Erythema multiforme
Gastrointestinal	Diarrhoea/vomiting
Endocrine	SIADH
Miscellaneous	Bullous myringitis

Answer 52

1. Hereditary angio-oedema.
2. Use fresh-frozen plasma or C1 esterase inhibitor concentrates.

Hereditary angio-oedema is inherited as an autosomal dominant trait. It is associated with C1 esterase inhibitor deficiency, resulting in high C1 esterase levels. Deficiency of C1 esterase inhibitor (which modulates complement) can lead to angio-oedema. A positive family history is very common, although there is a similar condition associated with an acquired lymphoproliferative disorder in which C1 esterase inhibitor levels are also low. Clinical features can occur late in adult life. Attacks are preceded with a painful macular rash, or even a rash simulating erythema marginatum. Triggering factors include trauma to the skin. Laryngeal oedema can be life-threatening. Abdominal pain occurs due to visceral oedema. Attacks can exceed 72 hours. Treatment is supportive, although fresh-frozen plasma can be given to abort severe or prolonged attacks. Inhibitors of plasmin, such as danazol, are used for long-term treatment. Hydrocortisone and chlorpheniramine are not as effective in the management of this condition as they are in acute anaphylaxis. The diagnosis is made by quantifying the C1 esterase level (high) and C1 esterase inhibitor level (low). C2 and C4 levels are also low.

Question 53

A 30-year-old male presented with a four-day history of passing dark urine. He had passed dark urine intermittently for six months, though such passage had never exceeded 24 hours, except on this occasion. More recently, he complained of malaise, lethargy and weakness. His general practitioner thought he appeared pale, and prescribed iron tablets. Two days before coming to the hospital, the patient developed sharp right lower chest pain which was worsened on inspiration, and a cough productive of bright red sputum. On further questioning, he volunteered a six-month history of intermittent abdominal pain and episodes of abdominal distension.

He had never taken any regular medication and had not travelled abroad for a year. He consumed 5–7 l of lager on weekends, and occasionally had a glass of wine with a meal.

On examination, he was pale and slightly jaundiced. He had a temperature of 37.5°C (99.5°F). There was no lymphadenopathy. The JVP was not raised. Examination of the respiratory system revealed dullness of the right base associated with reduction of air entry. Abdominal examination demonstrated firm, palpable hepatomegaly 4 cm below the costal margin. There were no other palpable masses. There was no clinical evidence of peripheral oedema.

Investigations are shown.

FBC	Hb 7.3 g/dl
	WCC 2.8×10^9/l
	Platelets 200×10^9/l
	MCV 93 fl
	Reticulocyte count 15%
Direct Coomb's test	Negative
Chest radiograph	Atelectasis at the right lung base
Urinalysis	Urobilinogen +++
	Haemosiderin ++
	Cell 0
Biochemistry	Sodium 136 mmol/l
	Potassium 4.8 mmol/l
	Urea 5.3 mmol/l
	Bilirubin 33 µmol/l
	AST 40 u/l
	Alkaline phosphatase 94 u/l
	Albumin 36 g/l

1. What is the cause of the dark urine?
A. Bilirubinuria.
B. Urobilinogenuria.
C. Myoglobinuria.
D. Haemoglobinuria.
E. Haemosiderinuria.

2. What is the cause of jaundice?
A. Haemolysis.
B. Hepatitis.
C. Gall stones.
D. Hepatic metastases.
E. Pancreatitis.

Question 54

An 18-year-old male developed sharp left-sided chest pain on running up a flight of stairs, followed by slight breathlessness on exertion. On examination, he appeared relatively well. His heart rate was 90 beats/min, and the respiratory rate was 18/min. On auscultation of the heart there was a clicking sound synchronous with the heart sounds.

1. What is the most probable cause of his symptoms?
2. Which investigation would you perform to confirm the diagnosis?

Answer 53

1. D. Haemoglobinuria.
2. A. Haemolysis.

Bilirubinuria does not occur in haemolytic anaemia because bilirubin is in the unconjugated form and therefore is not water-soluble and cannot be excreted in the urine. Urobilinogen does stain urine, but not enough to give it a red colour of haemoglobinuria. Myoglobin is produced in large amounts in rhabdomyolysis, and while it may produce red discoloration of urine, there is no evidence for rhabdomyolysis in this case. Haemosiderinuria occurs in intravascular haemolyis but can only be detected on staining the urine with Prussian blue.

Hepatitis, gall stones and pancreatitis do not account for the severity of the anaemia. Although haemolyis and thrombotic episodes can be present in a patient with malignancy, it does not account for the dark urine which is present in the absence of red cells in the urine.

The diagnosis is PNH. This is an acquired disorder of the haematopoietic cells which usually occurs after an episode of aplastic anaemia, leading to increased susceptibility of red cells to complement lysis. White cells and platelets are also affected. The onset of the disease is often insidious. The disorder is characterized by non-immune haemolytic anaemia, variable pancytopenia and thrombotic episodes. The MCV may be normal, depending on the extent of reticulocytosis. The molecular basis of the membrane defect has recently been unfolded and attributed to abnormalities in the synthesis of the phospholipid GPI. GPI serves an anchoring function for important cell surface proteins such as CD59 on red cells which is a complement lysis inhibitor. Lack of GPI does not permit red cells to express the antigen CD59 on their cell surface, leading to complement lysis. The thrombotic tendency results from inappropriate activation of platelets which are abnormally sensitive to complement. Intravascular haemolysis is reflected by an increased reticulocyte count, raised bilirubin levels, reduced serum haptoglobins, methaemoglobinaemia, increased urinary urobilinogen, haemoglobinuria and haemosiderinuria. The latter is only detectable by staining the urine with Prussian blue agent. Haemolysis is increased during sleep, hence the term PNH. It is not clear why haemolysis should increase during sleep. Haemolysis is usually worse after infections, following inoculations, blood transfusions and surgery. Anaemia causes fatigue and dyspnoea. Some patients present with intermittent abdominal pain which is worse during episodes of active haemolysis. There is mild jaundice and intermittent passage of dark urine. On examination, the patient may be pale and jaundiced. The spleen is sometimes palpable and the liver may be enlarged. Complications include venous thrombosis, increased susceptibility to infection due to granulocytopenia, iron deficiency, pigment gall stones and transformation to acute myeloid leukaemia. Thrombosis is the most frequent complication. Small vessel thrombosis may be the cause of abdominal pain, and swelling may be due to intermittent ascites, as in this patient. Portal vein or hepatic vein thrombosis is a serious complication. Pulmonary embolism is a recognized complication. In this case, the pleuritic chest pain and haemoptysis may be due to pulmonary embolism or infection, the latter worsening the haemolytic event. Acute myeloid leukaemia complicates a few cases of PNH and is characterized by rapid pancytopenia and blast cells in the peripheral blood film.

The diagnosis of PNH is made by addition of acidified serum to the red cells, which will cause rapid haemolysis. This is known as the Ham's test. The reason for acidification of the serum is to activate the alternative complement pathway.

The definitive treatment is marrow transplantation. Leucocyte-depleted blood transfusions are often necessary.

Answer 54

1. Small left apical pneumothorax.
2. Chest X-ray in end expiration.

A systolic click which is synchronous with heart sounds is a rare but recognized sign of a small left apical pneumothorax. It is often referred to as Hamman's sign. A differential diagnosis of this sign is the systolic click of mitral valve prolapse; however, this is not consistent with chest pain and breathlessness on exertion of sudden onset in a young man.

An inspiratory X-ray alone may fail to detect small apical pneumothoraces. The management is conservative. Patients are advised not to engage in strenuous exertion for at least two weeks.

Question 55

A 33-year-old male returned from Mombassa, East Africa with a high fever, headaches and rigors. On examination, he had a temperature of 40°C (104°F). A blood film performed on admission is shown (**55a**).

1. What is the diagnosis?

Question 56

A 15-year-old female was investigated for short stature. She measured 1.22 m tall. Her sister aged 14 was 1.53 m tall. She was born three weeks prematurely, and was noted to have a divergent squint affecting her left eye in childhood. She had achieved her milestones in a normal manner, but school performance had been below average. On examination, the patient weighed 42 kg. She had a left-sided divergent squint. Her neck was short and her hands were small. Breast development had just begun and there was scanty pubic and axillary hair growth. The heart rate was 90 beats/min and regular, and the blood pressure was 110/70 mmHg. The heart sounds were normal and the chest was clear. Abdominal and neurological examination was also normal.

Initial investigations are shown.

1. List two possible causes for her short stature.
2. Give one test you would perform to confirm the diagnosis.

FBC	Hb 13 g/dl
	WCC 4.2 × 10⁹/l
	Platelets 410 × 10⁹/l
Biochemistry	Sodium 136 mmol/l
	Potassium 3.8 mmol/l
	Urea 5.1 mmol/l
	Creatinine 90 µmol/l
	Glucose 5.2 mmol/l
	Calcium 1.96 mmol/l
	Phosphate 1.3 mmol/l
	Alkaline phosphatase 310 u/l
	Albumin 39 g/l
	TSH 2 mu/l
	Thyroxine 87 nmol/l (normal 60–160 nmol/l
	LH 4 u/l (normal 1–12 u/l)
	FSH 6 u/l (normal 1–9 u/l)
	GH 2 mu/l
X-ray	Left wrist, lateral skull – normal bone age

Answer 55

1. *Plasmodium falciparum* malaria.

The two malaria parasites commonly shown on blood films in higher examinations are *P. falciparum* and *P. vivax* (for comparison, the blood films of both parasites are shown side-by-side [**55b, c**]). *P. falciparum* can be dif-

ferentiated from *P. vivax* by the following features:
- The parasite count is high, whereas in *P. vivax* it is low.
- The affected cells are small and/or crenated, whereas in *P. vivax* the cells are large.
- The ring form has two chromatin dots, whereas *P. vivax* has just one.
- The actual ring is thin, whereas in *P. vivax* it is thick.

Answer 56

1. i. Pseudohypoparathyroidism.
ii. Idiopathic hypoparathyroidism
2. Serum PTH level.

A low serum calcium, raised phosphate and normal alkaline phosphatase are suggestive of either idiopathic hypoparathyroidism or pseudohypoparathyroidism. The short stature, short neck and squint are characteristic of pseudohypoparathyroidism. In addition, the patient has small hands – presumably secondary to short metacarpals – which are also associated with pseudohypoparathyroidism. However, these morphological changes are also infrequently present in idiopathic hypoparathyroidism. Pseudohypoparathyroidism results from resistance of some target tissues to the actions of PTH. The disorder may be asymptomatic, present with lethargy, neuromuscular irritability or psychosis. Neuromuscular irritability is only present in profound hypocalcaemia, and consists of paraesthesia of the face and extremities, carpopedal spasm, and latent tetany. Convulsions are relatively common.

The serum PTH distinguishes between idiopathic hypoparathyroidism and pseudohypoparathyroidism. In idiopathic hypoparathyroidism, PTH level is extremely low or absent. The diagnosis of pseudohypoparathyroidism is also confirmed by measuring urinary cyclic AMP and phosphate concentration after infusion of PTH (Howard–Ellsworth test). The normal response is an increase in both cyclic AMP and phosphate in the urine after PTH. In patients with end organ resistance to PTH, i.e. pseudohypoparathyroidism, there is no such response. In a small proportion there is a normal response (type II pseudohypoparathyroidism). In these cases the diagnosis is based on the identification of a relatively high level of PTH in relation to the low serum calcium level.

Question 57

A 55-year-old West Indian male presented with severe anterior chest pain. On arrival, he was hypotensive. An ECG performed in accident and emergency is shown (**57a**). Shortly after admission, the patient had an echocardiogram (**57b**).

1. What is the complete diagnosis?
2. What would be the next step in your management?

Question 58

A 70-year-old male presents to the accident and emergency department in the morning with a painful swelling on the anterior aspect of his left thigh which he had noticed on the previous evening. The swelling had become bigger and he was having difficulty walking due to the pain. He denied any recent trauma to the leg. Apart from a past history of TB 30 years ago, there was no other history of note. He was widowed three years ago and lived alone. He took paracetamol infrequently for aches and pains in his limbs.

On examination, he appeared unkempt and was thin. There was no pallor or oedema. Vital parameters were normal and he was apyrexial. There was a 6 cm, tender swelling on the anterior aspect of the left thigh. There was also evidence of widespread bruising on his forearms and legs.

Investigations are shown.

FBC	Hb 11 g/dl
	WCC 5 × 10⁹/l
	Platelets 170 × 10⁹/l
	MCV 90 fl
Clotting	PT 14 s (control 14 s)
	APTT 45 s (control 45 s)
	BT 12 min (control <10 min)

1. What is the swelling?
2. What is the diagnosis?
3. Which investigation would you request to confirm the diagnosis?

Answer 57

1. Acute inferior myocardial infarction with complete heart block complicating an acute proximal aortic dissection. The echocardiogram demonstrates an enlarged aortic root with an obvious dissection flap. (See Echocardiography, page 223.)
2. Immediate referral to the cardiothoracic surgeons.

Conditions predisposing to aortic dissection
Hypertension in Negroid patients
Marfan's syndrome
Ehlers–Danlos syndrome
Pregnancy
Coarctation of the aorta

Patients with proximal dissections should undergo urgent surgical repair, but those with distal dissection are treated conservatively. Repair is by resection of the ascending aorta and replacement with Dacron. In the interim, it would be important to relieve the severe pain with opiates and insert a temporary pacing wire to treat the complete heart block and help maintain circulation as he is hypotensive. In acute dissection, hypotension is due to rupture of the proximal dissection into the pericardial space which is not present in this case; therefore complete heart block is contributing to the hypotension in this case. In contrast with this case, most patients presenting with acute dissection are hypertensive and in these circumstances it is prudent to treat the hypertension aggressively to obtain a systolic blood pressure equal to or less than 100 mmHg. Drugs most commonly used include intravenous beta blockers, for example, labetolol, or intravenous nitroprusside. It is very important to recognize that the cause of myocardial infarction is a proximal dissection, and not coronary thrombosis. While thrombolytic therapy has revolutionized the management of acute coronary thrombosis, it is an absolute contra-indication in a patient who has sustained a myocardial infarction secondary to aortic dissection.

Aortic dissection is catastrophic, with a mortality rate of 1% per hour for the first 48 hours in untreated patients. Some 95% of dissections originate at the site of the intimal tear. Most tears occur in the ascending aorta (65%), followed by the proximal descending aorta (20%), in the transverse arch (10%) and in the distal thoracic aorta (5%). Predisposing factors are tabulated above.

Clinical features of acute dissection include very sudden onset of chest pain, either in the chest or between the shoulder blades. Syncope from tamponade, neurological deficit from involvement of the carotid artery, abdominal pain from mesenteric ischaemia, ischaemic upper limbs from brachiocephalic and left subclavian involvement and acute renal failure from involvement of the renal arteries are other presentations.

The diagnosis may be made by transthoracic echocardiography; however, transoesophageal echocardiography is the 'gold standard' test in the diagnosis of suspected dissection. MRI scanning is superior to transoesophageal echocardiogaphy, but its main disadvantage is that it is not portable.

Answer 58

1. Intramuscular haematoma.
2. Vitamin C deficiency (scurvy).
3. Platelet or leucocyte ascorbate concentration.

The normocytic anaemia, bruising and abnormal bleeding time in an elderly patient point to the diagnosis of vitamin C (ascorbic acid) deficiency, or scurvy. Vitamin C is abundant in fresh greens, citrus fruits, liver and kidney. Nutritional deficiency is relatively common in the elderly, who eat predominantly tinned foods. Vitamin C is required for the hydroxylation of proline in collagen synthesis. Deficiency results in abnormal connective tissue, resulting in easy bruising, bleeding gums, periosteal haemorrhage and muscle haematomas. The characteristic signs of vitamin C deficiency are perifollicular haemorrhages, widespread bruising and 'corkscrewing' of the body hair. The latter may be normal in the elderly. Patients may have coexistent iron and folate deficiency. The marrow is megaloblastic when there is folate deficiency. The bleeding time is prolonged, although platelet function is normal. The diagnosis is made by the demonstration of a low platelet or leucocyte ascorbate concentration. Treatment is with high doses of ascorbic acid.

Question 59

A 48-year-old female was investigated for an 11-month history of abdominal cramps and diarrhoea. She moved her bowels twice daily; the stool was loose and foul-smelling. There was no history of bleeding per rectum or tenesmus. Her appetite was unchanged, but she had lost 8 kg in weight. Two years ago she had a total abdominal hysterectomy and salpingo-oophorectomy for carcinoma of the cervix, followed by a course of external radiotherapy. She had been followed-up regularly by her gynaecologist, and was free from recurrence of the malignancy. She was married with two sons aged 10 and 12, respectively. She worked as a secretary. She consumed 1 unit of alcohol daily and was a non-smoker. There was no history of travel abroad. Systematic enquiry revealed a long history of Raynaud's phenomenon. She took paracetamol for very infrequent headaches.

On examination, she was thin. There was no pallor, clubbing, lymphadenopathy or oedema. The temperature was normal. Inspection of the oral cavity revealed two small, non-tender, shallow ulcers.

The abdomen was thin. There was a lower, midline scar. Mild tenderness was elicited on palpation of the right iliac fossa. Rectal examination was normal.

Investigations are shown.

FBC	Hb 10g/dl
	WCC 8×10^9/l
	Platelets 199×10^9/l
	MCV 106 fl
ESR	16 mm/h
Serum B_{12}	98 pmol/l
Serum folate	18 µg/l
Biochemistry	Calcium 2.12 mmol/l
	Phosphate 0.9 mmol/l
	Alkaline phosphatase 112 u/l
	Albumin 38 g/l
Urea/electrolytes	Normal
Throid function tests	Total thyroxine 110 nmol/l
	TSH 1.9 mu/l
Abdominal X-ray	Normal
Chest X-ray	Normal

1. What is the diagnosis?
A. Crohn's disease.
B. Coeliac disease.
C. Small bowel lymphoma.
D. Radiation enteritis.
2. Which investigation would you perform to reach a diagnosis?
A. Schilling test.
B. Duodenal biopsy.
C. Small bowel meal.
D. $^{14}CO_2$ breath test.

Question 60

An 18-year-old female had blood tests as part of a routine medical (right).

1. Suggest two possible diagnoses.
2. Which two investigations could be performed to differentiate between the diagnoses?

Hb	10.5 g/dl
WCC	6×10^9/l
Platelets	300×10^9/l
MCV	61 fl
MCHC	28 g/l
MCH	19 pg
Red cell count	6.8×10^{12}/l
Blood film	Hypochromia, anisocytosis, poikilocytosis, target cells
Sodium	136 mmol/l
Potassium	4.1 mmol/l
Urea	4 mmol/l
Creatinine	72 µmol/l

Answer 59

1. D. Radiation enteritis.
2. C. Small bowel meal.

The patient has a malabsorption syndrome. The B_{12} level is low in the presence of a normal folate level. This suggests either selective B_{12} malabsorption due to terminal ileal disease (Crohn's disease, terminal ileal resection, ileal TB), pernicious anaemia or excess utilization of B_{12} within the gut itself (bacterial overgrowth which occurs in the presence of a structural abnormality of the small bowel, e.g. after Billroth II gastric surgery, jejunal diverticula, Crohn's disease, intestinal fistulae, radiation enteritis and small bowel involvement in systemic sclerosis, amyloidosis and diabetic autonomic neuropathy).

Symptoms of malabsorption are absent in pernicious anaemia. The differential diagnosis is, therefore, between terminal ileal disease or bacterial overgrowth. There is no mention of small bowel surgery in the question. Ileal TB is unlikely in the absence of a febrile illness, night sweats,

only slightly elevated ESR, absent past history or contact with TB, and a normal chest X-ray. Although Crohn's disease is a possibility, the most likely answer is radiation enteritis. Radiation enteritis can complicate radiotherapy to the abdominal region. In the acute phase this may remain silent or present as diarrhoea. The sequel is fibrotic strictures or adhesions causing cramp-like abdominal pain. Strictures predispose to bacterial overgrowth, which in turn leads to steatorrhoea due to deconjugation of bile salts. Vitamin B_{12} is metabolized by the bacteria, whereas folate absorption is left unhindered. Moreover, some bacteria actually produce folate, often leading to elevated levels in the blood. Investigation involves small bowel meal, which will demonstrate the structural abnormality. Hydrogen or carbon dioxide breath tests will confirm the diagnosis.

Small bowel meal is regarded as the investigation of choice in this question because it will detect Crohn's disease, ileal TB, radiation enteritis and small-bowel lymphoma. The latter occasionally complicates radiotherapy, but does not lead to a selective B_{12} deficiency.

Answer 60

1. i. β-thalassaemia trait.
ii. Iron-deficiency anaemia.
2. i. Hb electrophoresis.
ii. Serum ferritin.

The best answer is β-thalassaemia trait. The clue lies in the fact that the MCV is disproportionately low compared with the Hb. In β-thalassaemia trait, the cells are small due to defective globin synthesis and are removed relatively rapidly from the circulation by the spleen. As a consequence, the marrow produces large amounts of red cells and, provided that iron and folate stores remain replenished, the Hb is only modestly reduced but the cells are relatively small. The red cell count itself, however, may be high. In iron deficiency, the marrow is unable to produce red cells to maintain a normal Hb because haem synthesis is incomplete without iron. Therefore, the number of cells produced (and hence the red cell count) is small compared with β-thalassaemia trait; however, the size is similar. By the time the iron deficiency has become severe enough to cause a reduction in the MCV as low as 61 fl, the Hb is much lower than in β-thalassaemia trait.

In β-thalassaemia major the Hb, red cell count and MCV are all very low, and such patients require life-long

blood transfusions to maintain a Hb around 10 g/dl. α-thalassaemia trait may present with a similar picture as β-thalassaemia trait if two of the four genes which code for α-globin chains are defective. When only one gene is defective the Hb and MCV are usually normal.

The investigation of choice is Hb electrophoresis. This is normal in a patient with iron deficiency, revealing approximately 98% HbA (i.e. normal Hb comprising two α- and two β-globin chains) and 2% HbA2 (two α- and two δ-globin chains). In β-thalassaemiaa trait the HbA is reduced to approximately 90%, the HbA2 is slightly increased to 6%, and in addition may be the presence of some HbF (fetal Hb; two α- and two γ-globin chains). The reason for this is that in β-thalassaemia trait the deficiency of normal β-globin means that α-globin chains combine with either γ-globin or δ-globin. In β-thalassaemia major, where there is no normal β-globin production, almost all the Hb is HbF.

The serum ferritin is also useful because it is low in iron deficiency but normal or increased in β-thalassaemia trait, unless there is coexisting iron deficiency. The slightly elevated ferritin in some patients with β-thalassaemia trait may be explained by the fact that defective β-globin synthesis prevents the marrow utilizing all the iron which is absorbed from the gastrointestinal tract, resulting in some iron accumulation.

Question 61

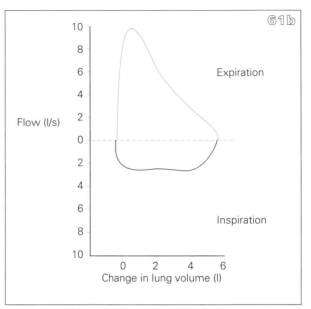

A 76-year-old female developed gradual onset of breathlessness over the past three weeks. On admission, she had stridor. Her respiratory rate was 30/min, and she was not cyanosed. Her trachea was slightly deviated to the right, and there was a mass just palpable in front of it, which moved slightly with respiration. The lower margins of the mass could not be defined Auscultation of the lungs revealed stridor-type sounds transmitted from the upper airways. She was managed with oxygen and saline nebulizers in the accident and emergency department, and felt considerably better. She mentioned having a problem with her thyroid gland, and over 20 years ago was told she did not need any treatment. She had lost 5 kg in weight over the past two months.

She had a chest radiograph (**61a**) in the accident and emergency department.

Lung function tests and a thyroid scan were performed the following day. Results of the flow loop curve (**61b**) and thyroid scan (**61c**) are shown.

1. What is the abnormality on the chest radiograph? List four possible causes for this appearance.
2. What is the abnormality on the flow loop curve and what does this suggest?
3. Give three possible causes for the abnormality in the flow loop curve in our patient.
4. What is the abnormality on the thyroid scan?
5. List two tests which would help confirm the cause of her breathlessness.

Question 62

The blood results shown were performed two months apart in a patient with HIV infection.

1. What is the most likely cause for the discrepancy between the results?

	October	December
Hb (g/dl)	11.8	7.6
WCC (× 10⁹/l)	3.0	3.1
Platelets (× 10⁹/l)	160	90
MCV (fl)	86	110
Reticulocyte count (%)	1.5	4
CD4	120	24

Answer 61

1. The lateral chest X-ray reveals a mass in the superior mediastinum. Possible causes of a superior mediastinal mass include retrosternal goitre, thymoma, lymphoma, malignant lymphadenopathy, teratoma, and aneurysm of the aortic arch. The most likely cause of the mass in this situation is a retrosternal goitre.
2. There is evidence of reduced airflow rate which is more pronounced in the inspiratory phase of respiration. This is suggestive of extrathoracic large airways obstruction. Typical examples include retrosternal goitre and its complications, compression by malignant lymph nodes and bilateral vocal cord paralysis.
3. i. Compression from a retrosternal multinodular goitre which has undergone malignant change.
ii. Compression from a retrosternal multinodular goitre due to spontaneous haemorrhage within the gland.
iii. Compression from locally metastasized lymphatic deposits from carcinoma of the thyroid.
4. A large 'cold nodule' in the left lobe of the thyroid gland.
5. i. CT scan of the neck and upper thorax.
ii. Fine-needle aspirate of the thyroid gland for histology.

There is a history of a chronic thyroid disorder in this elderly woman. She is clinically and biochemically euthyroid, and has a palpable mass in the suprasternal area which moves with swallowing. The most probable cause for the mass in the superior mediastinum is a retrosternal extension of a goitre. The reason for sudden deterioration is tracheal compression due to rapid enlargement of the goitre. This may occur as a result of haemorrhage or malignant change within the goitre. An additional cause of tracheal compression in this situation is compression from malignant lymph nodes. Tracheal compression causes stridor when it is severe. It is potentially a medical emergency requiring rapid relief of the compression, the speed of which is determined by the extent of respiratory embarrassment.

Carcinoma of the thyroid complicates approximately 4% of multinodular goitres. Most patients are asymptomatic, but some experience symptoms as a result of local compression of structures which include dysphagia, dysphonia, stridor and haemoptysis. Technetium scanning is the most widely used imaging agent of a goitre. Lack of uptake of technetium in parts of the thyroid gland is suggestive of hypofunction. Such 'cold' nodules are associated with carcinoma of the thyroid in 20% of cases. Cold areas can also occur with cysts, colloid adenomas, degenerative nodules and thyroiditis. The differentiation from a cyst is possible with US scanning. This patient has a very large area in the left lobe where there is no uptake (cold area). An US will confirm whether this is a cystic or a solid lesion; however, in this case the symptom of stridor raises the suspicion of sinister pathology and therefore a CT scan of the neck and thorax is more likely to provide extra information about the gland, its pathology and the extent of direct invasion from a probable malignant process. Fine-needle aspiration of the lesion is an invaluable means of making a histological diagnosis, provided an experienced cytopathologist is available to interpret the histology. The main limitation of this procedure is that it does not necessarily allow differentiation between a follicular adenoma and follicular carcinoma, and in a few cases false-negative results are generated due to sampling error. The results of the aspirate should be interpreted in the context of the patient's presentation and results from other imaging techniques.

Answer 62

1. Zidovudine toxicity.

The patient has become more anaemic, has developed a macrocytosis, thrombocytopenia and an increase in the CD4 count. The most likely cause of these abnormalities is treatment with AZT. AZT is a nucleoside analogue which inhibits the viral enzyme reverse transcriptase and is a DNA chain terminator. It is widely used in symptomatic HIV infection. In such patients it has been shown to reduce mortality by reducing the incidence of opportunistic infections due to a significant but transient improvement in the CD4 count. The drug has important haematological side effects which include a reduction in all cell lines and a megaloblastic change in the marrow. The general side effects of the drug include nausea, vomiting, myalgia, headaches, neuropathy and myopathy.

Other drugs which cause pancytopenia and macrocytosis in HIV patients are co-trimoxazole (used in the treatment of *Pneumocystis carinii*) and 2'3'-deoxynucleoside analogues other than AZT, such as dideoxyadenosine and dideoxyinosine. The latter drugs have less marrow toxicity.

Marrow suppression may occur in HIV as a direct result of the virus. Another important haematological manifestation of HIV in relation to the MRCP and similar examinations is the presence of a circulating anticoagulant in some cases.

Question 63

A 30-year-old Bangladeshi female was admitted to hospital with a two-month history of increasing lethargy and ankle swelling. One week before admission she developed right upper quadrant pain, nausea and anorexia. She immigrated from Bangladesh two years ago, and ever since coming to this country she had noticed a troublesome cough which was productive of yellow sputum and for which she had been prescribed several courses of oral antibiotics. She lived with her husband in a rented flat.

On examination, she was thin and slightly pale. Her temperature was 37.5°C (99.5°F). The heart rate was 110 beats/min and regular; the blood pressure was 95/55 mmHg. The JVP was grossly elevated. On examination of the precordium the apex was not palpable, and on auscultation both heart sounds were soft. On examination of the respiratory system there were harsh breath sounds on auscultation of the left upper zone. Abdominal examination demonstrated smooth and tender hepatomegaly palpable 6 cm below the costal margin. In addition, there was clinical evidence of moderate ascites. The lower limbs had pitting oedema to the shins.

Investigations are shown.

FBC	Hb 11 g/dl
	WCC 10 × 10⁹/l
	Platelets 180 × 10⁹/l
	MCV 85 fl
ESR	80 mm/h
Biochemistry	Sodium 129 mmol/l
	Potassium 4.3 mmol/l
	Urea 8 mmol/l
	Creatinine 90 µmol/l
	Glucose 5 mmol/l
Echocardiogram (**63a**)	
Sputum microscopy (**63b**)	

1. What is demonstrated on the echocardiogram?
2. What is the most probable cause for the abnormality on the echocardiogram?
3. List two therapeutic steps in your management of this patient.
4. What other step would you take after initiating therapy for the patient?

Question 64

The data are from cardiac catheter traces of a 14-year-old male, taken five years apart.

1. List three abnormalities in the catheter performed five years ago.
2. List three abnormalities in the catheter performed most recently.
3. What is the unifying diagnosis?

	5 years ago		Present	
	Pressure (mmHg)	Satn (%)	Pressure (mmHg)	Satn (%)
Superior vena cava		68		49
Right atrium	8	68	12	50
Right ventricle	40/5	94	120/20	50
Pulmonary artery	40/18	94	115/55	50
Pulmonary capillary wedge pressure	6		8	
Left ventricle	110/4	95	115/15	57
Aorta	115/60	95	100/50	50

Answer 63

1. The echocardiogram demonstrates a large pericardial effusion. (See *Table* for causes.) (See Echocardiography, page 223.)
2. Tuberculous pericardial effusion.
3. i. Pericardiocentesis.
ii. Empirical antituberculous therapy with rifampicin, isoniazid and ethambutol. In patients of ethnic origin, or where multi-resistant bacilli are suspected, there is a case for adding pyrazinamide.
4. Contact tracing.

Causes of pericardial effusion
Any infective pericarditis
Uraemia
Post myocardial infarction
Post cardiotomy
Dressler's syndrome
SLE
Rheumatoid arthritis
Malignancy
Hypothyroidism
Trauma
Aortic dissection
Drugs, e.g. practolol, phenylbutazone, procainamide, hydralazine

The most likely underlying cause is TB, considering that the woman has a productive cough and the sputum, which is stained with the Ziehl–Neelsen stain, reveals acid-fast bacilli. In the UK, the incidence of TB in immigrants from the Asian subcontinent is 40 times higher than in the native white population. Primary TB is usually without symptoms in the majority of individuals, although in a few cases there may be a cough, wheeze and fever. The primary complex heals with calcification; however, there may be reactivation of infection several years later due to malnourishment or conditions predisposing to immunosuppression resulting in pulmonary TB and possible dissemination to other organs via the lymphatics and the bloodstream.

The diagnosis is based on identifying the organism from pericardial fluid. In the simplest form this may be done by staining the fluid with Ziehl–Neelsen to reveal acid-fast bacilli, however, the yield is only 25% with this method. The organism may be cultured on Lowenstein-Jensen medium but this can take over 8 weeks. The quickest method of making the diagnosis in the event of a negative acid-fast stain is by PCR to tuberculous protein or by demonstrating evidence of the disease elsewhere, for example in the sputum.

Treatment is with empirical anti-tuberculous therapy. Because TB is spread from person to person, and effective tracing of close contacts helps limit spread of the disease, it is important to identify all individuals who may have come into close contact with the patient or those who share the same bathroom facilities. Individuals who are traced should have a chest X-ray and a tuberculin test. In adults, a normal chest X-ray positive test is a sign of immunity and nothing more needs to be done. In children who have not had a BCG vaccine, a positive tuberculin test is taken as evidence of infection, and treatment is instituted. If the test is negative, it is repeated again in six weeks and if remains negative the patient is given the BCG vaccine. In children under the age of one year who have a family member with TB, isoniazid is given as chemoprophylaxis for six months, together with immunization with a strain of BCG which is resistant to isoniazid.

Answer 64

1. i. Elevated right ventricular pressure.
ii. Elevated pulmonary artery pressure.
iii. Increase in oxygen saturation in the right ventricle, suggesting a left-to-right shunt at the level of the ventricle.
2. i. Huge increase in right ventricular pressure in the following five years.
ii. Huge increase in pulmonary artery pressure in the following five years.
iii. Reduction in oxygen saturation in the left ventricle, suggesting a right-to-left shunt at the level of the ventricles.
3. There has been a large increase in right ventricular pressure, leading to shunt reversal. The patient has developed Eisenmenger's phenomenon.

(See Guidelines for the Interpretation of Cardiac Catheter Data, page 220.)

Question 65

A 45-year-old male was referred to the local psychiatrist by his general practitioner with a three-month history of lethargy, loss of appetite, nausea, early morning wakening and loss of libido. He had recently lost his job as a clerk for making three serious errors in the space of a fortnight. There was no history of headaches or weight loss. He had experienced intermittent abdominal pain after meals which was investigated with upper gastrointestinal endoscopy four weeks earlier and attributed to a small gastric ulcer. Biopsy from the ulcer demonstrated an inflammatory infiltrate but there was no evidence of malignancy or *Helicobacter pyloris*. He had a long history of constipation which had not caused him any concern, and more recently complained of pains in his hands and feet. He was not sleeping well and awoke between two and three times a night to pass urine, which was extremely unusual for him. His wife was concerned that he was worried about loss of earnings and had become very depressed. He had no other significant past medical history. He was a non-smoker and consumed half a bottle of wine daily.

On examination, he had a reduced affect. There was no pallor, clubbing or lymphadenopathy. He was apyrexial. The heart rate was 96 beats/min and blood pressure 160/95 mmHg. Examination of his eye is shown (**65a**). On abdominal examination, a mass was identified in the right iliac fossa which was indentible. There was no tenderness and the bowel sounds were audible. A rectal examination was not performed. The examination of the cardiovascular and respiratory system was normal. He had painful hands, but there was no evidence of joint swelling or restriction of movements. Examination of his central nervous system, including his higher mental function was entirely normal.

Investigations are shown.

1. List two tests you would perform to come to a rapid diagnosis.
2. What is the definitive treatment?
3. How would you manage the patient after he has had the definitive treatment?

FBC	Hb 15 g/dl
	WCC 5 × 10⁹/l
	Platelets 306 × 10⁹/l
ESR	18 mm/h
Biochemistry	Sodium 136 mmol/l
	Potassium 4.2 mmol/l
	Bicarbonate 19 mmol/l
	Chloride 115 mmol/l
	Urea 7 mmol/l
	Creatinine 89 µmol/l
	Bilirubin 12 µmol/l
	AST 24 u/l
	Alkaline phosphatase 300 u/l
	Total protein 78 g/l
	Albumin 44 g/l
X-ray of hands (**65b**)	

Answer 65

1. **i.** Serum calcium.
ii. PTH level.
2. Parathyroidectomy.
3. Vitamin D supplements.

The symptoms of hypercalcaemia are rather non-specific, and include nausea, anorexia, weight loss, abdominal pain, bone pain, polyuria, polydipsia, lack of concentration, depression and occasionally acute psychosis. The abdominal pain may be non-specific or due to constipation, peptic ulcer disease, pancreatitis and renal colic, all of which are recognized complications of hyperparathyroidism. It is worth remembering that while nephrocalcinosis is also a complication of hyperparathyroidism, it is not associated with abdominal pain. This man has several of these symptoms, as well as recent peptic ulcer disease. The eye in **65a** reveals corneal calcification which occurs in hypercalcaemic states. The calcification is usually seen at the 3 and 9 o'clock positions. The hand X-ray (**65b**) demonstrates periosteal bone resorption which is characteristic of hyperparathyroidism. Hyperparathyroid-related bone disease is further supported by the raised alkaline phosphatase level. Bone changes are seen in 2% of cases of hyperparathyroidism. Cystic lesions may be present, and can result in pathological fractures. Extensive bone resorption affecting the skull gives it a characteristic 'salt-and-pepper' appearance on the skull X-ray.

Hyperparathyroidism is diagnosed by demonstrating elevated or normal levels of PTH in the presence of a high serum calcium. Primary hyperparathyroidism is usually secondary to a single, benign parathyroid adenoma. Hyperparathyroidism due to carcinoma of the parathyroid glands is extremely rare. Hyperparathyroidism can be part of MEN syndromes. Secondary hyperparathyroidism results from chronic calcium deficiency, and is a compensating mechanism whereby all four parathyroid glands undergo hyperplasia. In this situation, the calcium may be low or normal, but the PTH level is elevated. The condition is treated with vitamin D and calcium supplements. Tertiary hyperparathyroidism complicates some cases of secondary hyperparathyroidism where autonomous production of PTH occurs, leading to hypercalcaemia which is not controlled with vitamin D or calcium supplements. In this case, there is no underlying disorder to predispose to secondary or tertiary hyperparathyroidism, and so the most likely answer is primary hyperparathyroidism.

Other causes of hypercalcaemia are given below (*Table*). Myeloma is unlikely in the presence of a normal full blood count, ESR and globulin level. Sarcoidosis is associated with hypercalcaemia and band keratopathy, but is less likely in the presence of a normal chest X-ray. Moreover, it would not explain the X-ray changes in the hands. This patient is not taking regular antacids, which excludes the milk-alkali syndrome, a condition caused by chronic ingestion of calcium-based antacids and milk for the relief of dyspepsia or peptic ulcer disease. Metastatic bone disease is a possibility, but the majority of patients with bony metastases have overt metastatic deposits, particularly in areas where pain is experienced. In such cases, the albumin level is also low due to cachexia and the plasma bicarbonate is normal or high because bony destruction often releases bicarbonate from the bone. In hyperparathyroidism in the absence of renal disease, a mild metabolic acidosis is common. It is due to RTA and is reflected by a slightly low bicarbonate and a high chloride level.

In the past, other causes of hypercalcaemia – particularly malignancy – could be differentiated from hyperparathyroidism by the hydrocortisone suppression test, where high doses of hydrocortisone given daily for a week would fail to reduce the serum calcium level in hyperparathyroidism but not in other cases; however, the more sensitive PTH assays used nowadays have made this test obsolete.

Treatment of primary hyperparathyroidism is with total parathyroidectomy following transplantation of a small amount of parathyroid tissue into the forearm muscles. Following surgery, calcium levels have to be monitored because they fall rapidly and tetany can be precipitated. Hypocalcaemia can persist for several months during which time it is important to continue vitamin D supplements.

(See also Calcium Biochemistry table, page 217.)

Causes of hypercalcaemia	
1° hyperparathyroidism	Paget's disease (immobility)
3° hyperparathyroidism	Familial hypocalcuric hypercalcaemia
Sarcoidosis	
Multiple myeloma	
Thiazide diuretics	
Milk-alkali syndrome	
Addison's disease	
Acromegaly	
Phaeochromocytoma	
Thyrotoxicosis	
Vitamin D intoxication	

Question 66

A 44-year-old female was persuaded to come into hospital after she was seen in the out-patient clinic with jaundice. She was diagnosed as having autoimmune CAH five months ago and was successfully treated with high-dose steroids, which had gradually been withdrawn. She had not been taking any medication before admission and denied alcohol consumption.

On examination, she was thin and deeply jaundiced. She was alert and orientated, and did not demonstrate any signs of cognitive impairment. Abdominal examination was essentially normal.

Investigations on admission are shown.

Two days following admission, the patient became suddenly very aggressive, and soon after collapsed and was comatosed.

FBC	Hb 12.3 g/dl
	WCC 8×10^9/l
	Platelets 45×10^9/l
	MCV 109 fl
Clotting	PT 59 s (control 13 s)
	APTT 90 s (control 45 s)
LFT	Bilirubin 300 µmol/l
	AST 350 u/l
	Alkaline phosphatase 340 u/l
	Albumin 26 g/l

1. Which urgent investigation would be most useful in determining the cause of collapse?
A. CT scan of the head.
B. EEG.
C. Drug screen for sedatives.
D. Blood cultures.
E. Blood glucose.

Question 67

This pedigree chart (**67**) is from a family with a very rare condition.

1. What is the mode of inheritance?
2. What are the chances of A being affected?
3. What are the chances of B being affected?
4. What are the chances of C being affected?

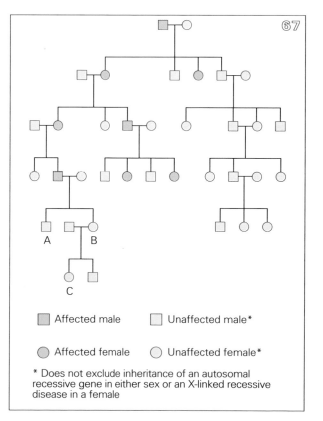

* Does not exclude inheritance of an autosomal recessive gene in either sex or an X-linked recessive disease in a female

Answer 66

1. E. Blood glucose.

The patient was admitted with gross hepatic dysfunction. She had previously been successfully treated with corticosteroids, and had a relapse after they were gradually withdrawn. She became aggressive and then comatosed. The most probable diagnosis is hepatic encephalopathy. Precipitating factors include gastrointestinal haemorrhage, sepsis, hypokalaemia, drugs promoting catabolism, sedatives and hypoglycaemia. In hepatic encephalopathy it is possible for both hypoglycaemia and hyperglycaemia to occur because glucose homeostasis is disturbed. Glycogen is neither efficiently stored nor mobilized and gluconeogenesis is impaireds. Early features of encephalopathy include confusion, irritation, aggressiveness or psychosis. Coma can ensue rapidly. The test which would be most useful in determining the cause of collapse is the serum blood glucose, because its correction and therapeutic effect are almost immediate. There is nothing in the history or examination to suggest sepsis, although it must be noted that patients with chronic liver disease do not always have a pyrexia. There is no history of sedative drug ingestion, and in practice screening for sedative drugs in unhelpful because it seldom influences the management. A cerebral haemorrhage is possible in the presence of a raised PT and low platelets. If the blood glucose is normal, a cerebral haemorrhage should be excluded by CT scanning of the head. If this is normal, the diagnosis is encephalopathy. An EEG is not necessary to diagnose encephalopathy, but at the onset of encephalopathy the EEG shows an alpha rhythm and as drowsiness worsens this is replaced by lower frequency theta activity. In deep coma, high-amplitude delta waves are present.

Answer 67

1. X-linked dominant.
2. Nil.
3. 100%.
4. 50%.

In X-linked conditions there is no male-to-male transmission. In X-linked dominant conditions, the female offspring of affected males have an abnormal phenotype, and in X-linked recessive conditions all female offspring are carriers but do not have the disease. In X-linked dominant conditions, an affected female will transmit the disorder to 50% of her daughters and 50% of her sons. In X-linked recessive conditions, an affected female will transmit the disease to 50% of her sons, and 50% of the daughters will be carriers i.e none will have the disease phenotype.

Examples of X-linked dominant condition include vitamin D-resistant rickets. Rett's syndrome, incontinentia pigmentii.

Question 68

A 65-year-old male was admitted with a six-week history of progressive dyspnoea. One week before admission he had developed dyspnoea at rest, orthopnoea and paroxysmal nocturnal dyspnoea. He had lost his appetite, and had lost over half a stone in weight in six weeks. He had a cough productive of yellow sputum initially which was treated with antibiotics; however, the cough persisted and three days before admission he had an episode of frank haemoptysis. The patient had enjoyed a very active and independent life and, apart from a truncal vagotomy and drainage procedure for a perforated duodenal ulcer 20 years ago, he had been very well. He was a non-smoker.

On examination, he appeared pale and was dyspnoeic. The heart rate was 144 beats/min and irregular; the blood pressure was 160/100 mmHg. The JVP was not raised. The respiratory rate was 30/min and temperature was 38°C (100.4°F). The heart sounds appeared normal; there were no audible murmurs. Auscultation of the lung fields revealed fine inspiratory crackles both anteriorly and posteriorly.

Examination of the abdomen and central nervous system was normal.

A subclavian line was inserted which revealed a CVP of 3 cm H_2O. A urinary catheter drained a residual urine volume of of 300 ml.

Investigations were as follows:

FBC	Hb 5.3 g/dl	Arterial blood gases	pH 7.32
	WCC 17×10^9/l	(on 40% oxygen)	pCO_2 5.6 kPa
	Platelets 249×10^9/l		pO_2 14 kPa
	MCV 89 fl		Bicarbonate 14 mmol/l
	MCHC 34 g/dl		O_2 saturation 99%
ESR	102 mm/h	Blood cultures	No growth
Biochemistry	Sodium 131 mmol/l	Urinalysis	Blood +++
	Potassium 5.7 mmol/l		Protein +++
	Urea 29 mmol/l		Pus cells +++
	Creatinine 560 µmol/l		Granular casts +++
	Calcium 2.1 mmol/l	Urine culture	No growth
	Phosphate 1.5 mmol/l	ECG	Atrial fibrillation; ventricular
	Albumin 33 g/l		rate of 154/min
	Bilirubin 14 µmol/l		Non-specific T-wave changes
	AST 19 u/l	Chest X-ray (**68**)	
	Alkaline phosphatase 113 u/l	Echocardiogram	Biatrial enlargement
	LDH 1320 u/l		Mild left ventricular
Thyroid function tests	Normal		hypertrophy with good
CRP	316 g/l		systolic function
PT	12 s (control 12 s)		The mitral valve appeared
APTT	43 s (control 41 s)		normal
Renal US	Normal-sized kidneys with		
	echogenic renal parenchyma		
	No evidence of obstruction		

The patient was treated with intravenous cefuroxime and erythromycin, and gently transfused with 3 units of packed cells. The temperature came down, CVP increased to 9 cm H_2O, and urine output averaged 420 ml/24 h. The Hb following transfusion was 6.4 g/dl. While on the ward, the patient had three episodes of frank haemoptysis.

Serial chest X-rays over four days remained unchanged. He reverted to sinus rhythm three days after commencing digoxin.

Serum biochemistry on day 4 is shown below.

Sodium 131 mmol/l
Potassium 6.0 mmol/l
Urea 35 mmol/l
Creatinine 780 µmol/l

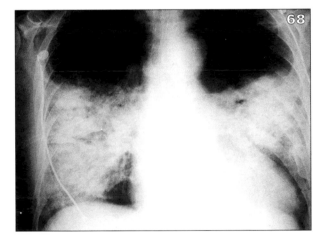

1. Describe the chest X-ray and give two possible pathological causes for this appearance.
2. List three possible diagnoses.
3. List at least four further tests which would be useful in confirming the diagnosis.
4. The patient was given 120 mg of intravenous frusemide, with no increase in urine output. What would be the next step in your management?

Answer 68

1. The chest X-ray reveals bilateral, widespread alveolar shadowing with sparing of the apices.

Possible causes of alveolar shadowing on the chest X-ray include:

i. Pulmonary oedema.
ii. Pulmonary haemorrhage.
iii. Pulmonary consolidation.

In this case, pulmonary oedema is unlikely if the apices are spared, and this could only be explained if there was pre-existing, severe bilateral apical emphysema.

2. The patient has a relatively acute illness involving the respiratory and renal system.

Possible cause of a systemic illness causing respiratory and renal impairment include:

The vasculitides (in order of decreasing frequency):
• Anti-GBM disease or Goodpasture's syndrome.
• Polyarteritis nodosa.
• Wegener's granulomatosis.
• Systemic lupus erythematosus.

Infection:
• Legionnaire's disease and secondary interstitial nephritis.
• Pneumococcal pneumonia with mycotic emboli to the kidneys.

3. i. Anti-GBM antibodies.
ii. ANCA.
iii. Renal biopsy with immunofluoresence studies.
iv. Transbronchial lung biopsy if the patient's respiratory status permits.
v. Anti-nuclear factor.
vi. *Legionella* antigen in the urine or *Legionella* RMAT on the serum.
vii. TLCO.
4. Haemodialysis.

The history of continuing haemoptysis and failure of the haemoglobin to rise sufficiently after blood transfusion strongly suggest that the chest X-ray appearances are secondary to pulmonary haemorrhage rather than any other cause. The presence of normal-sized kidneys is suggestive of an acute renal process. In chronic renal disease, the kidney size is usually small, although there are a few exceptions (see *Table A*). Pulmonary haemorrhage and acute renal failure are best explained by a systemic vasculitis. The best answers are, therefore, anti-GBM, polyarteritis nodosa or Wegener's granulomatosis in decreasing frequency. Anti-GBM disease is a rare condition where antibodies to the basement membrane of the glomeruli and alveoli lead to acute nephritis and pulmonary haemorrhage, respectively. The disease presents with cough, fatigue, dyspnoea or haemoptysis followed days, weeks or months later, by glomerulonephritis.

Wegener's granulomatosis would be the best answer if there was additional upper respiratory tract involvement. Although it is also possible, involvement of the upper respiratory tract is much more common in Wegener's than in any of the other vasculitides. SLE is rare in males and in this age group. Pulmonary haemorrhage is much less common in SLE than in the other vasculitides mentioned above. Although Legionnaire's disease is possible, there is no history of travel abroad or being in an environment with air conditioning, and it does not easily explain the pulmonary haemorrhage. Fever is a recognized feature of both infection and the vasculitides. The initial cough productive of yellow-brown sputum may have been secondary to a respiratory tract infection

---

Table A. Causes of chronic renal impairment with normal-sized kidneys

Myeloma
Diabetes mellitus
Amyloidosis
Polycystic kidney disease (kidneys are usually huge by the time renal impairment becomes apparent)

---

which is of interest because pulmonary haemorrhage is more common in anti-GBM disease if there has been a recent respiratory infection. Other factors predisposing to pulmonary haemorrhage in anti-GBM disease are smoking, coexisting pulmonary oedema and exposure to organic solvents.

Other conditions which affect the respiratory and renal system include IgA nephritis, which occurs following upper respiratory tract infections. Respiratory involvement can occur as an indirect consequence of glomerulonephritis if the ensuing renal failure is complicated by fluid overload, producing pulmonary oedema. A rare situation where a primarily renal disorder affects the respiratory system to produce haemoptysis is renal vein thrombosis complicated by pulmonary embolism.

The tests should be based around making the most probable diagnosis where two or three diagnoses are possible. The presence of anti-GBM antibodies will make the diagnosis of anti-GBM disease, which can be confirmed on renal biopsy, and immunofluorescence studies which will demonstrate IgG deposits around the GBM. A lung biopsy would be dangerous in the presence of frank pulmonary haemorrhage. High titres of serum ANCA may support a vasculitic process, particularly if the anti-GBM antibody is absent. Again, a renal or lung biopsy with immunofluoresence should help make the final diagnosis. The TLCO is raised in pulmonary haemorrhage. It is useful in the assessment of haemorrhage in the acute situation because the chest X-ray appearance takes several days to improve, even if the haemorrhage has ceased. The causes of raised TLCO are listed (*Table B*).

If Legionnaire's disease is suspected, and a rapid diagnosis is required, the best tests are estimation of the *Legionella* antigen and the RMAT. *Legionella* antigen is present in the urine of 90% of patients within 48 hours. The RMAT can be performed on the serum and respiratory secretions, and a result is available on the same day. Testing for raised levels of *Legionella* antibodies is possible in this case because the disease has been present for a little while, but if the illness had started in the previous week then this test would not be useful in making a rapid diagnosis as it can take up to 10 days for the *Legionella*

antibodies to rise appreciably.

The patient is oliguric, acidotic, has a rapidly rising creatinine, and has developed hyperkalaemia. Haemodialysis is indicated in all of these situations and when the patient shows evidence of fluid overload. It allows the opportunity for plasmapheresis, which is successful in some patients with anti-GBM disease, particularly with respect to pulmonary haemorrhage. However, results on the renal system are not very satisfactory if plasmapheresis is initiated after significant renal impairment has occurred. Subsequent management will be with high-dose steroids and cyclophosphamide.

Table B. Causes of raised TLCO

Pulmonary haemorrhage
Polycythaemia
Left-to-right shunts
Asthma

Question 69

An 18-year-old male was admitted following a collapse at a local night club. On examination he was drowsy. His temperature was 40°C (104°F), and he was sweating profusely. His heart rate was 120 beats/min, and regular. The blood pressure was 160/110 mmHg. His pupils were dilated and reacted poorly to light.

Investigations are shown.

1. What is the underlying cause of his presentation?
2. Explain his serum potassium and phosphate levels.
3. What is the cause of his abnormal clotting?
4. List two therapeutic steps in the management of his temperature.
5. Give two explanations for the hyponatraemia.

Hb	11 g/dl
WCC	11 × 10⁹/l
Platelets	100 × 10⁹/l
PT	20 s
APTT	70 s
TT	16 s
Sodium	125 mmol/l
Potassium	7.4 mmol/l
Urea	10 mmol/l
Creatinine	123 µmol/l
Phosphate	1.7 mmol/l
Urine	Blood +++

Answer 69

1. 'Ecstasy' (3, 4-methylenedioxymetamphetamine; MDMA) abuse.
2. Rhabdomyolysis.
3. DIC.
4. i. Cooling/tepid sponging.
ii. Intravenous dantrolene.
5. i. Syndrome of inappropriate antidiuretic hormone.
ii. Excess sodium loss from skin during profuse perspiration.

The history is of collapse at a local night club, and on examination the patient has a very high temperature, is sweating profusely, has dilated pupils, and is hypertensive. The blood tests reveal evidence of renal failure with a disproportionately high potassium and phosphate, hinting that the patient may have rhabdomyolysis; the haematological tests suggest underlying DIC. In this case, the most probable diagnosis is 'Ecstasy abuse'. The case would have been more difficult if he was hypotensive because then the differential diagnosis would have included septicaemia, encephalitis or meningitis, all of which must also be borne in mind when attending to a young patient with any of these features.

Ecstasy abuse has become an increasingly common problem over the past few years, and therefore knowledge of its recognition and management have become almost mandatory. The clinical features are basically those of a large concentration of circulating catecholamines in the blood. In the acute situation it may present as collapse, convulsions and hyperpyrexia, i.e a core temperature of 39–42°C (102.2–107.6°F) (see *Table* for causes of hyperpyrexia). Other features comprise profuse sweating, tachycardia, hypertension and dilated pupils.

The blood pressure may also be low due to shock from excessive fluid loss secondary to perspiration. Complications of Ecstasy abuse include rhabdomyolysis, acute renal failure (either from reduced renal perfusion or myoglobin-induced tubular damage), DIC, acute hepatitis, myocardial infarction and cerebrovascular accident.

Hyponatraemia is a common problem and may be due to excess sodium loss from the skin during perspiration. The problem is compounded because most Ecstasy abusers are advised to drink large amounts of water which may replenish fluid, but not the actual salt loss. Further-

more, Ecstasy is thought to cause SIADH which may exacerbate the hyponatraemia. In some cases the sodium concentration may be low enough to precipitate cerebral oedema and intractable seizures.

The management of the patient involves cooling with tepid sponging, and rectal paracetamol. Intravenous dantrolene is useful in controlling the hyperpyrexia. Diazepam is effective in controlling seizures. Fluid replacement will depend on the sodium concentration and the CVP. The general rule is to administer 1 litre of saline to all patients with a high temperature and low blood pressure before inserting a central venous catheter, irrespective of the sodium concentration. If the blood pressure goes up and the heart rate comes down, this is followed by another litre. After this, any further fluid replacement is determined by the CVP and the sodium concentration. If the sodium is low and the CVP is low, the patient is infused with normal saline until the CVP is normal. Following this, the sodium and fluid intake and output is observed carefully and fluid restriction is instituted to help combat possible SIADH. In the patient where the sodium is low and the venous pressure is high/normal, fluid restriction is instituted for the same reasons; however, if the sodium is low enough to cause coma and seizures, then therapy is with mannitol or hypertonic saline and frusemide. In patients who are hypertensive on admission, fluid replacement should be guided by the CVP from the beginning, and all other rules are the same as those for patients who are hypotensive at presentation.

Causes of hyperpyrexia

Septicaemia
Viral infections
Malaria
Neuroleptic malignant syndrome
Malignant hyperpyrexia
Ecstasy or other amphetamine abuse
Cocaine abuse
Malignancy
Aspirin toxicity
Prostaglandins

Question 70

70a

70b

1. What is shown on inspection of this patient's arm pit?
2. Comment on the dexamethasone suppression test.
3. What is the differential diagnosis for the patient's presentation?
4. Which single biochemical test would you perform to confirm the diagnosis?
5. What is demonstrated on the CT scan of the abdomen?
6. Which other condition does the patient have?
7. What is the management of this patient?

A 52-year-old male was investigated for obesity of recent onset, polydipsia and polyuria. On examination, he had a blood pressure of 180/105 mmHg, and was obese. Examination of the arm pit is shown (70a). He underwent routine investigations which are shown.

FBC	Hb 14 g/dl
	WCC 12 × 10⁹/l
	Platelets 230 × 10⁹/l
Biochemistry	Sodium 139 mmol/l
	Potassium 3.2 mmol/l
	Urea 7 mmol/l
	Bicarbonate 30 mmol/l
	Glucose 16 mmol/l

Serum cortisol (nmol/l)	9.00 a.m.	Midnight
	940	1,000
After dexamethasone 2 mg q.i.d. for 48 h	900	800

Chest X-ray   Normal
CT scan abdomen (70b)

Answer 70

1. The arm pit demonstrates acanthosis nigricans.
2. The high dose of dexamethasone fails to suppress the elevated cortisol down to normal.
3. The differential diagnosis is between ectopic ACTH and an autonomous glucocorticoid-secreting adrenal tumour (**70d**).
4. Plasma ACTH level, which will be elevated in ectopic ACTH secretion and suppressed in a cortisol-secreting tumour.
5. The CT scan demonstrates an adrenal tumour on the left side (see also detail, **70c,** arrowed).
6. Diabetes mellitus.
7. Surgical excision of the affected adrenal gland.

Acanthosis nigricans is characterized by velvety hyper-pigmentation and overgrowth of skin affecting the neck, axilla, groin or the face. The condition may be a normal variant in the Asian race. It is associated with internal malignancy, particularly carcinoma of the stomach and the lung and lymphoma. It is also associated with a variety of endocrine disorders causing insulin resistance and hyper-androgenic states (*Table A*). In this case, it is due to Cushing's syndrome.

The high-dose dexamethasone test suppresses the serum cortisol in over 60% of patients with Cushing's

Table A. Causes of acanthosis nigricans

Normal variant (Asian race)
Obesity
Carcinoma stomach, lung
Lymphoma
Cushing's syndrome
Acromegaly
Insulin-resistant diabetes
Polycystic ovary syndrome
Androgen-secreting tumours

Table B. Causes of Cushing's syndrome

Pituitary basophil adenoma
Ectopic ACTH secretion
Adrenal adenoma
Adrenal carcinoma
Iatrogenic

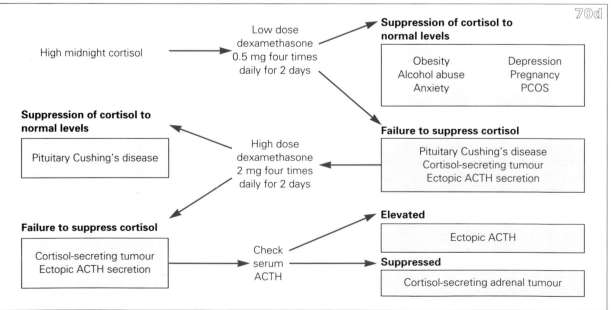

Table C. Complications of Cushing's syndrome

Obesity	Myopathy
Diabetes mellitus	Psychosis
Hypertension	Immunosuppression
Premature coronary artery disease	Poor wound healing
	Hypokalaemia
Osteoporosis	

The serum cortisol in patients with autonomous gluco-corticoid-secreting adenomas and those with ectopic ACTH production does not suppress to high-dose dexamethasone. In the normal clinical situation, the differential diagnosis between the three conditions, based on the dexamethasone suppression test, is not necessarily resolved; however, in the examination situation it is almost always assumed that suppression with high-dose dexamethasone excludes Cushing's disease.

disease (bilateral hyperplasia of the adrenal glands due to autonomous production of ACTH by a pituitary basophil adenoma); however, nearly 40% of cases fail to suppress.

Most tumours are benign; however, in rare instances adrenal carcinoma may result in Cushing's syndrome. Malignant tumours are highly aggressive and the prognosis is poor.

Question 71

71

A 69-year-old male was referred with a five-month history of pains in his shoulders and thighs, night sweats and weight loss of approximately 3 kg. The pain was worse in the mornings and during episodes of the night sweats. Two months previously the patient was seen in the accident and emergency department for ongoing testicular pain, but no obvious cause was found.

On examination, he appeared unwell and pale. He was apyrexial. There was no lymphadenopathy. His hands were examined (71). The heart rate was 104 beats/min and regular, and the blood pressure was 170/100 mmHg. The heart sounds were normal and the chest was clear. Abdominal examination was normal. On examination of the genitalia, there was testicular tenderness, but no swelling or erythema. There was no inguinal lymphadenopathy. Neurological examination demonstrated normal power, although hip extension was difficult due to painful quadriceps muscles. There was no fasciculation. Both ankle jerks, the left knee jerk and right supinator reflex were absent. There was loss of light touch sensation in both toes, extending to the medial border of the dorsal aspect of the left foot.

Investigations are shown.

FBC	Hb 9.5 g/dl
	WCC 15.1 × 10⁹/l
	Platelets 591 × 10⁹/l
	MCV 90 fl
ESR	104 mm/h
CRP	82 g/l
Biochemistry	Sodium 136 mmol/l
	Potassium 5.3 mmol/l
	Urea 6.5 mmol/l
	Creatinine 99 µmol/l
	Calcium 2.31 mmol/l
	Phosphate 0.9 mmol/l
	Albumin 35 g/l
	Bilirubin 7 µmol/l
	AST 22 u/l
	Gamma GT 43 u/l
	Alkaline phosphatase 162 u/l
	Total protein 77 g/l
	Glucose 5.4 mmol/l
Immunology	ANF negative
	Rheumatoid factor not detected
	Immunoelectrophoresis – polyclonal increase in gamma-globulin region
	No paraprotein
Blood cultures × 6	No growth
Urinalysis	Blood ++
	24 hour urine protein 2.4g
Urine culture	Negative. AAFB not detected on early morning urine specimens
Chest X-ray	Normal

1. Give at least two possible diagnoses.
2. List at least three useful investigations.

Answer 71

1. i. Polyarteritis nodosa (PAN).
ii. Polymyalgia rheumatica (PMR).
iii. Lymphoma.
iv. Testicular seminoma.
v. Post-primary TB.
2. i. Renal biopsy
ii Skin biopsy
iii. Muscle biopsy may help in the differentiation of vasculitis from polymyalgia rheumatica.
iv. Renal or hepatic angiography to demonstrate micro-aneurysms.
v. Serum ANCA lends support to a vasculitic process.
vi. CT scan thorax/abdomen to check for intra-abdominal malignancy, splenomegaly and para-aortic lymphadenopathy.
vii. Ultrasound of the testes.
viii. Bone marrow examination/culture for AAFB.
ix. Mantoux test.

This is a case where several diagnoses are possible. The patient is in his seventh decade and has evidence of general malaise, night sweats, weight loss and myalgia. There is clinical evidence of peripheral neuropathy. The inflammatory markers are elevated and the possible differential diagnoses in an elderly patient includes PAN, malignancy (including lymphoma), PMR and sepsis. TB is a possibility; however, a completely normal chest X-ray makes post-primary infection less probable. The main differentials are PAN and PMR. Factors differentiating between PAN and PMR have been tabulated below (*Table A*). Neuropathy can only be explained by PAN. The slide reveals livedo reticularis, which is a skin manifestation associated with connective tissue disease and the vasculitides. It is due to random spasm of cutaneous arterioles and secondary dilatation of capillaries and venules. The presence of livedo reticularis favours the diagnosis of PAN, which is a non-granulomatous vasculitis affecting medium-sized arteries. It is more common in males, and is most prevalent in the sixth and seventh decades. It may manifest with myalgia, night sweats and weight loss, and is a recognized cause of pyrexia of unknown origin. The disorder can affect the kidneys, cardiovascular system, gastrointestinal tract and nervous system. Arteritis leads to aneurysm formation, with subsequent thrombosis and infarction of the supplied organs. Clinical features include progressive glomerulonephritis, myocardial infarction, mesenteric ischaemia, peripheral neuropathy, CVA and vasculitic areas affecting the skin. Testicular pain is a recognized manifestation of PAN.

Inflammatory markers are elevated. ANCA may be detected and lend support for a vasculitic process, but it is not specific for PAN. The diagnosis is made by biopsying the affected organ or demonstrating micro-aneurysms on angiography. Treatment is with steroids.

Table A. Differentiation between PMR and PAN in this case

	PMR	PAN
Age	7th decade onwards	Middle age onwards
Sex	Male	Male
Symptoms	As above	As above
Neuropathy	Absent	Present
Testicular pain	Absent	Recognized
Livedo reticularis	Absent	Present
Raised ESR, CRP	Common	Common
Raised WCC, alkaline phosphatase	Common	Common
Raised ANF/Rh factor	Absent	Uncommon

Table B. American College of Rheumatology criteria for PAN

Weight loss of more than 4 kg
Livedo reticularis
Testicular pain
Myalgia, leg tenderness
Mono/polyneuropathy
Hepatitis B sAg positive
Arterographic abnormality
Positive biopsy

Table C. Causes of a very high (>100 mm/h) ESR

Multiple myeloma
Giant cell arteritis/polymyalgia rheumatica
Sepsis
Occult malignancy
SLE

Question 72

Hb	7.5 g/dl
MCV	95 fl
MCHC	34%
WCC	$10.5 \times 10^9/l$
Neutrophils	$8.4 \times 10^9/l$
Platelets	$290 \times 10^9/l$
Reticulocytes	9.8%
Blood film (72)	

A 45-year-old female on treatment for ulcerative colitis complained of increasing tiredness, while her bowel problems seemed well controlled.

Some of her results are shown.

1. What type of anaemia do these results suggest?
2. What is the likely cause?

Question 73

A 26-year-old male presented to the accident and emergency department with a stiff jaw and being unable to open his mouth. Three days previously he was immunized with tetanus toxin after lacerating his finger at work. On examination, he had evidence of 'lock jaw'. His injured finger was swollen, painful and exuding pus.

1. What is the immediate management?
A. Debridement and cleansing of the wound.
B. Injection of tetanus antitoxin into the wound.
C. Oral penicillin V.
D. Intramuscular human tetanus immunoglobulin.
E. Intravenous pancuronium.

Answer 72

1. Oxidative haemolytic anaemia.
2. Therapy with sulphasalazine.

The patient has a low Hb and a high reticulocyte count, suggesting either haemolysis or recent blood loss. The blood film is diagnostic. It is stained with methyl violet to reveal small inclusions within red cells termed Heinz bodies, which are essentially precipitated Hb. They occur in patients with genetic Hb abnormalities (unstable Hb), or when the iron within the haem molecule is oxidized from the ferrous state (Fe^{2+}) to the ferric state (Fe^{3+}) to produce methaemoglobin. Causes of methaemoglobinaemia are discussed in Answer **120**, page 156. In this case, therapy for ulcerative colitis with sulphasalazine (sulphonamide) is the culprit. Patients taking sulphonamides may develop a chronic haemolytic anaemia due to the oxidative action of the drugs on the Hb. Haemolysis is particularly severe in patients with glucose-6-phosphate dehydrogenase deficiency. Management involves drug withdrawal; however, if this is not possible then a lower dosage should be prescribed, together with iron and folate supplements.

Answer 73

1. D. Intramuscular injection of human anti-tetanus immunoglobulin.

Tetanus is caused by the anaerobic, Gram-positive bacillus *Clostridium tetani*. The organism produces spores which are commonly found in soil and faeces of domestic animals. Soil is the natural habitat for *Cl. tetani*. The organism gains entry into the body through traumatic wounds, where it multiplies under anaerobic conditions and produces tetanospasmin, a potent neurotoxin. The toxin reaches the spinal cord via the blood or by retrograde axon transport and increases excitability in motor neurones by interfering with the function of inhibitory neurones. The toxin may also produce overactivity of the sympathetic nervous system. The incubation period after injury is less than 14 days and can be as early as 2 days.

The dominant features of tetanus are rigidity and reflex spasms. Rigidity may affect any muscle, including the jaw muscles so that the mouth cannot be fully opened as in this case. This is known as 'trismus' or 'lock jaw'. Stiffness may affect the facial muscles, altering facial appearance. Risus sardonicus (pursing of the lips with retraction of the angles of the mouth) is a characteristic feature of this phenomenon. Pharyngeal involvement may produce dysphagia early in the disease. Rigidity of the muscles of the back cause the body to curve back excessively with the head fully retracted (ophisthotonus). Reflex spasms are a sudden exacerbation of underlying rigidity which last 1–2 seconds. The time of onset of spasms from the first symptoms of rigidity is know as the 'period time'. This is usually within 72 hours. The shorter the period time, the worse the prognosis. Large groups of muscles are affected at any one time. Relaxation may take a few seconds, which is particularly hazardous when thoracic muscles are involved because respiration is impeded until relaxation of the muscles occurs. Laryngeal spasm is probably the most dangerous event in tetanus.

Autonomic overactivity has effects on the cardiovascular system. Tachycardia, massive swings in blood pressure and cardiac arrhythmias are recognized complications. Haemodynamic instability may produce hypoperfusion of vital organs leading to multisystem failure and death. Most deaths are from respiratory failure, either due to laryngeal spasms, respiratory muscle fatigue and paralysis, or pulmonary aspiration.

The mainstay of treatment in an affected individual is to give intramuscular human immunoglobulin immediately. Human immunoglobulin will remove circulating tetanospasmin from the blood. Fixed neurotoxin has to be removed from the wound by aggressive cleansing and, if necessary, by surgical debridement of the wound. Despite such measures the organism may not be entirely removed from the wound and added protection with intravenous penicillin is mandatory. Diazepam is useful in controlling spasms. In severe cases total paralysis with curarization (using intravenous pancuronium) and artificial ventilatory support are necessary to reduce mortality from respiratory failure.

Prevention is by active immunization and meticulous wound cleansing as soon as possible after trauma.

Question 74

A 33-year-old Indian male presented with a four-week history of a painful swollen knee which he attributed to a fall during a game of tennis. The knee was painful after the fall, but over the next two weeks he developed swelling and increasing pain which was only partially relieved by paracetamol. He had never had a similar problem in the past. Apart from feeling slightly more breathless than usual while playing tennis over the past three months, he had no other complaints. There was no significant family history except that his grandparents had both had TB. He could not ever recall having had a BCG vaccine, but did have several chest X-rays in his early teenage years. On examination, he appeared well. He had a temperature of 37.5°C (99.5°F). Examination of his upper arms did not reveal a BCG scar. Examination of the left knee demonstrated a painful erythematous joint with a large synovial effusion. On examination of the respiratory system there were some harsh breath sounds in anterior aspect of the chest. The attending rheumatologist requested some investigations which are shown.

On the basis of these investigations, the patient was commenced on empirical antituberculous therapy. He was reviewed four months later and had an ESR check which measured 57 mm/h. The swelling in the left knee had subsided, but the changes on the chest X-ray persisted. Six months later he presented to the accident and emergency department with swelling in his right knee and both ankles. In addition, he complained of pain in the cervical area and lower back pain which radiated into the buttocks and was worse in the mornings.

1. What is the diagnosis?
2. How would you explain the changes on the chest X-ray?
3. Give two diagnostic tests.
4. Apart from diagnostic tests, which other investigation would you perform to help his further management?
5. What is the management of his condition?

74a

FBC	Hb 12 g/dl
	WCC 7 × 10⁹/l
	Platelets 308 × 10⁹/l
ESR	107 mm/h
Chest X-ray (**74a**)	
Rheumatoid factor	Negative
X-ray of left knee	Soft-tissue swelling
	No bony involvement
Aspirate of knee joint	Yellow fluid; low viscosity; WCC 50/mm³; culture sterile
Synovial biopsy	Thickened synovium macroscopically with histological evidence of increased inflammatory infiltrate

Answer 74

1. Ankylosing spondylitis.
2. Bilateral apical fibrosis.
3. i. X-ray of the sacroiliac joints, which will demonstrate sacroiliitis and may demonstrate squaring of the lumbar vertebrae with thickening and calcification of the interspinous ligaments.
ii. HLA typing for B27, however, one must remember that this found in 5% of the general population.
4. Respiratory function tests given the history of breathlessness on exertion and the lung fibrosis.
5. NSAID and physiotherapy.

While the inflamed knee joint in association with the abnormal chest X-ray may be highly suggestive of TB in an Asian patient, the failure to improve with anti-tuberculous therapy is against this diagnosis. In a young male with a synovitis of the knee joint followed by pain in the ankle joints and in the lumbar and cervical area, the differential diagnosis is between rheumatoid arthritis, adult Still's disease and a seronegative arthropathy, particularly ankylosing spondylitis. The absence of rheumatoid factor is against the diagnosis of rheumatoid arthritis. Still's disease is not sufficient to explain the chest X-ray abnormalities, which in this case are due to apical fibrosis

(**74b**) (*Table A* lists other causes), a well-recognized complication of ankylosing spondylitis. Other complications of ankylosing spondylitis are listed below (*Table B*). In addition, there is an increased incidence of scleritis and scleromalacia.

Ankylosing spondylitis is a chronic inflammatory disorder which predominantly affects the spinal joints. It is strongly associated with the presence of HLA B27, which is present in 95% of all cases, and the disease is more prevalent in males in their second and third decades. The exact aetiology for the disorder is unknown. Most patients present with a sacroiliitis causing back pain and stiffness which is worse in the mornings. There is a characteristic loss of lumbar lordosis and a reduced ability to flex the spine. An asymmetric peripheral large joint arthropathy may be the presenting feature in some patients as in this case. Enthesopathy causes pain in the tendons, particularly the Achilles tendon. Weight loss, low-grade fever and high inflammatory markers in the blood are recognized. Extra-articular complications occur in approximately 15% of patients. The diagnosis is a clinical one, but is helped by the demonstration of sacroiliitis on the X-ray of the pelvis and the demonstration of thickening and calcification of the interspinous ligament which may give the appearance of a bamboo spine.

Table A. Causes of apical lung fibrosis
TB
Extrinsic allergic alveolitis
Ankylosing spondylitis
Allergic bronchopulmonary aspergillosis
Radiation
Sarcoidosis
Histiocytosis X

Table B. Ankylosing spondylitis is easily remembered as the 'A' disease
Arthritis
Atlano axial subluxation
Arachnoiditis (spinal)
Apical fibrosis
Anterior uveitis
Aortitis
Aortic regurgitation
Atrioventricular block
Amyloidosis
Ig**A** nephropathy
Achilles tendinitis
Plantar f**A**sciitis

Table C. Causes of sacroiliitis
Ankylosing spondylitis
Reiter's syndrome
Psoriatic arthropathy
Enteropathic arthritis (inflammatory bowel disease)
Whipple's disease
Osteoarthritis

Question 75

A 21-year-old female developed a sudden left hemiparesis followed by loss of vision in her left eye 24 hours afterwards. For three months she had felt generally listless, experienced frequent night sweats and had lost 4 kg in weight. Over the past two weeks she had become breathless on exertion and could not sleep unless she was propped up on three pillows. She lost consciousness on two occasions and was seen in the local accident and emergency department with a suspected epileptic seizure three days earlier, but was not admitted. The medical officer had arranged an out-patient appointment with a cardiologist because he had heard an interesting murmur. The patient had enjoyed a healthy life before this illness and had never travelled abroad.

On examination, she was unwell. The temperature was 37.6°C (98.6°F). She had a heart rate of 110 beats/min, which was regular, and the blood pressure was 90/60 mmHg. The JVP was elevated 4 cm above the sternal angle. The cardiac apex was not displaced. On auscultation, the heart sounds were normal but there was a soft mid-diastolic murmur in the mitral area, as well as a mitral regurgitant murmur. Auscultation of the lung fields revealed fine inspiratory crackles at both lung bases. Neurological examination demonstrated a left hemiparesis. The speech was intact. Examination of the left fundus is shown (**75a**).

Investigations are shown.

FBC	Hb 10 g/dl
	WCC 8×10^9/l
	Platelets 360×10^9/l
ESR	90 mm/h
Biochemistry	Sodium 135 mmol/l
	Potassium 4.1 mmol/l
	Urea 8 mmol/l
	Glucose 5 mmol/l
ECG (**75b**)	
Chest X-ray	Cardiac silhouette slightly enlarged
	Upper lobe vein distension and bibasal interstitial lung shadowing

1. List three abnormalities on the ECG.
2. What information can be gained regarding the chambers of the heart from the ECG?
3. What is the cause of loss of vision in her left eye?
4. What is the diagnosis?
5. Which test would you perform to confirm the diagnosis?

Question 76

A 15-year-old male is admitted for parathyroidectomy. His father had a parathyroidectomy 20 years previously.

Pre-operative blood and post-operative blood (two months later) results are shown.

1. What is the diagnosis?
2. How would you confirm the diagnosis?

Pre-operative	Calcium 2.8 mmol/l
	Phosphate 0.8 mmol/l
	Albumin 44 g/l
	PTH 40 ng/l
Post-operative	Calcium 2.9 mmol/l
	Phosphate 0.9 mmol/l
	Albumin 43 g/l
	PTH undetectable

Answer 75

1. **i.** Right axis deviation.
ii. P mitrale.
iii. Voltage criteria for right ventricular hypertrophy.
2. Left atrial enlargement; right ventricular hypertrophy.
3. Embolic central retinal artery occlusion.
4. Left atrial myxoma.
5. Transthoracic echocardiogram (**75c**).

The differential diagnosis is between atrial myxoma and endocarditis affecting a stenosed mitral valve. The latter is less likely for three main reasons: (i) there is no past history of rheumatic fever to account for mitral stenosis (congenital mitral stenosis is rare and would have presented at a much younger age); (ii) endocarditis is rare in mitral stenosis due to the low pressure proximal to the valve surface; and (iii) it is unusual for a patient with mitral stenosis to be in sinus rhythm in the presence of symptomatic mitral stenosis. Left atrial myxoma (**75c**) would explain the dyspnoea, constitutional upset, fever, cardiac signs and the cerebral emboli.

Atrial myxomata are the most common tumours of the heart, with 75% being found in the left atrium. The tumours are benign and characteristically attached to the fossa ovalis by a pedicle. They are highly mobile and prolapse to and fro through the mitral valve orifice. The movement through the valve produces an added sound in diastole known as a 'tumour plop', which sounds like a third heart sound, and a mid-diastolic murmur which may be confused for mitral stenosis. However, third heart sounds do not occur in mitral stenosis. Breathlessness due to increased left atrial pressure is common. Mechanical obstruction of the mitral valve orifice may cause syncope or even sudden death. Constitutional upset and pyrexia is common, as are raised inflammatory markers and hypergammaglobulinaemia. Haemolysis is also recognized. Systemic emboli from the gelatinous tumour may complicate atrial myxoma. Arrhythmias, including atrial fibrillation are uncommon. The diagnosis is made by echocardiography and the management is surgical excision.

Answer 76

1. Familial benign hypocalcuric hypercalcaemia.
2. 24-hour urinary calcium estimation or a urinary calcium clearance to creatinine clearance (CaCl/CrCl) ratio.

Familial benign hypocalcuric hypercalcaemia is an autosomal dominant disorder which is characterized by life-long, asymptomatic hypercalcaemia. However, some patients develop acute pancreatitis, gall stones and chondrocalcinosis. The abnormality is in the calcium-sensing receptor, a G-protein-coupled receptor. It may be difficult to distinguish from primary hyperparathyroidism, and in 20% of cases the PTH is mildly elevated. The serum phosphate values are usually normal or slightly reduced. In contrast to other causes of hypercalcaemia, the 24-hour urinary calcium is reduced; 75% of patients have values <2.5 mmol/l, and 95% have values <5 mmol/l. The serum calcium level may vary from mild elevation to marked hypercalcaemia with values exceeding 3.5 mmol/l. The CaCl/CrCl ratio can be used to improve differentiation between hyperparathyroidism and familial benign hypocalcuric hypercalcaemia:

$$CaCl/CrCl = Ur_{Ca} \times P\,Cr/P\,Ca \times Ur_{Cr}$$

Some 80% of patients with familial benign hypocalcuric hypercalcaemia have a ratio of <0.01, whereas more than 70% of those with primary hyperparathyroidism have values above this cut-off.

The management is conservative.

Question 77

A 29-year-old male presented with a three-hour history of severe epigastric pain and profuse vomiting. The pain radiated into his back, and was not relieved by any of the antacid therapies which he had tried at home. There was no previous history of abdominal pain. He was a non-smoker and consumed 1–2 units of alcohol on an infrequent basis.

On examination, he was distressed with pain. On inspection of the trunk there were several raised lesions (77). There was no pallor. His heart rate was 100 beats/min and blood pressure 140/80 mmHg. On examination of the abdomen, he was very tender in the epigastrum but there was no abdominal rigidity. Bowel sounds were reduced.

Investigations are shown.

FBC	Hb 15 g/dl
	WCC 16 × 10⁹/l
	Platelets 200 × 10⁹/l
Biochemistry	Sodium 128 mmol/l
	Chloride 98 mmol/l
	Potassium 3.6 mmol/l
	Urea 6 mmol/l
	Creatinine 100 µmol/l
	Calcium 2.1 mmol/l
	Albumin 42 g/l
	Glucose 6 mmol/l
Chest X-ray	Normal
Abdominal X-ray	Normal

1. Which urgent test would you request to confirm the diagnosis?
2. Which two other investigations would you request to aid your management?
3. What is the full diagnosis?
4. Give two possible explanations for the low sodium.

Question 78

A patient collapsed during an ECG (78a).

1. What is the cause of collapse?
2. What is the immediate management?

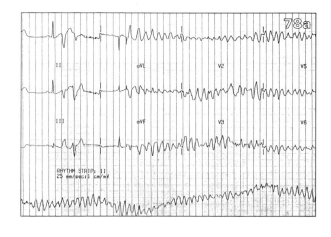

Answer 77

1. Serum amylase.
2. i. Arterial blood gases.
ii. Clotting studies.
3. Acute pancreatitis secondary to hypertriglyceridaemia.
4. i. Vomiting.
ii. Pseudohyponatraemia secondary to hyperlipidaemia.

Causes of acute pancreatitis
Alcohol abuse
Cholelithiasis
Coxsackie and mumps virus
Hypercalcaemia
Hypertriglyceridaemia
Drugs: thiazides, steroids, azathioprine
ERCP
Trauma

The history of acute abdominal pain radiating to the back and associated with profuse vomiting is consistent with acute pancreatitis, although a perforated duodenal ulcer and cholecystits may present similarly. The slightly low serum calcium supports the diagnosis of acute pancreatitis because the associated rise in serum lipase resulting from pancreatic damage leads to an increase in the free fatty acid concentration in the blood, which has the effect of binding calcium and thus reducing the 'free calcium' in the serum.

A very high serum amylase is usually diagnostic of acute pancreatitis, but acute parotitis may cause similarly high levels. However, in the latter case the history is of painful parotid glands. A modestly elevated level is seen in perforated duodenal ulcer, cholecystitis, aortic aneurysm.

A neutrophil leucocytosis is common. The serum calcium may be low for reasons explained above. It is mandatory to check urea, electrolytes, glucose, arterial blood gases, chest X-ray and clotting. The most common cause of mortality is renal failure and respiratory failure due to hypovolaemia and ARDS, respectively. The latter is thought to be due to the effects of high levels of trypsin which have leaked from the pancreas, on lung surfactant. DIC is another important cause of mortality.

In this case, the cause of pancreatitis is hypertriglyceridaemia, as evident by the multiple eruptive xanthomata on the trunk of this young male patient. Causes of acute pancreatitis are tabulated below. In the UK, the most common cause of acute pancreatitis is alcohol abuse, followed by cholelithiasis ('gall stones').

The low sodium is either due to vomiting or is a result of pseudohyponatraemia resulting from hyperlipidaemia. In hyperlipidaemia and paraproteinaemias, the serum sodium is falsely low because only the sodium in free water space is measured. True hyponatraemia can be differentiated from pseudohyponatraemia by measuring the plasma osmolality which is low in the former, and normal in the latter.

Answer 78

1. Ventricular fibrillation precipitated by the 'R on T' phenomenon.
2. DC cardioversion using 200 J.

The rhythm is broad complex, and the QRS-complexes are very irregular and are of varying amplitude and duration. This is typical of ventricular fibrillation.

There is only one effective method of reverting ventricular fibrillation to sinus rhythm, and that is DC cardioversion using a high-energy shock. The quicker this is given, the higher the chance of reverting to sinus rhythm. The window for success is around 2 minutes, following which reversion becomes increasingly difficult. The most common cause of ventricular fibrillation is myocardial infarction; however, the cardiomyopathies, ventricular aneurysms, electrolyte imbalances (particularly hypokalaemia) and certain drug overdoses (e.g. cocaine or tricyclic antidepressant drugs) are also recognized causes. Following myocardial infarction, multiple ventricular

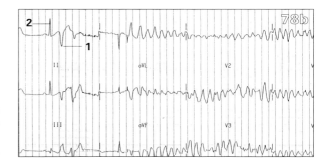

ectopics occurring on the preceding T-wave may cause monomorphic ventricular tachycardia which can degenerate into ventricular fibrillation. Post-myocardial infarction patients with 'R on T' ventricular ectopics are treated prophylactically with a lignocaine infusion to reduce the frequency of the ectopics.

In this case (78b), there is clear evidence of the R-wave of an ectopic beat (1) on the T-wave of the preceding sinus beat (2).

Question 79

A 24-year-old basket ball player was referred to the local cardiologist after experiencing two episodes of dizziness while playing basket ball in one week. During the last episode he almost lost consciousness. There were no other associated symptoms. He had similar dizzy episodes one month previously, but attributed these to a coryzal illness. There was no history of headaches. He had no past medical history of significance. His father died in Mexico at the age of only 27 years but the patient was not sure about the cause of death. He had a step brother and sister who were well.

On examination, he appeared well. He weighed 90 kg and was 1.85 m tall. His heart rate was 68 beats/min and his blood pressure was 130/60 mmHg. The JVP was not raised. On examination of the precordium, he had a double apical impulse. On auscultation, there was a loud pansystolic murmur in the mitral area, and an ejection systolic murmur at the left lower sternal edge. His chest was clear. Examination of his peripheral pulses was normal, as was examination of the central nervous system.

The patient had a 12-lead ECG, echocardiogram and 24-hour ECG (79a–d).

1. What is the significance of the double apical impulse?
2. With respect to auscultation, what other manoeuvres could you have performed to try and ascertain the cause of the murmurs?
3. What are the abnormalities on the ECG and how would you interpret them?
4. What are the abnormalities on the two-dimensional and M-mode echocardiograms?
5. What is the significance of the abnormality on the 24-hour ECG?
6. What is the diagnosis?
7. What implications (if any) does this have on the patient's career?

Answer 79

1. A double apical impulse is the result of a palpable fourth heart sound which occurs when there is forceful left atrial contraction against a non-compliant left ventricle. This sign is often present in conditions which produce significant left ventricular hypertrophy. Examples include aortic stenosis, hypertrophic cardiomyopathy and occasionally severe left ventricular hypertrophy due to hypertension.

2. In the absence of hypertension, the differential diagnosis is between aortic stenosis and hypertrophic cardiomyopathy. In hypertrophic cardiomyopathy, an obstructive element is present in approximately 30% of patients. The obstruction is variable and thought to be due to anterior motion of the mitral valve towards the hypertrophied interventricular septum in systole, thus narrowing the left ventricular outflow tract. The exact mechanism for this is not clearly understood. The obstruction is worsened by manoeuvres which reduce LVEDP, and in these circumstances the murmur is louder. The Valsalva manoeuvre (blowing against a closed glottis) increases intrathoracic pressure and therefore reduces venous return to the heart, reducing LVEDP. Standing from a squatting position has similar consequences. In aortic stenosis these manoeuvres reduce the intensity of the systolic murmur.

3. The ECG reveals sinus rhythm with voltage criteria for left ventricular hypertrophy and deep S-waves in the septal (V2–V3) leads. In addition, there is T-wave inversion in the inferior leads. Regular physical training can also produce left ventricular hypertrophy; however, the extent of hypertrophy seldom exceeds the upper limit of normal. While it is common to have voltage criteria of left ventricular hypertrophy in athletes, accompanying T-wave inversion in any lead other than V1–V2 should raise the suspicion of organic heart disease and the need for further investigation.

4. The two-dimensional echocardiogram reveals asymmetrical left ventricular hypertrophy. The septum is grossly hypertrophied. The left ventricular cavity size is small. Both these features suggest the diagnosis of hypertrophic cardiomyopathy. The M-mode study demonstrates systolic anterior motion of the mitral valve, which is also suggestive of hypertrophic cardiomyopathy. Other echocardiographic features of hypertrophic cardiomyopathy include an enlarged left atrium and evidence of diastolic dysfunction on Doppler studies. The systolic function is usually excellent.

5. The 24-hour ECG demonstrated a run of non-sustained ventricular tachycardia. This occurs in approximately 25% of patients with hypertrophic cardiomyopathy, and is a high-risk marker of sudden death. Other markers of high risk include syncopal episodes and a family history of sudden death. The patient is experiencing syncopal episodes. The patient's father died aged 27, and in this context we have to assume that he may have had hypertrophic cardiomyopathy. This combination classifies the patient into the high-risk category for sudden death. These patients are treated with amiodarone and/or implantable automatic cardiovertor defibrillator.

6. Hypertrophic cardiomyopathy.

7. The diagnosis of hypertrophic cardiomyopathy in an athlete leads to disqualification from competitive sport, in order to minimize the risk of sudden death.

Hypertrophic cardiomyopathy (HCM) has a prevalence of 0.1–0.2%. It is inherited as an autosomal dominant trait in over 70% of cases, but sporadic cases are recognized. It is a genetically heterogeneous condition which is caused by mutations within genes encoding the sarcomeric proteins. The disease has been assigned to eight separate chromosomal loci (*Table*). Mutations within genes encoding β-myosin heavy chain and troponin T account for over half of all patients with HCM. Some 50% of patients have chest pain and breathlessness; 20% present with dizziness or syncope. Sudden death is frequently the first presentation, particularly in adolescents, young adults and athletes. The overall mortality rate is 3%. Sudden death commonly occurs during or immediately after strenuous exertion. The diagnosis is made using echocardiography to demonstrate left ventricular hypertrophy, which is usually asymmetric, but can be concentric in up to 40% of cases.

Molecular genetics of hypertrophic cardiomyopathy

Chromosome	Gene affected	Chromosome	Gene affected
14	β-myosin heavy chain	11	Myosin-binding protein C
1	Troponin T	7	?
19	Troponin I	3	Myosin essential light chain
15	α-tropomyosin	12	Myosin regulatory light chain

Question 80

A 68-year-old male was admitted for investigation of increasing weakness and recent onset of jaundice. There was no other relevant past medical history. In particular, there was no travel abroad and he was not taking any medication.

On examination, he had non-tender lymphadenopathy in the cervical, axillary and inguinal areas. Abdominal examination revealed an enlarged spleen 6 cm below the costal margin.

Investigations are shown.

1. List three abnormalities on the blood film.
2. Explain the cause of the phenomenon indicated by the arrow.
3. What is the cause for the jaundice?
4. Give two possible explanations for the raised MCV.
5. Which single investigation would you perform to ascertain the cause of this patient's anaemia?

FBC	Hb 10.1 g/dl
	WCC 60 × 10⁹/l
	Platelets 190 × 10⁹/l
	Reticulocyte count 12%
	MCV 101 fl
Blood film (**80**)	
Biochemistry	Bilirubin 39 µmol/l
	AST 20 u/l
	Alkaline phosphatase 70 u/l
	Albumin 36 g/l
	Total protein 56 g/l
Chest X-ray	Normal
Urinalysis	Urobilinogen ++
	Bilirubin 0

Question 81

A 19-year-old medical student was admitted to the accident and emergency department with headache and drowsiness on a cold winter's morning. He shared a house with three fellow students, who found him in bed after he failed to answer several wake-up calls to attend an anatomy viva.

On examination, he was flushed and drowsy. He was apyrexial. There was no evidence of a skin rash. His heart rate was 100 beats/min and regular, and the blood pressure was 120/80 mmHg. Neurological examination revealed a Glasgow coma score of 11/15. There was no nuchal rigidity. The cranial nerves, motor and sensory systems were normal. Examination of all other systems was normal.

Investigations are shown.

1. What is the diagnosis?
2. Which investigation would you perform next?
3. What is the management?

FBC	Hb 14 g/dl
	WCC 9 × 10⁹/l
	Platelets 370 × 10⁹/l
Biochemistry	Sodium 135 mmol/l
	Potassium 4.4 mmol/l
	Urea 4 mmol/l
	Creatinine 80 µmol/l
Arterial blood	pH 7.37
gases	pO₂ 7.2 kPa
	pCO₂ 3.8 kPa
	Bicarbonate 23 mmol/l
	O₂ saturation 98%
Chest X-ray	Normal
ECG	Sinus tachycardia

Answer 80

1. i. Numerous mature lymphocytes.
ii. Smudge or smear cell.
iii. Red cell agglutination.
2. Smudge or smear cells are an artefact phenomenon which arises during blood film preparation due to the fragility of lymphocytes in chronic lymphatic leukaemia.
3. Warm autoimmune haemolytic anaemia (see *Table* for other causes).
4. i. Reticulocytosis secondary to haemolysis.
ii. Megaloblastic anaemia due to folate deficiency from increased cell turnover.
5. Direct Coomb's test.

Causes of autoimmune haemolytic anaemia for higher examinations	
Warm (IgG antibody attaches to red cells at 37°C (98.6°F))	
SLE	Chronic lymphatic leukaemia
Lymphoma	Methyl dopa
Carcinoma	
Cold (IgM antibody attaches to red cells below 37°C (98.6°F))	
Mycoplasma pneumonia	
Infectious mononucleosis	
Paroxysmal cold haemoglobinuria (IgG)	
Lymphoma	

Chronic lymphatic leukaemia usually affects the middle-aged and the elderly. It is a malignancy of B-cell lymphocytes. The clinical features are insidious, and the diagnosis may be made incidentally on a blood film. The main features are lethargy, night sweats, weight loss and recurrent infections due to hypogammaglobulinaemia. Physical examination reveals generalized lymphadenopathy and hepatosplenomegaly. The characteristic blood picture is of a lymphocytosis and a mild normochromic normocytic anaemia. Smudge or smear cells are common. As disease progresses, the anaemia becomes more severe, partly due to marrow suppression and partly due to an autoimmune haemolytic anaemia, and a thrombocytopenia becomes evident. Patients presenting with low platelets have advanced disease and a poor prognosis. Folate deficiency may occur secondary to increased cell turnover and haemolysis. Therapy is commenced in symptomatic patients. The drug of choice is chlorambucil. Severely immunosuppressed individuals may be treated with intravenous gamma-globulin preparations.

Answer 81

1. Carbon monoxide poisoning.
2. Arterial carboxyhaemoglobin.
3. 100% oxygen.

The clue for the diagnosis of carbon monoxide poisoning comes from the arterial blood gases which reveal hypoxia, but a normal oxygen saturation. Carbon monoxide displaces oxygen from Hb and displaces the oxygen dissociation curve to the left. It also inhibits cellular respiration by inhibiting the cytochrome oxidase system. This results in tissue hypoxia which may manifest as headaches, dizziness, convulsions, nausea and vomiting. On examination, patients may have tachycardia, tachypnoea, ataxia and cherry red discoloration of the lips; however, the latter is a relatively rare and late manifestation of the condition. Retinal haemorrhages are a recognized complication of carbon monoxide poisoning. Late complications include basal ganglia infarction and parkinsonism, and sometimes neuropsychiatric symptoms. Oxygen saturation is normal because automated analysers cannot differentiate between oxyhaemoglobin and carboxyhaemoglobin; however, pO_2 is low when there is significant carbon monoxide poisoning. It is worth noting that arterial pO_2 is often normal in patients with carbon monoxide poisoning; therefore, a high index of suspicion is needed to diagnose the condition. Carbon monoxide poisoning is caused by combustion engines, faulty stoves or paraffin heaters when facilities for ventilation are poor.

The diagnosis is made by direct measurement of arterial carboxyhaemoglobin level. Levels of 40–60% are associated with neurological symptoms and signs (described above), as well as cardiac brady- and tachyarrhythmias. Levels above 60% are associated with coma and death.

The management of carbon monoxide poisoning involves administration of 100% oxygen by a tight-fitting mask. This reduces the half-life of carboxyhaemoglobin from 4 hours to approximately 90 minutes. During this period, carboxyhaemoglobin levels should be measured 2-hourly, and the oxygen continued until the carboxyhaemoglobin level is below 10%. Patients with neurological signs and symptoms, ECG abnormalities, myocardial ischaemia, pulmonary oedema and shock require hyperbaric oxygen (3 atm) at a specialized centre. Some would agree that any individual with a carboxyhaemoglobin level exceeding 25% should also be considered for hyperbaric oxygen, even if symptoms are absent.

Question 82

A 38-year-old businessman was admitted to hospital with nausea, vomiting and drowsiness. He had been in Thailand for 10 days and returned back to England two days previously. He was well in Thailand, but on arrival to England developed general malaise and a headache. He attributed his symptoms to excess alcohol ingestion while abroad, and attempted to relieve his symptoms with two paracetamol tablets. He continued to have a headache the following morning, and took another two tablets of paracetamol, without much relief of his symptoms. Following this, he took two paracetamol tablets every four hours. He gradually became more unwell, nauseous and started vomiting. There was no neck stiffness, photophobia or diarrhoea. He normally consumed two bottles of wine and occasional spirits per day and smoked 30 cigarettes a day. While abroad, he had drunk more alcohol than usual. There was no significant past medical history.

On examination, he was tanned and had a flushed face. He was mildly icteric. He had a fever of 39°C (102.2°F). He was slightly drowsy, but could hold a normal, coherent conversation. There was no evidence of asterixis. Examination of the fundi was normal. The heart rate was 110 beats/min and blood pressure 105/70 mmHg. Examination of the precordium revealed a very soft third heart sound. His chest was clear. Abdominal examination revealed a slightly tender palpable liver edge 4 cm below the costal margin. The spleen was not palpable.

Investigations are shown.

FBC	Hb 15.8 g/dl
	WCC 9×10^9/l
	Platelets 105×10^9/l
	MCV 102 fl
Clotting	PT 20 s (control 14 s)
Malaria parasite	Not detected
Biochemistry	Sodium 133 mmol/l
	Potassium 3.5 mmol/l
	Urea 5 mmol/l
	Creatinine 98 µmol/l
	Bilirubin 30 µmol/l
	AST 1500 u/l
	Alkaline phosphatase 110 u/l
Serum ferritin	500 µg/l
Chest X-ray	Normal

1. Which test would you perform immediately?
A. Blood cultures.
B. Hepatitis serology.
C. Blood ethanol level.
D. Serum paracetamol level.
E. Liver biopsy.
2. What is the cause of the deterioration of his symptoms?
A. Paracetamol poisoning/viral hepatitis.
B. Paracetamol poisoning/alcohol abuse.
C. Haemochromatosis/hepatoma.
D. Viral hepatitis/paracetamol intoxication.
E. Haemochromatosis/paracetamol poisoning.

Question 83

A 42-year-old female presented with increasing dyspnoea on exertion. She had a past history of rheumatic fever. Left and right cardiac catheter data were as follows:

Chamber	Pressure (mmHg)	Oxygen saturation (%)
Right atrium	10	68
Right ventricle	40/10	68
Pulmonary artery	40/22	68
PCWP	16	
Left ventricle	160/10	96
Aorta	110/70	96

1. List three diagnoses.

Answer 82

1. D. Serum paracetamol level.
2. B. Paracetamol poisoning and alcohol abuse.

There is a history of alcohol abuse and consumption of 6–7 g of paracetamol in 24 hours. Ingestion of 15 g of paracetamol is regarded as a significant overdose in normal healthy individuals; however, the dose of paracetamol required to cause hepatotoxicity in individuals with chronic, heavy alcohol ingestion is much lower. This is explained by the ability of alcohol to induce hepatic microsomal enzymes and to deplete hepatic intracellular levels of glutathione. Paracetamol itself is not hepatotoxic, but it is usually metabolized to NAPQI which is a potent oxidative agent with potential to cause massive hepatic necrosis. The metabolite is normally rapidly conjugated with glutathione, which renders it inactive and is excreted. In patients with heavy alcohol ingestion the detoxifying microsomal enzyme concentration is increased to metabolize alcohol. Although this is a beneficial effect when dealing with alcohol, it can have serious consequences when large amounts of paracetamol are ingested because it leads to rapid metabolism of the drug to NAPQI. The hepatocytes are relatively depleted of glutathione due to hepatic damage from alcohol and soon become completely depleted in an attempt to conjugate NAPQI. The result is an excess of NAPQI, causing hepatic necrosis which can have profound effects if hepatic reserve has already been severely affected by alcohol abuse. Alcohol abusers are more likely to develop massive hepatic necrosis and have a worse prognosis from paracetamol overdose.

Hepatitis A infection is possible and in the early stages does produce general malaise, fever, nausea and elevated hepatic transaminases. Hepatitis A has an incubation period of two weeks and has a hepatitic and a cholestatic phase. It is feasible that the patient contracted the virus abroad and is now in the hepatitic phase; however, given the history of alcohol abuse and self-administration of a significant amount of paracetamol, this is less likely than the answer given above.

The diagnosis of haemochromatosis is raised due to the high serum ferritin level of 500 µg/l; however, high ferritin levels and deposition of iron in the liver also occur in alcohol-related disease and patients with regular blood transfusions (secondary haemochromatosis). Liver biopsy is the main way of distinguishing between primary and secondary haemochromatosis. In secondary haemochromatosis the biopsy will reveal changes of alcoholic hepatitis (Mallory bodies) as well as iron deposition. Moreover, primary haemochromatosis is not usually associated with significant derangement of LFT unless the disease is very advanced or there is development of hepatocellular carcinoma, which is a recognized complication of cirrhosis of the liver due to any cause, but particularly haemochromatosis. In this case there would be a history of poor health before travelling abroad, as well as other features of haemochromatosis such as diabetes mellitus and hypogonadism, which are absent. The LFT usually demonstrate a high alkaline phosphatase and a raised bilirubin in the presence of hepatocellular carcinoma.

Answer 83

1. i. The right ventricular pressure and pulmonary artery pressures exceed 35 mmHg, indicating pulmonary hypertension.
ii. The PCWP exceeds the LVEDP by 6 mmHg, indicating significant mitral stenosis.
iii. There is a pressure drop of 50 mmHg across the aortic valve, indicating moderate to severe aortic stenosis.

(See Guidelines on the Interpretation of Cardiac Catheter Data, page 220.)

Question 84

A 15-year-old male was admitted with sudden onset of rapid palpitations which were not associated with chest pain or dizziness. On examination, he was well-perfused and his blood pressure was 110/65 mmHg. An ECG performed in the accident and emergency department is shown (**84a**). He was treated by the medical officer, and his ECG afterwards is shown (**84b**).

1. What is shown in the 12-lead ECG while the patient is having palpitations?

2. List four forms of treatment with which the medical officer may have attempted to treat the palpitation.

3. Which cardiac condition does this patient have?

4. List four forms of drug therapy which could be safely used to prevent the patient's symptoms.

5. What is the definitive treatment in a young patient with this disorder?

Question 85

A 33-year-old male with recently diagnosed acute schizophrenia was referred the accident and emergency department after he was found collapsed on the psychiatric ward. On examination, the patient was very drowsy and appeared rigid. The heart rate was 120 beats/min, and regular; blood pressure was 110/60 mmHg.

The temperature was 40°C (104°F). Examination of the cardiovascular, respiratory and abdominal system was normal. Neurological examination demonstrated generalized rigidity of all muscle groups.

Investigations are shown.

FBC	Hb 15 g/dl
	WCC 10 × 10⁹/l
	Platelets 300 × 10⁹/l
Urinalysis	Protein +
Biochemistry	Sodium 138 mmol/l
	Potassium 4 mmol/l
	Urea 10 mmol/l
	Creatinine 160 µmol/l

1. What is the diagnosis?

2. Which investigation would you perform to confirm the diagnosis?

3. Briefly, list three management steps.

Answer 84

1. An atrioventricular tachycardia with LBBB.
2. i. Vagotonic manoeuvres such as carotid sinus massage, Valsalva manoeuvre, compression of the eyeball.
ii. Intravenous adenosine.
3. Wolff–Parkinson–White syndrome (type A).
4. i. Sotalol.
ii. Flecanide.
iii. Disopyramide.
iv. Amiodarone.
5. Radiofrequency ablation of the accessory pathway.

Wolff–Parkinson–White syndrome (WPW) is a congenital condition with a prevalence of 1 in 1,500 and is characterized by an accessory conduction pathway between the atria and ventricles (bundle of Kent) which predisposes to an electrical re-entrant circuit and tachycardia. During sinus rhythm the electrical impulse conducts rapidly over the accessory conduction pathway and depolarizes the ventricles prematurely. This results in a short PR-interval and a wide QRS-complex with a slurred upstroke, commonly referred to as a delta wave. Anterograde conduction through the accessory pathway and retrograde conduction via the atrioventricular node may predispose to two types of tachyarrhythmias which are atrioventricular re-entrant tachycardia or atrial fibrillation. Two variants of WPW are recognized: type A (left-sided pathway which is characterized by an upright (positive) delta wave in V1, as in this case; and type B (right-sided pathway) which is characterized by a negative delta wave in V1 (**84c**). The former is more common.

In atrioventricular tachycardia the ventricular rate is between 140–280 beats/min and the P-wave is seen just after the QRS-complex, usually in the ST-segment.

In atrial fibrillation, there is a rapid irregular rhythm with some QRS-complexes exhibiting delta waves.

Management of atrioventricular re-entrant tachycardia involves either vagotonic manoeuvres such as carotid sinus massage, Valsalva manoeuvre, compression of the eyeball, or intravenous adenosine. Atrial fibrillation does not usually respond to vagotonic manoeuvres, but may be abolished by adenosine. DC cardioversion is reserved for those patients who are haemodynamically unstable and unresponsive to adenosine. Drugs which may be used to prevent arrhythmias include the class I and class III anti-arrhythmic agents, of which the most popular is sotalol. Both digoxin and verapamil are contraindicated in WPW because they increase conduction through the accessory pathway and increase the risk of malignant ventricular arrhythmias. Radiofrequency ablation of the accessory pathway is the definitive treatment in patients with atrial fibrillation or frequent atrioventricular re-entrant tachycardia.

Answer 85

1. Neuroleptic malignant syndrome secondary to the use of phenothiazines.
2. Serum creatinine kinase.
3. i. Stop drug.
ii. Intravenous diazepam.
iii. Adequate hydration to prevent renal failure.

The neuroleptic malignant syndrome is a rare but life-threatening condition that can occur with any antipsychotic drug, irrespective of dose. It is most common when starting treatment or increasing the dose. Symptoms include fever, muscle rigidity, confusion and impaired consciousness. Autonomic instability is well-recognized and is associated with excessive sweating, labile blood pressure and tachycardia. The diagnosis is made by demonstrating a grossly elevated creatinine kinase. Rhabdomyolysis may precipitate renal failure, which can be avoided by adequate hydration. Other complications include aspiration pneumonia and respiratory failure. The management of this condition involves stopping the neuroleptic drug immediately, antipyretics and rehydration. The drug dantrolene may be useful in some cases.

Question 86

A 59-year-old male presented with a three-week history of cough and progressive breathlessness and three episodes of haemoptysis in 24 hours. At the onset of the initial symptoms he visited his general practitioner, who diagnosed a respiratory tract infection and prescribed a course of broad-spectrum antibiotics. The cough persisted and the patient remained breathless. His effort tolerance had become significantly reduced from walking two miles daily to being breathless at rest. He had felt increasingly lethargic and nauseous for a week before being seen in the accident and emergency department. Twenty-four hours previously he had coughed an egg-cup-full of fresh clots of blood on three separate occasions. There was no history of sore throat or night sweats. Prior to a week previously, his appetite was good. There was no history of weight loss. He had a past history of haemorrhoids which were surgically ligated two years ago.

The patient was married with one son and worked as a mechanic. He smoked 10 cigarettes per day and consumed 2–3 units of alcohol per week. There was no history of travel abroad. There was no family history of note, with the exception that his mother had been treated for pulmonary TB 16 years ago.

On examination, he appeared pale and centrally cyanosed. There was no evidence of clubbing or lymphadenopathy. There was bilateral pitting ankle oedema. The heart rate was 110 beats/min, and regular, and blood pressure was 176/105 mmHg. The JVP was raised 4 cm above the sternal angle. On examination of the respiratory system chest expansion was symmetrically reduced. The trachea was central. Percussion note was dull at both bases, and on auscultation there was widespread bronchial breathing at both mid zones and bases. Precordial and abdominal examination was normal.

Investigations are shown.

FBC	Hb 7.2 g/dl
	WCC 12×10^9/l
	Platelets 500×10^9/l
Biochemistry	Sodium 137 mmol/l
	Potassium 5.2 mmol/l
	Urea 19 mmol/l
	Creatinine 400 µmol/l
	Calcium 2.1 mmol/l
	Phosphate 2 mmol/l
	Albumin 40 g/l
ECG	Sinus tachycardia. Partial RBBB
Chest X-ray	Alveolar shadowing affecting both lower zones
Urinalysis	Blood +++
	Protein ++
	Numerous blood cells and red cell casts
Lung function	FEV$_1$ 65%predicted
	FVC 60%predicted
	TLC 68%predicted
	RV 66% predicted
	TLCO 110% predicted

1. Comment on the respiratory function tests.
2. What is the most likely diagnosis?
3. List two tests you would request to confirm the diagnosis.
4. What are the four predisposing factors for producing the changes seen in the chest?

Question 87

A 60-year-old male presents with an episode of amaurosis fugax. On examination, apart from splenomegaly, there are no abnormal neurological or other clinical findings.

Investigations are shown.

1. What is the diagnosis ?
2. List at least three haematological investigations that are indicated.

Hb	14.2 g/dl
PCV	0.55
MCV	69 fl
MCH	18.2 pg
WCC	15×10^9/l
Neutrophils	88%
Lymphocytes	8%
Monocytes	4%
Platelets	475×10^9/l
Blood film	Hypochromia ++

Answer 86

1. Restrictive lung defect with a raised KCO. (See Respiratory Function Tests, page 221.)
2. Goodpasture's syndrome. Other possible diagnoses include microscopic polyarteritis nodosa and Wegener's granulomatosis.
3. i. Renal biopsy.
ii. Anti-GBM disease.
4. i. Smoking.
ii. Lower respiratory tract infection.
iii. Pulmonary oedema.
iv. Inhalation of organic solvents.

The patient has evidence of acute glomerulonephritis. The breathlessness, haemoptysis, raised KCO and bilateral alveolar shadows on the chest X-ray are highly suggestive of pulmonary haemorrhage. The combination of acute nephritis and pulmonary haemorrhage may occur in anti-GBM disease, Wegener's granulomatosis, microscopic polyarteritis nodosa and SLE. In anti-GBM disease, patients who are smokers are more predisposed to lung haemorrhage, as are patients who are exposed to hydrocarbons. The patient is both a smoker and has been exposed to hydrocarbons from his occupation as a garage mechanic. The most probable diagnosis is anti-GBM disease.

Anti-GBM disease is rare, with prevalence 1 case per million. The male to female ratio is 2:1. The age of onset has two peaks which are the third and the seventh decades. There is a strong association between HLA DR2 and anti-GBM disease, the antigen being present in approximately 80% of affected patients. Other HLA associations include HLA DR4 and HLA DR2. Circulating anti-GBM antibodies are responsible for both the nephritis and pulmonary haemorrhage.

Clinical features are those of rapidly progressive nephritis and/or pulmonary haemorrhage. Fatigue and breathlessness may pre-date the onset of nephritis or frank haemoptysis. Glomerulonephritis is of the rapidly progressive type, and renal function may be completely lost within a week. Some 60% of patients have pulmonary haemorrhage. Smokers, patients with coexisting lower respiratory tract infections and pulmonary oedema, and patients exposed to hydrocarbons are more prone to haemorrhage.

The chest X-ray may reveal alveolar shadowing in the presence of pulmonary haemorrhage. The differentiation from pulmonary oedema (which looks the same) requires determination of the KCO, which is raised in haemorrhage and reduced in oedema.

Investigations include renal biopsy with immuno-fluorescent which demonstrate rapidly progressive glomerulonephritis and linear IgG deposits along the basement membrane. Transbronchial lung biopsy may be useful, but has a lower histological yield.

Management is with early plasmapharesis, methylprednisolone and cyclophosphamide.

Answer 87

1. Polycythaemia rubra vera (PRV) complicated by iron-deficiency anaemia.
2. i. Red cell mass estimation.
ii. Leucocyte alkaline phosphatase score.
iii. Bone marrow aspiration.
iv. Serum ferritin.

The patient has a normal Hb but the PCV and the red cell count are elevated. Furthermore, he has associated leucocytosis, thrombocytosis and splenomegaly, which should raise the suspicion of PRV. The normal (as opposed to high Hb) is due to co-existing iron deficiency. The diagnosis of iron deficiency is supported by the low MCV.

PRV has an insidious onset. It rarely occurs before the fifth decade. Symptoms include lethargy, depression, vertigo, tinnitus and amaurosis fugax. On examination, the patient may have a plethoric facial complexion, hypertension, and a palpable spleen in approximately 70% of cases. Complications include bleeding due to thrombocythaemia, stroke from hyperviscosity, and gout from increased cell turnover. Bleeding is most commonly from the upper gastrointestinal tract. PRV may progress to myelofibrosis or acute myeloid leukaemia.

Management is by venesection, although this may result in iron deficiency. Busulphan or hydroxyurea are effective in controlling the thrombocytosis.

Question 88

A 54-year-old Turkish male was admitted to hospital with a three-week history of malaise, headaches, pain in his arms, legs and lower back and night sweats. His appetite was poor, and he had lost almost half a stone in three weeks. He worked as a butcher. He had returned from a holiday in Turkey six weeks ago where he lived on his brother's farm for two weeks.

On examination, he was unwell. He had generalized cervical lymphadenopathy. His temperature was 38.5°C (101.3°F). The blood pressure was 120/60 mmHg. Cardiovascular examination revealed a soft systolic murmur at the apex. Examination of the respiratory system was normal. On examination of his abdomen he had a palpable spleen 4 cm below the costal margin. The liver edge was also palpable 3 cm below the costal margin. Genital examination demonstrated an erythematous scrotum with a swollen, tender left testicle. Examination of the central nervous system, including the fundi, was normal. His lower back was tender, but movements were not restricted. Similarly, his limbs were tender but there was no fasciculation and power was preserved. He had tender, red, macular lesions on his shins which varied between 2–5 cm in diameter.

Investigations are shown.

FBC	Hb 11.8 g/dl
	WCC 2 × 10⁹/l (neutropenia)
	Platelets 440 × 10⁹/l
ESR	66 mm/h
CRP	210 mg/l
U&E	Normal
LFT	Normal
Chest X-ray	Few calcified paratracheal lymph nodes

1. What is the diagnosis?
2. List three tests you would perform to help confirm the diagnosis.
3. What is the management?

Question 89

A 13-year-old Scottish female was admitted with acute colicky central abdominal pain associated with vomiting. The only past history was that of a viral illness associated with a rash two weeks previously. On examination, she appeared pale. The heart rate was 110 beats/min and the blood pressure 140/90 mmHg. The abdomen was generally tender, but there was no guarding, and bowel sounds were infrequent. Examination of the central nervous system revealed reduced power and tone in the lower limbs, and absent ankle and knee reflexes.

Investigations are shown.

FBC	Hb 10 g/dl	Biochemistry	Sodium 134 mmol/l
	WCC 7 × 10⁹/l		Potassium 3.2 mmol/l
	Platelets 170 × 10⁹/l		Bicarbonate 15 mmol/l
	MCV 63 fl		Chloride 115 mmol/l
	MCHC 28 g/dl		Urea 7 mmol/l
Blood film (**89**)			Creatinine 80 μmol/l
Urinary δ-ALA	100 mmol/day (normal range 11–57 mmol/day)		Glucose 4 mmol/l
		CT of brain	Normal

1. What is the diagnosis?
2. Which investigation will you perform to confirm the diagnosis?
3. What is the most probable cause for the abnormal electrolytes?
4. What is the management?

Answer 88

1. Brucellosis.
2. i. Blood culture.
ii. Marrow culture.
iii. *Brucella* agglutination test or *Brucella* immunoglobulins (ELISA).
3. Tetracycline and rifampicin; co-trimoxazole.

The history of malaise, myalgia, headaches and weight loss in association with neutropaenia, hepatosplenomegaly and erythema nodosum is highly suggestive of brucellosis.

Brucellosis is caused by *Brucella*, a Gram-negative bacillus, which may be contracted from cows, goats, pigs or sheep. It has a wide animal reservoir. Three main species cause infection in man: *B. abortus* (cattle), *B. melitensis* (goats/sheep), and *B. suis* (pigs). The organism usually gains access into the human body through the gastrointestinal tract as a result of consuming unpasteurized milk; however, contact with animal carcasses may also increase risk of oral ingestion of the bacterium. Brucellosis is virtually eliminated in the UK due to the strict policy of pasteurization of milk. Once in the gastrointestinal tract, the bacilli travel to the lymphatics and infect lymph nodes, and eventually there is haematogenous spread to many other organs.

The onset is usually insidious. General malaise, headaches, myalgia, weakness and night sweats are common. There is an undulant high fever. Lymphadenopathy is common. Hepatosplenomegaly may be present, but an acute hepatitis is rare. Splenomegaly usually indicates severe infection. Spinal tenderness is relatively common. Haematogenous spread may be complicated by arthritis, orchitis, endocarditis, osteomyelitis, and meningoencephalitis.

Brucellosis may become chronic when it is undiagnosed and is associated with fatigue, myalgia, depression, and occasionally fever. Palpable splenomegaly is characteristic. In a few cases the infection may be localized to specific organs such as the bones, heart or central nervous system. In these circumstances, systemic features are absent in over 60% of cases and antibody titres are low.

The diagnosis is based on positive blood cultures and rising anti-*Brucella* immunoglobulin titres. Blood cultures are positive in only half the cases. The *Brucella* agglutination test is positive within four weeks of the onset of illness. Treatment is with tetracycline and rifampicin for six weeks, although co-trimoxazole is also effective.

Answer 89

1. In a young girl with abdominal pain, vomiting, neuropathy and anaemia, the most likely diagnosis is lead poisoning, although several other conditions may also cause the same symptoms (*Table*).
2. Serum lead level; a lead concentration above 4 mmol/l is toxic.
3. The electrolytes demonstrate hypokalaemia and a metabolic acidosis with a normal anion gap, or in other words a hypokalaemic, hyperchloraemic acidosis.
4. D-penicillamine therapy.

Causes of abdominal pain and neuropathy
AIP
Lead poisoning
Arsenic poisoning
Guillain–Barré syndrome
Polyarteritis nodosa
Diabetic ketoacidosis
Intra-abdominal malignancy
Sarcoidosis
Alcohol abuse

Acute lead poisoning is rare, but chronic poisoning may occur in scrap metal workers or plumbers, in individuals ingesting water from lead pipes, and in children ingesting old lead-based paint in the house. Lead interferes with haem and globin synthesis (see Answer **44**, page 64). The effects are a microcytic anaemia and raised precursors of haem synthesis. The latter cause abdominal symptoms, autonomic and motor neuropathy which are identical to those seen in AIP. In both lead poisoning and AIP the δ-ALA is elevated; however, lead poisoning is differentiated from AIP by the relatively severe anaemia, basophilic stippling affecting the red cells and the elevated proto- and coproporphyrins. Basophilic stippling is caused by aggregates of RNA resulting from inhibition of the enzyme pyrimidine-5-nucleotidase. Other features include haemolytic anaemia, lead encephalopathy (which is characterized by a high CSF protein), a blue line on the gums, and dense metaphyseal bands at the end of long bones in children (known as lead lines). Proximal RTA is recognized and comprises a hypokalaemic, hyperchloraemic acidosis, as well as loss of amino acids in the urine.

Question 90

A 52-year-old obese hypertensive female was seen in the accident and emergency department with sudden onset of palpitations and breathlessness. She had a history of hypertension, congestive cardiac failure and non-insulin-dependent diabetes mellitus. She was taking captopril 50 mg twice daily, nifedipine slow release 20 mg twice daily, metformin 500 mg three times daily, and frusemide 80 mg daily. The frusemide dose had recently been doubled by her general practitioner to control her persistently elevated blood pressure and help her breathlessness. She had previously undergone several investigations to exclude a secondary cause for the hypertension.

On examination, the patient appeared breathless, but was not cyanosed. She was well perfused. The heart rate was 100 beats/min, and regular; blood pressure was 150/100 mmHg. The JVP was not elevated. On examination of her precordium, the apex was not palpable, but the heart sounds were normal. There were no murmurs. Respiratory examination revealed good chest expansion. The trachea was central and percussion was normal. Auscultation of the lung fields was normal. There was no evidence of peripheral oedema, but she had an erythematous skin rash on her shins.

Blood results are shown.

1. Interpret the blood gases.
2. What is the single most likely explanation for the abnormal blood gas results?

Biochemistry	Sodium 134 mmol/l
	Potassium 4.3 mmol/l
	Creatinine 120 µmol/l
	Urea 8 mmol/l
ECG	Sinus tachycardia
Chest X-ray (**90**)	
Arterial blood gases	pH 7.5
	pCO_2 1.8 kPa
	pO_2 15 kPa
	Bicarbonate 19.3 mmol/l
	Base excess +7

Question 91

A 25-year-old Malaysian male was admitted to hospital as an emergency when he noticed that he was completely paralysed for two hours after waking from his sleep in the early hours of the morning. He had experienced this type of severe weakness on four occasions over the past few months, and remarked how they always occurred during sleep and on waking he could not move. He drank four units of alcohol every night. He had recently seen his general practitioner for anxiety attacks and was being counselled. He emigrated to England in 1994 and worked as a chef. He was single. All his family members were in Malaysia and were well.

On examination, he was thin; otherwise, physical examination was normal.

Investigations are shown.

FBC	Normal
Biochemistry	Sodium 136 mmol/l
	Potassium 2 mmol/l
	Urea 5 mmol/l
	Bicarbonate 23 mmol/l
	TSH <0.1 mu/l
	Thyroxine 190 nmol/

1. What is the diagnosis?
2. List two important steps in the management of this patient.

Answer 90

1. The blood gases demonstrate a partially compensated respiratory alkalosis.
2. Hyperventilation.

Respiratory alkalosis is characterized by a low pCO_2 and a high pH. Respiratory alkalosis may be seen in hyperventilation and artificial ventilation. In these situations it is associated with a high or normal pO_2. It is also seen in conditions predisposing to ventilation/perfusion mismatch such as pneumonia, pulmonary oedema, pulmonary embolus and parenchymal lung disease. In this particular case, the patient has a normal pO_2 and clear lung fields on the chest X-ray, suggesting that she is hyperventilating (see *Table* for causes of respiratory alkalosis).

In all chronic respiratory alkalotic states the kidneys compensate by excreting excess bicarbonate to produce a relative metabolic acidosis in an attempt to normalize the blood pH. Therefore, in compensated respiratory alkalosis the plasma bicarbonate is low.

Acute salicylate poisoning also produces a combined respiratory alkalosis and metabolic acidosis. In toxic doses, salicylates stimulate hyperventilation through effects on the respiratory regulatory system. Renal compensation leads to increased excretion of bicarbonate, resulting in metabolic acidosis. In addition, salicylates interfere with oxidative phosphorylation and lead to lactic acidosis, further exacerbating the metabolic acidosis.

(See Acid–base Disturbance, page 228.)

Causes of respiratory alkalosis

Due to stimulation of the central nervous system:
Anxiety
Hypoxia
Salicylate poisoning
Encephalitis
Brain stem injury

Due to pulmonary disease:
Asthma
Pneumonia
Lung fibrosis
Pulmonary oedema
Pulmonary embolus

Answer 91

1. Hypokalaemic periodic paralysis associated with thyrotoxicosis.
2. i. Correct the hypokalaemia.
ii. Treat the thyrotoxicosis.

Hypokalaemic periodic paralysis is a rare condition which is often inherited as an autosomal dominant trait. It is characterized by episodic paralysis which classically occurs at night while the patient is asleep. The cause of hypokalaemia is not clear, but shifts in potassium from the extracellular fluid to the intracellular fluid are thought to be responsible. Symptoms can be precipitated by administering intravenous glucose and insulin into such patients, which would lend support to the potassium shift theory. Other precipitating factors include alcohol, large carbohydrate meals, anxiety and tension. Recovery is usually rapid, but can be expedited by intravenous potassium supplements. Long-term treatment is with potassium supplements or potassium-sparing diuretics.

In oriental males, aged between 20 and 50 years, the condition is associated with thyrotoxicosis. The symptoms of thyrotoxicosis may precede the paralysis, or may not be apparent. Paralysis occurs during sleep and periods of prolonged rest. Arrhythmias associated with hypokalaemia are a recognized feature in this condition. Treatment of the thyrotoxicosis prevents further attacks of paralysis. In the meantime, the potassium needs to be corrected. Propranolol is successful in preventing attacks in approximately 60% of cases. Although thyrotoxicosis is more common in females, periodic paralysis only affects males. The mechanism of hypokalaemia is the same as in familial periodic paralysis.

An important differential diagnosis when the patient is in the paralysed state is Guillain–Barré syndrome and acute myaesthenia gravis.

Question 92

A 39-year-old male was admitted with malaise, lethargy and bleeding gums. Investigations on admission were as follows:

FBC	Hb 4 g/dl
	WCC 70 × 10⁹/l
	(predominantly blasts)
	Platelets 26 × 10⁹/l
Blood film (**92**)	
Biochemistry	Sodium 137 mmol/l
	Potassium 3.7 mmol/l
	Urea 4 mmol/l
	Creatinine 74 µmol/l

The patient received chemotherapy which he tolerated well, but on the second day post-chemotherapy he complained of severe nausea. Biochemical results were as follows:

Biochemistry	Sodium 136 mmol/l
	Potassium 7.2 mmol/l
	Urea 23 mmol/l
	Creatinine 300 µmol/l
	Urate 1.2 mmol/l
	Phosphate 3 mmol/l

1. What was the haematological diagnosis?
2. How do you account for the abnormal biochemistry?
3. What is the cause for the renal failure?
4. State two steps which should have been taken to prevent this complication.

Question 93

A 59-year-old headmaster was referred to a chest unit with a six-month history of progressive breathlessness. His effort tolerance one year previously was very good, allowing him to jog 10 km, twice a week. Since then he has had to give up running due to fatigue and breathlessness. His condition had continued to deteriorate, despite the use of steroid and salbutamol inhalers prescribed by his general practitioner. He was now breathless after walking just 200 m. He was a non-smoker. He had been a headmaster in a London public school for nearly 25 years. There was no family history of lung disease. He had never worked with asbestos, and did not keep pets.

On examination, the patient was cyanosed and tachypnoeic. His hands and feet were clubbed. The JVP was not raised, and heart sounds were normal. On auscultation of the lung fields there were bilateral fine end-inspiratory crackles at both lung bases.

Investigations are shown.

FEV₁ (% predicted)	50	Blood gases on air
FVC (% predicted)	52	pH 7.45
FEV₁/FVC (%)	89	pCO₂ 3.5 kPa
TLC (% predicted)	56	pO₂ 6.4 kPa
KCO (% predicted)	60	Bicarbonate 22 mmol/l

Bronchoalveolar lavage revealed increased number of cells which were predominantly neutrophils
Chest X-ray (**93**)

1. What is the diagnosis?
2. Which two investigations will you perform to confirm the diagnosis?

Answer 92

1. Acute myeloid leukaemia. Myeloblasts are large round cells with a round nucleus and prominent nucleoli. In addition, they may contain cytoplasmic inclusions known as Auer rods which are almost pathognomonic of the condition.
2. Tumour lysis syndrome. The large numbers of blasts destroyed by chemotherapy liberate large amounts of intracellular contents into the bloodstream, as evidenced by the high potassium and phosphate concentrations. The nucleic acid from the cell nuclei is metabolized to produce urate which is excreted by the kidney.
3. Hyperuricaemic nephropathy. High concentrations of urate may cause crystallization within renal tubules and acute renal failure.
4. The condition is prevented by pre-hydration and allopurinol, which inhibits synthesis of urate.

Answer 93

1. i. Restrictive lung defect with reduced KCO.
ii. Cryptogenic fibrosing alveolitis.
2. i. High-resolution CT scan.
ii. Transbronchial lung biopsy.

In the absence of an obvious underlying cause (occupational, drugs, connective tissue disorder) for the symptoms and signs, the most likely diagnosis is CFA, which is a disorder of unknown aetiology which usually occurs in middle age. It is characterized by progressively worsening dyspnoea, eventually leading to respiratory failure and cor pulmonale from pulmonary hypertension. The cardinal signs include cyanosis, clubbing and fine inspiratory crackles at both lung bases. The chest X-ray demonstrates a ground-glass appearance in the mid zones and bases of the lung which progresses to nodular shadows and streaky fibrosis. The end result is a 'honeycomb appearance of the lung on the chest X-ray'.

Lung function tests demonstrate a restrictive lung defect and a low KCO.

Blood gases demonstrate a low arterial oxygen content and a normal CO_2 content unless the patient develops end-stage respiratory failure. The quality of high-resolution CT scans obviate the need for lung biopsy to diagnose the condition in the majority of patients, but in younger patients biopsy may be useful in differentiating the condition from other causes of a similar chest X-ray appearance. Bronchoalveolar lavage reveals large numbers of neutrophils, and transbronchial biopsy will demonstrate cellular infiltration and thickening and fibrosis of the alveolar walls.

Some 50% patients are positive for rheumatoid factor, and 33% are positive for ANF.

CFA is associated with other autoimmune conditions such as coeliac disease, primary biliary cirrhosis, ulcerative colitis and RTA.

The management is with prednisolone. Azathioprine or cyclophosphamide may be used as steroid-sparing drugs. Most patients also require oxygen therapy. The median survival is five years.

Causes of lung fibrosis

CFA	Pneumoconiosis
Extrinsic allergic alveolitis (farmer's lung; bird-fancier's disease)	Asbestosis
	Neurofibromatosis
Sarcoidosis	Tuberous sclerosis
Connective tissue disease (SLE, rheumatoid arthritis, systemic sclerosis)	Histiocytosis
	Ankylosing spondylitis
Vasculitides	TB
Drugs (busulphan, bleomycin, cyclophosphamide)	Radiation

Question 94

A 76-year-old female was admitted after being found on the floor by the home help. She complained of frequent dizzy spells, particularly after standing from a recumbent position. She had experienced several falls at home, but never required hospital admission. She had become housebound due to the dizzy spells and falls and was increasingly dependent on the social services. She also complained of lethargy, hoarse voice, intermittent confusion, and weight gain of almost 7 kg over the past seven months. She had a history of arthritis for which she took paracetamol when in pain. She was not taking any other regular medications.

On examination, she was pale and frail. The heart rate was 60 beats/min and regular. The blood pressure was 200/60 mmHg when lying, and 90/50 mmHg when standing. The JVP was not raised. The apex was displaced slightly. Auscultation of the heart revealed soft first and second heart sounds. There were no added sounds or murmurs. Auscultation of the lungs was normal, as was examination of the abdomen. Central nervous system examination was essentially normal, with the exception of bilateral absence of the ankle jerks.

Investigations are shown.

1. What is the most likely explanation for the dizzy spells and falls?
2. What is the explanation for the electrolyte abnormality?
3. Which single test would you request to confirm this?
4. What is the unifying diagnosis?

FBC	Hb 10 g/dl
	WCC 6 × 10⁹/l
	Platelets 149 × 10⁹/l
	MCV 87 fl
Biochemistry	Sodium 118 mmol/l
	Potassium 5.3 mmol/l
	Urea 3 mmol/l
	Creatinine 69 µmol/l
	Bilirubin 12 µmol/l
	AST 20 u/l
	Alkaline phosphatase 100 u/l
	Albumin 36 g/l
	Total protein 63 g/l
Chest X-ray (94)	
ECG	Normal rhythm and complexes

Question 95

A 69-year-old male was seen by his general practitioner with pain in his wrist after a fall. He complained of generalized weakness and pains in his lower limbs over the past few months. Several investigations were ordered, the results of which are as follows:

1. Give two possible diagnoses.
2. Give three reasons to support the cause of this patient's raised IgG level.

FBC	Hb 13 g/dl	Biochemistry	Phosphate 0.7 mmol/l
	WCC 7 × 10⁹/l	(continued)	Alkaline phosphatase 240 u/l
	Platelets 350 × 10⁹/l	Immunology	IgG 23 g/l
ESR	55 mm/h		IgM 2 g/l
Biochemistry	Sodium 136 mmol/l		IgA 2.4 g/l
	Potassium 4 mmol/l		Paraprotein 6 g/l
	Urea 6 mmol/l	X-ray of wrist	Fracture radius, small
	Creatinine 90 µmol/l		radiolucent area adjacent to
	Calcium 2.0 mmol/l		fracture

Answer 94

1. Postural hypotension.
2. Addison's disease.
3. Short synacthen test.
4. Polyendocrine deficiency type 2 (Schmidt's syndrome).

> **The polyendocrine deficiency syndromes**
>
> *Polyendocrine deficiency syndrome (type 2) comprises any two of the following:*
> Autoimmune hypoadrenalism
> Autoimmune hypothyroidism
> Insulin-dependent diabetes mellitus
>
> *Polyendocrine deficiency syndrome (type 1) comprises any two of the following:*
> Autoimmune hypoparathyroidism
> Autoimmune hypoadrenalism
> Mucocutaneous candidiasis, alopecia, pernicious anaemia
>
> Vitiligo and hypogonadism may occur in both forms

The postural hypotension and hyponatraemia suggest the diagnosis of Addison's disease. For causes and further details on Addison's disease, see Answer **112**, page 146. The additional history of weight gain, croaky voice, and enlarged heart on the chest X-ray suggest coexistent hypothyroidism. (Note: in pure Addison's disease the heart is characteristically small due to chronic hypovolaemia; however, if hypothyroidism is also present the heart may be enlarged due to a consequent cardiomyopathy or a pericardial effusion.) Approximately 10% of cases of Addison's disease due to autoimmune adrenalitis are associated with other endocrine deficiencies (*Table*). The association of autoimmune adrenalitis with autoimmune hypothyroidism or insulin-dependent diabetes mellitus is termed Schmidt's syndrome or polyendocrine deficiency type 2.

The patient's confusion could be explained by either Addison's disease or hypothyroidism. Absent ankle jerks are not uncommon in the elderly. In hypothyroidism, the ankle jerk characteristically demonstrates slow relaxation; however, there may be absent reflexes due to a secondary peripheral neuropathy. Other neurological manifestations of hypothyroidism include cerebellar syndrome and coma.

Answer 95

1. i. Osteomalacia.
ii. Monoclonal gammopathy of undetermined significance.
2. i. Not anaemic.
ii. No evidence of immune paresis.
iii. Paraprotein level below 20 g/l.

The diagnosis of osteomalacia is relatively straightforward on the bone biochemistry, which classically reveals hypocalcaemia, hypophosphataemia and a raised alkaline phosphatase, the latter being secondary to an increase in PTH release in response to hypocalcaemia. Skeletal manifestations of osteomalacia include Looser's zones, which are linear radiolucent areas seen most commonly in the bones of the forearms, scapulae, femurs and the pelvis. The raised ESR and IgG level associated with a very mild paraproteinaemia will confuse some readers, and commit them to make the erroneous diagnosis of multiple myeloma. However, there are a few pointers to suggest that the cause for the raised IgG level is MGUS rather than myeloma.

MGUS affects a very small proportion of the elderly. It is characterized by benign monoclonal proliferation of lymphocytes, resulting in a modest increase in IgG levels and an associated paraprotein of <2 g/l (in myeloma, the paraprotein level is usually >20 g/l). In contrast with patients suffering from myeloma, these patients are not anaemic, they do not have immune paresis, i.e. the other immunoglobulins are not reduced because of monoclonal proliferation, Bence Jones proteins are classically absent (may be present in <10%), and the skeletal survey is normal. The condition was originally termed benign monoclonal gammopathy, but it is now recognized that 10% of patients develop multiple myeloma, hence the relatively new term, MGUS.

Question 96

A 42-year-old male presented with a four-month history of headaches, generalized weakness, and polyuria. On examination, the physical examination was normal with the exception of a blood pressure of 190/105 mmHg.

Initial investigations are shown.

The patient was treated with a calcium antagonist, and underwent further investigations which led to him having abdominal surgery to cure his hypertension. The full macroscopic specimen of the abnormality removed is shown (96b).

Biochemistry	Sodium 142 mmol/l
	Potassium 3.3 mmol/l
	Urea 4.0 mmol/l
	Creatinine 100 μmol/l
	Bicarbonate 36 mmol/l
	Chloride 107 mmol/l
ECG (96a)	

1. What is the electrolyte abnormality?
2. List four abnormalities on the ECG, and two inferences you would make from these abnormalities.
3. What was the cause of his hypertension?
4. Which two investigations would he have had to confirm the diagnosis before surgery?
5. With all of the above information at hand, which anti-hypertensive agent should he have been prescribed?

Answer 96

1. Hypokalaemic alkalosis. (see Answer **114**, page 148).
2. i. First-degree atrioventricular block. The PR-interval in much greater than 200 ms. There are many causes of first-degree atrioventricular block (*Table A*); however, in this case the most likely cause is hypokalaemia.
ii. There is voltage criteria of left ventricular hypertrophy. The sum of the S-wave in V1 and the R-wave in V5 or V6 exceeds 0.35 mV (each small square on the ECG is 0.1 mV) which conforms with the Sokolow criteria for left ventricular hypertrophy.
iii. There is ST-segment depression in the lateral leads which may be secondary to left ventricular hypertrophy or to hypokalaemia. Although myocardial ischaemia is also a recognized cause of ST-segment depression, it is unlikely in the context of this question.
iv. There are prominent U-waves (upright waves immediately following the T-wave, **96c** arrowed) which are suggestive of hypokalaemia. Other ECG changes in relation to metabolic abnormalities are tabulated below (*Table B*).
3. Primary hyperaldosteronism or Conn's syndrome secondary to an adrenal adenoma. Conn's tumours are bright yellow as opposed to phaeochromocytomas, which are a greyish-purple colour (**96d**).
4. i. Lying and standing plasma renin and aldosterone levels.
ii. High-resolution abdominal CT scan.
5. High doses of spironolactone, an aldosterone antagonist.

Hypokalaemic alkalosis and hypertension in the MRCP and similar examinations is highly suggestive of primary hyperaldosteronism, which is often referred to as Conn's syndrome. The syndrome is caused by excessive secretion of aldosterone by the adrenal gland. This leads to increased salt and water retention, causing hypertension and clinical symptoms of hypokalaemia which include muscle weakness, polyuria and polydipsia from nephrogenic diabetes insipidus, and paraesthesia. Accelerated hypertension may complicate primary hyperaldosteronism, and cardiac arrhythmias may result from hypokalaemia. The serum renin level in primary hyperaldosteronism is suppressed, whereas in conditions causing secondary hyperaldosteronism the renin is elevated. Primary hyperaldosteronism may be caused by an autonomous aldosterone-secreting adrenal adenoma or bilateral hyperplasia of the adrenal gland.

The diagnosis is made by simultaneous measurement of serum renin and aldosterone levels in the lying and standing positions. The renin is low, and the aldosterone level is high, in the supine position. On standing suddenly, there is a paradoxical drop in the aldosterone level in patients with an adenoma and an exaggerated rise in aldosterone levels in patients with hyperplasia. Imaging with CT scanning is very useful in distinguishing between adenoma and hyperplasia. Adrenal adenomas >0.5 cm in diameter can be diagnosed by high-resolution CT scan. Adrenal vein sampling is only useful when there is doubt about the existence of an adenoma.

Iodolabelled cholesterol scintiscan is not a very sensitive method for identifying Conn's tumours.

The management of adrenal adenoma is surgical excision, and the management of hyperplasia is with a high-dose aldosterone antagonist, such as spironolactone.

Table A. Causes of first-degree atroventricular block

Ischaemic heart disease
Cardiac conduction tissue disease (sinoatrial disease)
Rheumatic fever
Myocarditis
Drugs
Hypokalaemia
Athlete's heart

Table C. Endocrine causes of hypertension

Conn's syndrome
Cushing's syndrome
Phaeochromocytoma
Acromegaly
Thyrotoxicosis
Hyperparathyroidism
11-β- and 17-β-hydroxylase deficiency

Table B. ECG changes in relation to metabolic abnormalities frequently encountered in the MRCP and similar examinations

Hypokalaemia
Peaked P-waves
Long PR-interval
Increased duration of the QRS-complex
U-waves
Long QT-interval
Flattened T-waves
ST-segment depression

Hyperkalaemia
Flat P-waves
Peaked T-waves
Increased duration of the QRS-complex
Sinusoidal QRS-complexes (pre-arrest)

Hypocalcaemia
Long QT-interval

Hypercalcaemia
Short QT-interval

Question 97

A 15-year-old farmer's daughter was admitted to the infectious diseases unit with a five-day history of right upper quadrant pain. On examination, she was pyrexial with a temperature of 38.4°C (101.1°F). She appeared unwell and jaundiced.

Investigations are shown.

1. Suggest at least two possible diagnoses.
2. Give three possible causes for the anaemia.

FBC	Hb 8 g/dl
	WCC 18.8 × 10⁹/l
	Platelets 140 × 10⁹/l
	Reticulocyte count 20%
Blood film	No fragmented red cells seen
Clotting	PT 36 s (control 12 s)
	APTT 59 s (control 45 s)
Biochemistry	Sodium 136 mmol/l
	Potassium 4.9 mmol/l
	Urea 26 mmol/l
	Creatinine 400 µmol/l
	Bilirubin 50 µmol/l
	AST 900 u/l
	Alkaline phosphatase 300 u/l
	Albumin 33 g/l
Hepatitis B sAg	Absent
HCV Ab	Absent
CMV serology	Absent
Monospot test	Negative

Answer 97

1. i. Leptospirosis (Weil's disease).
ii. Acute hepatitis A infection.
iii. Paracetamol overdose.
iv. Iron overdose.
2. i. Blood loss from endothelial damage resulting in haemorrhage.
ii. Haemolysis.
iii. Disseminated intravascular coagulation causing blood loss.

The patient has evidence of hepatitis together with renal failure and a coagulation disorder. The clinical scenario which would fit this triad is fulminant hepatic failure complicated by the hepatorenal syndrome. The majority of cases are due to viral hepatitis (hepatitis A, B, C and D, although EBV, CMV, Coxsackie and herpes simplex virus have been implicated; Lassa fever, Ebola virus and Marburg virus should be considered in a patient who has recently returned from Africa), and drugs (paracetamol, iron, tetracycline, isoniazid, rifampicin, halothane). Other recognized causes include toxins (alcohol, carbon tetra-chloride), leptospirosis (Weil's disease), Wilson's disease, and pregnancy. In a farmer's daughter, leptospirosis causing hepatic and renal failure (Weil's disease) is a distinct possibility, but hepatitis A and drug overdose should also be borne in mind.

Leptospirosis is caused by the spirochaete *Leptospira icterohaemorrhagica*. Rodents, particularly rats, are the most important reservoir of infection. Other hosts include cattle, pigs, goats, hamsters, mice, hedgehogs, foxes and skunks. The organism is excreted in the urine and may survive in the soil for several weeks. Entry into the human host is through cuts and abrasions on the skin, or through intact mucous membranes. Occupations most susceptible are sewage workers, fishermen, vets and farmers. Replication occurs in the blood and tissue and multisystem involvement may occur. The kidneys and liver are most affected. Glomerular injury occurs first causing an acute interstitial nephritis and tubular necrosis. In the liver there is evidence of centrilobular necrosis in severe cases.

The incubation period is 7–12 days. The initial (septi-caemic) phase is 4–7 days in duration. It is characterized by fever, headaches, myalgia, abdominal pain, vomiting, skin rash (macular, maculopapular or haemorrhagic) or conjunctival injection. Fever is high, myalgia is present in over 85% of cases and a major hallmark of the disease, and the headache may be severe. Persistent headache is suggestive of meningitis. Proteinuria and haematuria may be present during this phase, and renal failure is evident in just over 50% of patients. Jaundice and impairment of liver function is present only in severe cases. Some 90% of cases are anicteric. Hepatosplenomegaly is present in approximately 20%. Respiratory involvement is common, and manifests as a dry cough, haemoptysis and confluent shadow on the chest X-ray. The second phase of the disease (immune phase) varies between 4–30 days. The patient is afebrile. Antibody titres to *Leptospira* are rising. Deterioration in liver and renal function may continue. Meningism, uveitis and a rash are common. Haematological manifestations include thrombocytopenia, haemolytic uraemic syndrome characterized by fragmented red cells on the blood film, and intravascular haemolysis. Endothelial injury may cause blood loss from the gastrointestinal tract and the lung.

Blood cultures are positive in the first week, and by the second week the urine culture is also positive. IgM antibodies to *Leptospira* are detectable in the first week. There is a rising titre in the second week. Treatment is with high-dose penicillin.

Brucellosis is also recognized in farmers. The bacterium (Gram-negative bacillus) infects mammals, particularly cows, and can be contracted from contact with infected urine or drinking unpasteurized milk. Acute brucellosis is also characterized by fever, headache and myalgia; however, it is unlikely in this case due to the absence of a high fever, leucopenia, and assumed absence of hepatosplenomegaly, which is common in brucellosis. In addition, abnormal liver function or jaundice are extremely rare in brucellosis. Chronic brucellosis is associated with lassitude, headaches, depression, night sweats, skeletal, cardiovascular, neurological, genitourinary, pulmonary and intra-abdominal complications. Brucellosis has been eradicated in the UK due to mandatory pasteurization of milk.

Question 98

These ECG traces are from 40-year-old men. One is breathless on exertion (**98a**) and the other has a systolic murmur (**98b**).

For **98a**:
1. What information does the ECG give you with respect to cardiac morphology?
2. Give four acquired causes and three inherited causes for the ECG abnormalities.

For **98b**:
1. List two abnormalities.
2. Suggest two possible diagnoses.

Question 99

A 17-year-old male was referred to the local paediatrician because his mother was concerned that he was considerably shorter than his peers. He was well in himself. He had never required to shave, and had just recently noticed some pubic hair in his genital area. On examination, he measured 1.58 m. He had slight bilateral gynaecomastia. His voice had not broken. There was no facial hair. There was scanty pubic hair in the genital region and his testes were small. His father and mother were 1.83 m and 1.68 m tall, respectively.

Results of dynamic pituitary function testing with 0.2 units/kg insulin, 100 μg of LHRH and 200 μg of TRH were as follows:

Time (min)	Glucose (mmol/l)	GH mu/l	Cortisol (nmol/l)	TSH (mu/l)	LH (u/l)	FSH (u/l)	Testosterone (nmol/l)
0	4.0	1.4	400	2.0	29	16	34
20	2.8	12.0	860	5.2	40	24	60
30	1.6	28	1270	-	-	-	-
40	1.5	32	1450	-	-	-	-
60	2.2	20	1120	8	34	20	60

1. What is the most probable diagnosis?
A. Prader–Willi syndrome.
B. Kleinfelter's syndrome.
C. Onset of puberty.
D. Kallman's syndrome.
E. Testicular feminization syndrome.

Answer 98

For **98a**:
1. The ECG demonstrates voltage criteria for right atrial enlargement and right ventricular hypertrophy.
2. Acquired causes include:
i. Fibrotic lung disease.
ii. Bronchiectasis.
iii. Thromboembolic pulmonary disease.
iv. Chronic obstructive airways disease.
Inherited causes:
i. Cystic fibrosis.
ii. α-1 antitrypsin deficiency.
iii. Ostium secundum atrial septal defect (may be inherited as an autosomal dominant trait).

Information regarding atrial enlargement is gained from leads II and V1 (**98c**). Right atrial enlargement is characterized by a tall P-wave in both II and V1 which exceeds 0.25 mV (or two-and-a-half small squares). Voltage criteria for left atrial enlargement are a little more complicated. In lead II, the P-wave has a bifid appearance and the duration of the P-wave is 120 ms (three small squares). In V1, the P-wave is biphasic with a terminal (negative) portion of the P-wave exceeding or equal to 40 ms in duration (one small square) and more than or equal to –0.1 mV (one small square) in depth. The presence of a biphasic P-wave in V1 which does not satisfy these criteria cannot be diagnosed as left atrial enlargement on the ECG.

Information regarding voltage criteria for ventricular hypertrophy is gained from leads V1 and V5, particularly if the Sokolow's criteria (most commonly used) are to be applied. Right ventricular enlargement is suggested by the sum of the R-wave in V1 and the S-wave in V5 or V6 exceeding 1.25 mV (12.5 small squares). In addition, there may be ST-segment depression and T-wave inversion in leads V1–V3 and right axis deviation. Left ventricular hypertrophy is characterized by the sum of the S-wave in V1 and the R-wave in V5 or V6 exceeding 40 mm. The additional presence of ST-segment depression and/or T-wave inversion in V5 and V6 is more suggestive of the diagnosis.

For **98b**:
1. i. Voltage criteria for left atrial enlargement.
ii. Left ventricular hypertrophy (see explanation above).
2. i. Aortic stenosis.
ii. Hypertrophic cardiomyopathy.

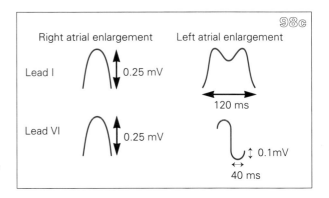

98c
Right atrial enlargement — Left atrial enlargement
Lead I — 0.25 mV — 120 ms
Lead VI — 0.25 mV — 0.1mV — 40 ms

Answer 99

1. D. Kallman's syndrome.

The findings are consistent with recent onset of puberty. The basal gonadotrophins and testosterone levels are generally high during puberty. The patient has scanty pubic hair and gynaecomastia, both markers of puberty. Prader–Willi and Kleinfelter's syndrome are recognized causes of primary hypogonadism; however, the high testosterone level is against this. Testicular feminization syndrome would be associated with a similar testosterone and gonadotrophin level; however, patients affected with the testicular feminization syndrome are phenotypically female (see Answer **158**, page 208). Kallman's syndrome is rare and often inherited as an X-linked recessive trait. It is characterized by deficient gonadotrophin production by the pituitary, anosmia, cleft palate and colour blindness. These patients may also have congenital renal and cerebral defects. Other causes of primary hypogonadism in males are given (*Table*).

Causes of primary hypogonadism in the male
Testosterone biosynthetic enzyme deficiencies
Kleinfelter's syndrome
Prader–Willi syndrome
Lawrence–Moon–Biedel syndrome
Noonan's syndrome
Rubella
Mumps orchitis
Castration
Cystic fibrosis
Sickle cell anaemia
Cirrhosis
Chemotherapy
Alcohol

Question 100

A 47-year-old female visited her general practitioner to request hormone replacement therapy. She had been amenorrhoeic for four months, and has complained of sweating excessively and fatigue. She had also noticed an increase in the size of her hands such that her wedding ring was very tight, her shoe size had increased recently, and her head appeared larger. Three years ago she had an episode of haemoptysis, following which she had a chest X-ray that revealed a small opacity in the right lung. She was subsequently lost to follow-up.

On examination, she had large, spade-shaped hands and broad feet. There was a palpable smooth thyroid goitre. The heart rate was 96 beats/min and the blood pressure was 160/90 mmHg. On examination of the respiratory system there was dullness and reduced air entry at the right lung base.

The patient was referred to an endocrinologist for further investigations:

Initial investigations were as follows:

FBC	Hb 13 g/dl	Biochemistry	Calcium 2.5 mmol/l
	WCC 9 × 10 ^{9}/l	(continued)	Phosphate 1 mmol/l
	Platelets 210 × 10 ^{9}/l		Albumin 40 g/l
	MCV 89 fl		Alkaline phosphatase 100 u/l
Biochemistry	Sodium 135 mmol/l		Bilirubin 10 µmol/l
	Potassium 4 mmol/l		AST 20 u/l
	Urea 6 mmol/l		ALT 25 u/l
	Creatinine 98 µmol/l	Chest X-ray (100)	

CT scan of thorax   Bulky mediastinum due to lymphadenopathy (mediastinal views)
MRI of pituitary   Normal
Endocrine investigations: Thyroid function   TSH 3 mu/l (normal range 0.5–5.0 mu/l)
   Thyroxine 110 nmol/l
Gonadotrophins   FSH 60 u/l   LH 30 u/l

Oral glucose tolerance test with 75 g glucose after an overnight fast:

Time (min)	0	30	60	120
Blood glucose (mmol/l)	8	15	20	10.5
GH (mu/l)	60	64	94	58

Insulin tolerance test: 0.3 units/kg:

Time (min)	0	30	45	60	90	120
Blood glucose (mmol/l)	8	4	1.8	3	8	11
Cortisol (nmol/l)	180	260	700	620	500	400

Serum calcitonin	Normal	Serum PTH	Normal
Serum glucagon	Normal	Serum noradrenaline	Normal
Serum VIP	Normal	Urinary VMA	Normal

1. List two inferences you can make from the oral glucose tolerance test.
2. Comment on the insulin tolerance test.
3. Comment on the abnormal gonadotrophin levels, and give the most likely explanation.
4. Comment on the chest X-ray.
5. What is the connection between the chest X-ray and the endocrine abnormality?

Answer 100

1. The patient has diabetes mellitus and acromegaly. The fasting blood glucose is over 6.7 mmol/l and the 2-hour blood glucose level is 10.5 mmol/l. Impaired glucose tolerance is diagnosed when fasting blood glucose is above 6.7 mmol/l and the 2-hour blood glucose is under 10 mmol/l. The resting growth hormone level of above 4 mu/l is highly suggestive of acromegaly. In normal people, growth hormone secretion is suppressed to below 2 mu/l with hyperglycaemia; however, in acromegaly there is failure of growth hormone secretion suppression and there may be a paradoxical rise in growth hormone levels with hyperglycaemia.

2. There is adequate hypoglycaemia (blood glucose under 2.2 mmol/l) and there is an appropriate rise in serum cortisol (>550 nmol/l), suggesting adequate pituitary ACTH reserve.

3. The patient is aged 47 and has amenorrhoea. The grossly elevated gonadotrophin reflects menopause. The low circulating oestrogen level (lack of negative feedback of oestrogen on the pituitary) is the stimulus for hypersecretion of the gonadotrophins.

4. The chest X-ray demonstrates a large, well-defined circular mass situated in the lower lobe of the right lung which may be consistent with a carcinoma, adenoma or a large secondary metastasis.

5. The endocrine tests are suggestive of acromegaly. The most common cause of acromegaly is autonomous secretion of growth hormone by an acidophil adenoma in the pituitary. In this case, the pituitary appears normal on the MRI scan and there is no other pituitary endocrine abnormality. It is highly possible that the cause of acromegaly is due to ectopic growth hormone or GHRH secretion. Ectopic growth hormone or GHRH secretion is a very rare but recognized characteristic of certain tumours, particularly those affecting the lung, pancreas or ovary. Small cell lung carcinoma or bronchial carcinoid, and ovarian teratomas are capable of growth hormone or GHRH secretion. More common examples of ectopic hormone production include ACTH (small cell carcinoma lung), ADH (small cell carcinoma lung), PTH-related peptide (hypernephroma, squamous cell lung carcinoma), erythropoietin (hepatocellular carcinoma, hypernephroma) and 5-HIAA (carcinoid tumours).

Question 101

A 29-year-old male living in a hostel presented with a three-week history of reduced visual acuity and a six-week history of watery diarrhoea. There was no history of headaches or abdominal pain. On further questioning, he mentioned he had a sore mouth and throat, and found it difficult to swallow. He had not been on any medications in the past six months.

On examination, he was thin. Inspection of his tongue and oral cavity are shown (**101a, 101b**). Examination of his fundi is shown (**101c**). Examination of the abdomen and central nervous system was normal.

Investigations are shown.

1. What is the cause of his reduced visual acuity?
2. Why does he have dysphagia?
3. What is the cause of the abnormality on his tongue?
4. Give two possible explanations for his diarrhoea.
5. Which two drugs should the patient take for his diarrhoea and reduced visual acuity?

FBC	Hb 10 g/dl
	WCC 4 × 10⁹/l
	Platelets 170 × 10⁹/l
Biochemistry	Sodium 134 mmol/
	Potassium 4.1 mmol/l
	Urea 4 mmol/l
	Creatinine 67 µmol/l
	Glucose 4 mmol/l
Chest X-ray	Clear
Upper gastrointestinal endoscopy	Oesophagitis
Oesophageal washings (**101d**)	
Stool microscopy (**101e**)	
Rectal biopsy (**101f**)	

Answer 101

1. CMV retinitis.
2. Oesophageal candidiasis.
3. Oral hairy leukoplakia.
4. i. Cryptosporidial infection.
   ii. CMV colitis.
5. i. Ganciclovir.
   ii. Paromomycin.

The patient has evidence of several AIDS-defining conditions. The fundal appearance is consistent with CMV retinitis, which is the most common cause of visual impairment in these patients. The diagnosis is clinical. Early retinal changes include narrowing of the lumen of the retinal vessels. This is followed by vascular occlusion and perivascular haemorrhages (red areas), resulting in retinal ischaemia (white areas). Without therapy, the condition progresses to bilateral blindness. Treatment is with intravenous ganciclovir, followed by oral maintenance therapy. CMV may also cause encephalitis, colitis and cholangitis, all of which are best treated by the same drug. In the gastrointestinal tract CMV is diagnosed histologically by the demonstration of round intranuclear inclusion bodies within epithelial cells of the intestinal mucosa, as shown in the rectal biopsy (**101f**).

Oral candidiasis is common in patients with HIV and is treated with nystatin or fluconazole. Gastric washings in this patient reveal *Candida* hyphae. Oesophageal *Candida* may cause severe dysphagia, but responds to the same treatment. Hairy leukoplakia affects the lateral borders of the tongue. Unlike *Candida*, it cannot be scraped off the tongue with ease. The condition is painless and is due to infection with EBV. Its presence is highly suggestive of HIV infection. Acyclovir may be of some benefit in its management.

The stool reveals evidence of *Cryptosporidium*, which is the most common cause of diarrhoea in patients with HIV infection. The diarrhoea may be transient or persistent, and may be mild or profuse. The diagnosis is made by staining stool with modified Ziehl–Neelsen stain (**100e**) to demonstrate red cysts of *Cryptosporidium*. Treatment may be difficult and usually involves anti-diarrhoeal agents and fluid replacement. Definitive drugs in the management of cryptosporidial infection include spiramycin and paromomycin.

The neurological complications of HIV are discussed in Answer **116**, page 152. Other complications are shown (*Table*).

Complications of HIV

Respiratory	*Gastrointestinal*
Pneumocystis carinii pneumonia	HIV enteritis
CMV pneumonia	CMV colitis
Cryptococcal pneumonia	Giardiasis
TB (including *Mycobacterium avium* intracellulare)	*Cryptosporidium*
Histoplasmosis	*Isospora belli*
Lymphoma	*Salmonella enteritidis*
Kaposi's sarcoma	*Shigella* dysentery
	Candida infection
Skin	*Mouth*
Seborrhoeic dermatitis	Herpetic stomatitis
Molluscum contagiosum	Aphthous ulcers
Folliculitis	Kaposi's sarcoma
TB	
Candida infection	
Tinea infection	
Pityriasis versicolor	
Kaposi's sarcoma	

Question 102

A 16-year-old Nigerian male presented to hospital with severe pain affecting his left knee and right elbow. He required admission to another hospital with similar pain three years ago, and was treated with painkillers. He had experienced milder pains at home for which he had required paracetamol. He was one of four siblings and had an older sister who was known to have a form of anaemia.

On examination, he was distressed with pain. His temperature was 38°C (100.4°F). The left knee and right elbow joints were extremely painful, but joint movement was not restricted. The rest of the physical examination was normal.

Investigations are shown.

1. What is the mechanism of joint pain in this patient?
2. List two investigations you would perform to help with the diagnosis.
3. What is the underlying diagnosis?

FBC	Hb 10.2 g/dl
	WCC 11 × 10⁹/l
	Platelets 190 × 10⁹/l
	MCV 69 fl
	MCHC 29 g/dl
	Reticulocyte count 7.7%
Blood film	Numerous target cells and polychromasia
Biochemistry	Sodium 135 mmol/l
	Potassium 3.7 mmol/l
	Urea 6 mmol/l
	Aspartate aminotransferase 48 u/l
	Bilirubin 40 µmol/l
	Alkaline phosphatase 130 u/l

Question 103

A 35-year-old Irish nurse returns from Baltimore and is admitted with sharp right lower chest pain which is worse on inspiration. The following day she develops similar pain in the left lower chest. On examination, she has a temperature of 39°C (102.2°F) and reduced air entry at the base of the right lung. There are pleural rubs at the base of both lungs.

Investigations are shown.

Twenty-four hours afterwards, the patient developed substernal pain and on auscultation had an audible soft clicking synchronous with the heart sounds.

1. List two possible diagnoses which account for all her symptoms and signs.
2. List at least two tests you would perform to confirm each diagnosis.

FBC	Hb 12 g/dl
	WCC 3.5 × 10⁹/l
	Platelets 300 × 10⁹/l
ESR	33 mm/h
Chest X-ray	Normal lung fields and cardiac size
Arterial gases	pH 7.4
	pO₂ 11.5 kPa
	pCO₂ 4.5 kPa
	Bicarbonate 25 mmol/l

Answer 102

1. Bone infarction.
2. i. Hb electrophoresis.
ii. Family screening.
3. Sickle cell anaemia. It is also possible that he may have another sickel syndrome such as HbSC disease or HbS/β-thalassaemia trait.

Complications of sickle cell anaemia
Hand and foot syndrome. Usually seen in infancy
Painful bony crises. Seen later in life. Precipitated by cold, dehydration, fever or hypoxia
Aplastic crises. May follow infection from parvovirus B19
Splenic sequestration. Common in infancy. Severe anaemia and splenic enlargement
Hepatic sequestration. As with splenic sequestration
Pulmonary syndromes (thrombotic and sequestration)
Cerebral syndromes (usually thrombotic)
Infections from capsulated organisms (autosplenectomy)
Gall stones (pigment). Usually in adults
Progressive renal failure (papillary necrosis). Usually in adults
Chronic leg ulcers. Usually in adults
Recurrent priapism
Avascular necrosis of femoral heads
Salmonella osteomyelitis

Sickle cell anaemia (HbSS) is the most common sickling disorder which is inherited as an autosomal recessive trait. It is due to a point mutation in both β-globin genes, which results in the substitution of the amino acid glutamine for valine on position 6. Other sickling disorders include HbSC disease (where one β-globin chain is similar to that seen in HbSS and the other β-globin chain is similar to that seen in HbC, another haemoglobin variant), and HbS/β-thalassaemia trait. Patients with HbSC make equal quantities of HbS and HbC, whereas those with HbS/β-thalassaemia trait make predominantly HbS. The amino acid substitution in HbS causes red cell sickling during deoxygenation, leading to increased rigidity and aggregation in the microcirculation. This results in a haemolytic anaemia and episodic tissue infarction – 'the sickle cell crises' (see *Table*).

The sickle cell gene is spread widely throughout Africa, some Mediterranean countries, the Middle East and parts of India. It confers protection to malaria.

Patients with sickle cell anaemia are anaemic (Hb 6–10 g/dl) and have a high reticulocyte count (10–20%). The blood film demonstrates polychromasia, target cells and variable numbers of sickle cells. In general, patients with HbSC disease have a less severe form of anaemia, more target cells and less sickle cells. They have fewer crises; however, retinal damage, aseptic necrosis of neck of femur and recurrent haematuria are important complications. Pulmonary emboli may occur, particularly during and after pregnancy. Individuals who are carriers, i.e. those with just one abnormal β-globin gene (sickle cell trait) are not anaemic and do not have clinical abnormalities, but may rarely develop a sickling crisis in conditions of extreme hypoxia. Renal papillary necrosis and an inability to concentrate urine is recognized in a very small proportion of individuals with sickle cell trait.

The diagnosis is made by Hb electrophoresis. A definitive diagnosis requires the demonstration of sickle cell trait in both parents.

Answer 103

1. i. Systemic lupus erythematosus.
ii. Bornholm's disease (Coxsackie virus).
2. i. Double-stranded DNA antibody.
ii. Antinuclear antibody.
iii. CRP.
iv. Serum complement.
v. Electron microscopy of stool for Coxsackie virus.
vi. Acute and convalescent titres for Coxsackie virus.
vii. Echocardiogram.

The patient has symptoms suggestive of polyserositis (pleurisy and pericarditis), a high temperature, a slightly elevated ESR, and a relative leucopenia. The most probable diagnosis is SLE, although epidemic myalgia or Bornholm's syndrome due to Coxsackie virus (A or B) infection may present in a similar fashion. The patient has returned from Baltimore, where there may have been an epidemic of Coxsackie virus infection. Familial Mediterranean fever is also characterized by polyserositis and a fever; however, her place of origin is against the diagnosis.

SLE is a multisystem disorder due to a vasculitic process. The disease is thought to have a genetic and autoimmune basis, although a viral aetiology has been proposed by some. It usually affects patients below 40 years, is more common in Negroes, and has a female:male ratio of 10:1. The disease often presents with fatigue, arthralgia, and arthritis. Pyrexia is common. In addition, there may be renal, pulmonary, cardiac, neurological, haematological and cutaneous involvement. Renal disease is either due to acute diffuse, diffuse proliferative, membranous or focal segmental glomerulonephritis. Pleurisy, pleural effusions and fibrotic lung disease are well recognized (30–40%). Pericarditis is the most common cardiological manifestation of the condition, affecting 30% of patients. Pericardial constriction or tamponade are rare complications. Non-infective endocarditis (Libman–Sacks endocarditis) is extremely rare and is rarely of clinical significance. It is usually a post-mortem finding. Neurological manifestations include peripheral and cranial neuropathy, aseptic meningitis, seizures, chorea, neuropsychiatric disorders, and a syndrome resembling multiple sclerosis. Haematological manifestations are common, especially in active disease, and include mild normochromic, normocytic anaemia, leucopaenia, thrombocytopenia and autoimmune haemolysis. Leucopenia occurs in 65% of patients, which is in contrast with the other vasculitidies where the WCC is elevated. Skin manifestations include the characteristic malar butterfly rash on the face in acute SLE or chronic discoid lesions in areas exposed to sunlight. Livedo reticularis, vasculitic skin nodules, alopecia and Raynaud's phenomenon may also occur.

The collection of symptoms affecting different systems should raise suspicion in a young woman, and the diagnosis is confirmed by detection of antibodies to double-stranded DNA which is relatively specific for SLE. However, the test is positive in only 60% of patients. Antinuclear antibody is present in 90% of patients. It is less specific for SLE and may be present in other vasculitidies. The ESR is usually high and may exceed 100 mm/h. The CRP is characteristically normal unless there is underlying infection, a feature common to patients taking immunosuppressant medication for management of disease. Complement levels, particularly C3 are depressed. Circulating lupus anticoagulant, an antiphospholipid antibody is detected in 30–40% of patients.

Management includes NSAIDs for musculoskeletal problems. Chloroquine is useful where cutaneous manifestations predominate. Corticosteroids and other immunosuppressants (azathioprine, cyclophosphamide and chlorambucil) are used when disease is severe.

Epidemic myalgia due to Coxsackie A or B (Bornholm's disease) is also possible. Despite the name, sporadic cases do exist. Children and young adults are affected most commonly. The symptoms are usually sudden and comprise abdominal or thoracic pain. Myalgia affecting the chest muscles, fever and headaches are usually present. Pleurisy and pericarditis are recognized features, and both pleural and pericardial rubs may be present. The diagnosis is clinical, but the virus may be isolated in faeces. Acute and convalescent sera for Coxsackie virus antibodies will confirm the diagnosis if there is a four-fold rise in antibody titres between the two samples.

Question 104

An 8-year-old male with a known history of haemophilia A presented with a 10-hour history of pain in the left groin which radiated to the back. He described this as a dull pain which was constant in nature. He was given factor VIII concentrate and admitted for observation; however, the pain persisted and a few hours later was radiating into the anterior aspect of the left thigh.

On examination, he appeared unwell. He was afebrile. The heart rate was 90 beats/min and the blood pressure was 100/55 mmHg. The patient's left hip was held in flexion. Power testing revealed that he was unable to extend his left hip from the flexed position and knee extension on the left side was weak. The left knee jerk was absent, and sensory testing demonstrated reduced sensation in the anterior and medial aspect of the left thigh. Examination of the abdomen was normal.

1. Which of the following cannot explain why he failed to respond?
A. Inadequate dose of factor VIII.
B. Antibodies to factor VIII.
C. Factor VIII may have expired.
D. Factor VIII stored at 4°C (39.2°F).
E. Deficiency of other clotting factor due to chronic active hepatitis.
2. What is the cause of the neurological signs?
A. Occlusion of the femoral artery.
B. Allergic reaction to Factor VIII.
C. Femoral nerve compression.
D. Prolapsed L3/L4.
E. Spinal cord tumour.

3. What is the diagnosis?
A. Psoas abscess.
B. Psoas haematoma.
C. Necrosis of the quadriceps muscle.
D. Haemarthrosis affecting the left hip joint.
E. Spinal cord arachnoiditis.
4. Which investigation would be least useful in the management of this patient?
A. CT scan of the abdomen.
B. Factor VIII antibody level.
C. Factor VIII estimation.
D. APTT.
E. Bleeding time.

Answer 104

1. D. Factor VIII stored at 4°C (39.2°F).
2. C. Femoral nerve compression.
3. B. Psoas haematoma.
4. E. Bleeding time.

Haemophilia A is inherited as an X-linked recessive condition. The incidence is between 30–120 per million. It is due to the deficiency or low levels of Factor VIII, which results in abnormal clotting and a tendency to spontaneous bleeding or bleeding after minor injury. Important sites of bleeding are the joints, the psoas muscle, sublingual and pharyngeal areas, renal and gastro-intestinal tract. Cerebral haemorrhage is an important cause of death.

The question requires knowledge regarding important bleeding sites in haemophilia and the management of such an emergency. The presentation comprises pain in the left groin, hip held in flexion, absent knee jerk (L3,L4) and reduced sensation in the anterior and medial aspect of the thigh (L2,L3). All these features are typical of femoral nerve compression (L2–L4). A femoral nerve lesion actually causes weakness of hip flexion, and therefore in this case the flexed hip implies irritation of the nerve. In the context of the history of haemophilia this almost certainly represents a psoas haematoma. (The femoral nerve crosses the iliac fossa between the psoas muscle and the iliacus muscle before entering the thigh deep to the inguinal ligament.) A psoas abscess may present with similar neurological signs; however, the absence of fever or rigors is against this. Haemarthrosis is common in haemophilia, and although it is possible for a patient to have haemorrhage into the hip bone, this would not explain the sensory signs or the absence of the knee reflex. Spinal cord arachnoiditis generally presents with root pain and gradual paraplegia. Muscle haematomas may cause necrosis, but in this case the muscle at risk is the psoas, not the quadriceps muscle. Femoral artery thrombosis would be most unusual in a haemophiliac, and the presentation would consist of sudden onset of pain and paralysis of the left lower limb.

Failure to manage the bleed may be due to a variety of reasons which have been listed in the stems in the first part of the question. Patients with Factor VIII antibodies are those who are completely deficient in Factor VIII, or have very low (<5%) levels. In this case, possible therapeutic remedies are very high doses of Factor VIII, purified porcine Factor VIII, Factor IX concentrates or activated prothrombin complex (contains activated X). An inadequate dose of Factor VIII is a very important cause of continued bleeding. Factor VIII which has been held at a temperature exceeding 4°C (39.2°F) for more than a couple of hours is not very effective. In the past, up to 50% of patients had CAH, and it is possible that underlying chronic liver disease may prevent early haemostasis due to several other clotting factor deficiencies.

Further useful investigations should consist of a CT scan of the abdomen to confirm the psoas haematoma. The APTT is an indicator of the severity of the clotting abnormality and a good guide to adequate replacement of Factor VIII levels. Factor VIII levels are useful in determining the amount of Factor VIII which should be replaced to correct the APTT. Estimation of Factor VIII antibodies is very useful because it calls for other therapeutic applications which have been mentioned above. The BT is of no use because it is unchanged in haemophilia, but is elevated in Von Willebrand's disease (*Table*).

Clotting abnormalities	PT	APTT	TT	BT
Haemophilia A	N	↑	N	N
Haemophilia B	N	↑	N	N*
Von Willebrand's disease	N	↑	N	↑
Vitamin K deficiency	↑	N	N	N
Heparin therapy	↑	↑	↑	(↑)**
DIC	↑	↑	↑	(↑)**

* Can be differentiated from haemophilia A, by measuring Factor VIII and IX levels. In haemophilia A, Factor VIII is low, and in haemophilia B, Factor IX is low
** Increased if the platelet count is low

Question 105

This is an ECG (**105**) from an 18-year-old male with a single episode of syncope. He had no past medical history of note. His mother died suddenly while swimming at the age of 29, but no obvious cause was found at post-mortem examination.

1. What is the ECG diagnosis?

Question 106

A 37-year-old man was admitted to hospital with a three-day history of a generalized headache and photophobia. He gave a five-day history of a dry cough before the onset of headache. On examination, he was unwell. The temperature was 37.7°C (99.9°F). Kernig's sign was absent. There was no evidence of papilloedema or any neurological deficit. There was no history of travel abroad. He was married with two children. He was a non-smoker and consumed 4–8 units of alcohol per week. The following day his condition deteriorated. He became drowsy and developed weakness in his lower limbs.

On examination, he was drowsy and his temperature was 38°C (100.4°F). He had a left facial nerve palsy and had failure of lateral gaze on the same side. The upper limbs were normal. The lower limbs had diminished power. Lower-limb reflexes were brisk. The left plantar was upgoing and the right plantar was equivocal. Abdominal reflexes were diminished.

Investigations are shown.

CSF analysis	
Cells	White cells 80/mm^3 (40% lymphocytes) Red cells Absent
Protein	0.8 g/l
Glucose	3 mmol/l (blood glucose 4.4 mmol/l)
Gram stain	Negative
EEG	Slow waves

1. What is the diagnosis?
A. Viral encephalomyelitis.
B. *Listeria* meningoencephalitis.
C. Tuberculous meningitis.
D. Lyme disease.
E. Cortical vein thrombosis.

Answer 105

1. LQTS (see Examination Answer **2**, page 239).

Answer 106

1. A. Viral encephalomyelitis.

The most likely diagnosis is viral encephalomyelitis. There is a prodrome of dry cough in an otherwise fit, relatively young healthy male with no past history or history of travel, followed by drowsiness and signs consistent with brainstem involvement. Most cases of viral encephalitis are self-limiting and may present as a febrile illness associated with headache and photophobia. In a small proportion of patients the illness is more severe and is accompanied by progressive drowsiness, coma, seizures and focal neurological signs, particularly affecting the brain and spinal cord. Demyelination of the spinal cord and brainstem is characteristic. The patient has left-sided 6th and 7th cranial nerve palsies, which are suggestive of pontine involvement. In addition, he has brisk lower-limb reflexes, upgoing plantars, and absent abdominal reflexes suggestive of spinal cord involvement. The CSF reveals a modestly elevated WCC with a significant number of lymphocytes and a modestly elevated protein count. The CSF sugar content is normal, which excludes tuberculous and bacterial meningitis. Other causes of high lymphocyte count and elevated protein are shown in *Table A*. The EEG demonstrates the characteristic slow waves seen in viral encephalitis, although this appearance may also be seen in metabolic encephalopathies and cortical vein thrombosis. The most commonly implicated viruses in viral encephalitis are measles, herpes, influenza and pertussis.

Lyme disease may also cause neurological involvement. It is caused by the spirochaete, *Borrelia burgdoferi*, which is transmitted by tick bites. The initial illness (stage 1) is characterized by a fever and a typical erythematous indurating rash at the site of the tick bite, known as erythema chronicum migrans. The second stage of the disease occurs between two and three weeks afterwards, and is characterized by cardiac and neurological involvement. Cardiac manifestations include pericarditis, myocarditis and heart block of varying degrees. Neurological involvement is characterized by symptoms of meningitis, focal neurological signs including cranial nerve palsies and a radiculopathy. There is no history of tick bites or travel to North America; however, the history of tick bites is not always elicited. It is only remotely possible that the patient may have been in contact with ticks. CSF findings include lymphocytosis and a modestly elevated protein count (*Table B*). The CSF sugar is normal. The diagnosis is made by demonstrating elevated titres of IgG to the spirochaete.

The diagnosis of *Listeria* meningoencephalitis is less likely for several reasons. First, listerosis usually affects neonates, elderly patients, pregnant women and the immunosuppressed. Second, the CSF usually demonstrates features of a bacterial meningitis (high neutrophil count, high protein and low sugar), but Gram stain is positive in a very few cases. The condition is characterized by a febrile illness. Cerebral involvement is characterized by features of meningitis and drowsiness. Focal neurological signs and cranial nerve palsies are recognized features.

Cortical vein thrombosis is characterized by rapid onset of headache, drowsiness and focal neurological signs and epilepsy. The EEG reveals slow waves. The CSF is characterized by high content of neutrophils and lymphocytes and a high protein. It may complicate bacterial meningitis or tuberculous meningitis. It usually occurs in young children following serious illness and dehydration. It is a recognized complication of myeloproliferative disorders, pregnancy and the contraceptive pill. There is a possibility that the sudden deterioration in

---

Table A. Causes of lymphocytosis and elevated CSF protein

Infections
Viral meningitis
Tuberculous meningitis
Listeria meningoencephalitis
Neurosyphilis
Leptospirosis
Lyme disease
Brucellosis
Toxoplasmosis
Cryptococcal meningitis
Partially treated bacterial meningitis
Cerebral abscess

Non-infectious
Cerebral lymphoma/leukaemia
Sarcoidosis
SLE
Behçet's disease
Multiple sclerosis
Cortical vein thrombosis

Table B. CSF findings in infectious meningitis

	Pressure	WCC (mm³)	Protein g/l	Sugar
Viral meningitis or encephalitis*	Normal Slightly raised	10–100 (lymphocytes)	0.4–0.8	>1/2 blood glucose
Bacterial meningitis**	Raised	200–3,000 (neutrophils)	0.5–2.0	<1/3 blood glucose
TB meningitis	Raised	50–500 (lymphocytes)	0.5–3.0	<1/3 blood glucose
Lyme disease	Normal Slightly raised	50–500 (lymphocytes)	0.4–0.8	>1/2 blood glucose
Cryptococcal meningitis	Normal Slightly raised	50–300 (lymphocytes)	0.5–3.0	Usually low

* Similar findings may be seen in cerebral toxoplasmosis, leptospiral meningitis, brucellosis, *Listeria* meningitis.
** In partially treated bacterial meningitis there may be evidence of a pleiocytosis (presence of both lymphocytes and neutrophils) where the predominant cells are lymphocytes. The sugar content of the CSF may be only slightly reduced.

the patient's condition may be due to this complication. However, CSF features are not in keeping with bacterial or tuberculous meningitis, the prodromal illness was short and did not seem severe, and his past good health is against a coexisting disorder which may have predisposed to cortical vein thrombosis.

Question 107

A 20-year-old female is admitted to hospital with a 12-hour history of weakness in her arms and legs. This was accompanied by paraesthesia in her hands and feet. Five days before admission she experienced severe pain between her shoulder blades, and shortly afterwards developed blurred vision. The back pain had persisted but was less severe on admission. There was no history of headaches or nausea, but she had been constipated for two days and had intermittent lower abdominal pain. At the age of eight years she suffered a bout of viral meningitis for which she was in hospital for a week. At the age of 15 years she took an overdose of sleeping tablets while her parents were undergoing a divorce. She had enjoyed good health otherwise.

On examination, the patient was not distressed but had an expressionless face and found it difficult to close her eyes. She was afebrile. Examination of her fundi demonstrated blurred discs but no haemorrhages. Power in all her limbs was markedly diminished. She found it difficult to raise her arms above her shoulders, and could not move her legs. The tone in the legs was diminished and the reflexes in all her limbs were absent. Abdominal reflexes were present and the plantar response was normal. On examination of the abdomen she had a smooth palpable mass just above the symphysis pubis.

Investigations were as follows:

FBC	Hb 13 g/dl
	WCC 7 × 10⁹/l
	Platelets 300 × 10⁹/l
CT scan of brain	Normal

1. What four investigations (apart from CSF examination) would affect your management?
2. What is the diagnosis?
3. List three poor prognostic factors in this disease.

Answer 107

1. i. Blood pressure measurement.
ii. 24 hour tape.
iii. Bed-side spirometry.
iv. Arterial blood gases.
2. Post-infectious polyneuropathy (Guillain–Barré syndrome).
3. Poor prognostic markers for the disease are listed below (*Table B*).

The patient presents with generalized muscle weakness following severe pain in the mid-thoracic area. She also complained of diplopia before the weakness, and has evidence of papilloedema and generalized motor neuropathy on examination. The patient has no sensory level to suggest spinal cord compression, therefore the constipation and the palpable bladder indicate an underlying autonomic neuropathy. The diagnosis which fits best with the symptoms and signs is Guillain–Barré syndrome or post-infectious polyneuropathy.

Guillain–Barré syndrome is a polyneuropathy which may develop over a few days or even a few weeks after an infectious illness, usually involving the respiratory tract. Enterovirus, EBV, *Mycoplasma*, *Campylobacter jejuni* and *Chlamydia* have been implicated, but the condition may occur following surgical conditions. In the majority of cases the underlying cause is never identified. The onset is often heralded by severe lumbar or interscapular pain, as in this case, and is followed by proximal, distal or generalized

muscle weakness due to a motor neuropathy; however, some sensory loss is also present. Sensory loss commonly manifests as distal paraesthesiae and loss of vibration and positional sensation. The latter results in a sensory ataxia. The cranial nerves may also be involved, particularly those innervating the extraocular muscles of the eye. In the context of the history above, the diplopia is almost certainly due to cranial nerves supplying the extraocular muscles. Bulbar involvement is also recognized. Autonomic neuropathy may complicate some cases, and may present as accelerated hypertension, tachyarrhythmias, abdominal pain, and bladder atony. Death may occur from respiratory failure due to respiratory muscle paralysis, or from arrhythmias and haemodynamic instability due to autonomic neuropathy. Aspiration may also cause death in patients with bulbar muscle involvement. The differential diagnosis and prognostic markers of the disease are listed below (*Tables A* and *B*).

The disease is characterized by a significantly elevated protein content in the CSF in the presence of a normal WCC. However, cases due to infectious mononucleosis may be associated with a mild pleiocytosis. The differential diagnosis of a high CSF WCC and a high protein content is tabulated below (*Table C*). Papilloedema may develop either due to accelerated hypertension or to impaired CSF resorption because of the elevated CSF protein content. The presence of papilloedema in this case makes it mandatory to measure the blood pressure. Histologically, there is segmental demyelination – possibly due to a cell-mediated delayed hypersensitivity. In the form of Guillain–Barré which accompanies *Campylobacter jejuni* infection there is an acute, purely axonal motor neuropathy with rapid progression and a mortality rate as high as 5%.

Management of the disease is by intravenous Sandoglobulin. The use of corticosteroids remains controversial.

Variants of Guillain–Barré include the Miller–Fisher syndrome, which comprises external ophthalmoplegia, ataxia and areflexia. The condition is highly suggested by the presence of antibodies to the sphyngomyelin component GQ1b.

Table A. Differential diagnoses of Guillain–Barré syndrome

Acute polymyositis
Myaesthenia gravis
Acute intermittent porphyria (motor and
    autonomic neuropathy)
Lead poisoning
Hypokalaemic periodic paralysis

Table B. Poor prognostic markers in Guillain–Barré syndrome

FVC <1.1 litres
Arterial blood oxygen <8 kPa
Arterial blood carbon dioxide >6 kPa
Coexistent lower respiratory tract infection
Coexistent pulmonary oedema
Accelerated hypertension
Arrhythmias
Bulbar muscle involvement
Guillain–Barré syndrome following *Campylobacter*
    infection

Table C. Causes of a high CSF protein in the presence of a normal CSF cell count

Guillain–Barré syndrome
Spinal cord tumour causing spinal block (Froin's
    syndrome)
Acoustic neuroma
Lead encephalopathy
Subacute sclerosing panencephalopathy

Question 108

This pedigree chart (**108a**) is from a family with a bleeding disorder.

1. What is the mode of inheritance?
2. What is the most probable diagnosis?
3. What are the chances of A being a carrier?
4. What are the chances of B being affected?
5. What are the chances C of being affected?
6. What are the chances of D being a carrier?
7. What are the chances of E being affected?
8. What are the chances of E being a carrier?
9. What are the chances of F being a carrier?

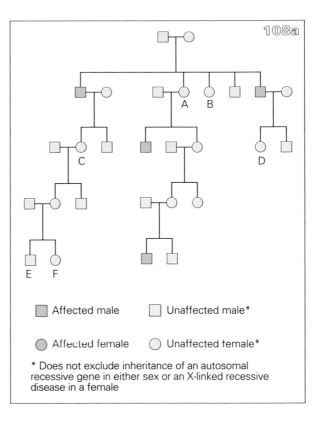

108a

| ■ Affected male | □ Unaffected male* |
| ● Affected female | ○ Unaffected female* |

* Does not exclude inheritance of an autosomal recessive gene in either sex or an X-linked recessive disease in a female

Question 109

The following are cardiac catheter data from an 18-year-old female with breathlessness on exertion.

Chamber	Pressure (mmHg)	Oxygen saturation (%)
Superior vena cava	–	68
Inferior vena cava	–	67
Right atrium	a = 14	
	v = 20	
		(high) 68
		(mid) 69
		(low) 83
Right ventricle	92/20	83
Pulmonary artery	94/42	82
PCWP	a = 14	
	v = 22	
Left ventricle	160/20	96
Aorta	100/70	96

1. List at least four physical signs that you would elucidate on examination of this patient.
2. List at least three abnormalities which may be seen on the ECG?
3. What is the diagnosis?

Answer 108

1. X-linked recessive.
2. Haemophilia A or haemophilia B.
3. 100%.
4. 0.
5. 0.
6. 100%.
7. 25%.
8. 0.
9. 25%.

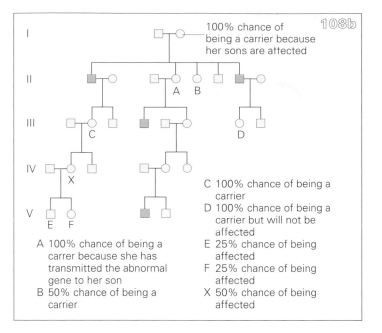

A 100% chance of being a carrer because she has transmitted the abnormal gene to her son
B 50% chance of being a carrier
C 100% chance of being a carrier
D 100% chance of being a carrier but will not be affected
E 25% chance of being affected
F 25% chance of being affected
X 50% chance of being affected

The answer is illustrated (**108b**).

In this pedigree, only males are affected. Therefore, the condition must be X-linked recessive. In X-linked recessive conditions, only males will be affected; females will be carriers. In this pedigree, the female in generation 1 is a definite carrier because she has two affected sons (who have inherited the X-chromosome with the abnormal gene from their mother). Female A in generation 1 is also a definite carrier because she has an affected son. There is a 50% chance that female B is a carrier because a female carrier (her mother) will transmit the abnormal gene to 50% of her sones and 50% of her daughters. A female harboring an X-linked recessive genetic abnormaility will not be affected assuming her other X-chromosome is free of the genetic mutation. Female C is a definitive carrier because her father is affected. In X-linked conditions the male passes his X-chromosome (with the abnormal genetic mutation) to all his daughters. In contrast none of the sones receive the abnormal gene from the father becuase they inherit his Y chromosome. For the same reasons, female D is also a definite carrier.

There is a 50% chance that female X in generation IV is a carrier, therefore half of her sons will be affected and half of her daughters will be carriers, that is, there is a 25% chance of male E being affected and a 25% chance of female F being a carrier.

Answer 109

1. i. A right ventricular heave. The right ventricle must have hypertrophied to generate such a high systolic pressure.
ii. A pansystolic murmur of mitral regurgitation at the apex. The large 'v'-wave in the PCWP suggests mitral regurgitation.
iii. Fixed splitting of the second heart sound from the ASD.
iv. Pansystolic murmur of tricuspid regurgitation at the left sternal edge. The large 'v'-wave in the right atrial pressure suggests tricuspid regurgitation.
v. Systolic flow murmur in the pulmonary area.
2. i. Partial RBBB.
ii. Right ventricular hypertrophy.
iii. Left atrial enlargement.
iv. Right atrial enlargement.
v. Left axis deviation. The ECG in ostium primum defects characteristically reveals partial or complete RBBB and left axis deviation (**101**). In contrast, patients with ostium decundum defects have partial RBBB and right axis deviation.

3. There is a step up in the oxygen saturation in the low right atrium, suggesting an ostium primum ASD. The defect is associated with mitral and tricuspid ring defects, causing both mitral and tricuspid regurgitation.

A step up in oxygen saturation in the upper right atrium would indicate a sinus venosus defect, and a step up in the mid right atrium would indicate an ostium secundum ASD.
(See Interpretation of Cardiac Catheter Data, page 220.)

Question 110

A 19-year-old dustman was admitted to hospital with severe retrosternal chest pain associated with belching and vomiting. He was a non-smoker. He had been celebrating a friend's birthday and had consumed a considerable amount of alcohol the night before. He was diagnosed as having epilepsy 12 years ago and was on regular anticonvulsant medication. There was no family history of ischaemic heart disease or epilepsy. He had an older brother who was fit and well. He had been in hospital eight months previously with an axillary vein thrombosis which had been treated with warfarin for six months. He wore glasses for being short-sighted.

On examination, he was thin and tall measuring 1.9 m. He had a kyphoscoliotic spine. Examination of his hands, oral cavity and left eye is shown (**110a–110c**, respectively). The findings on fundoscopy are also shown (**110d**). A cardiovascular examination was normal. The patient had pectus excavatum; the chest was clear on auscultation. An abdominal examination revealed mild tenderness in the epigastrum.

Investigations are shown.

FBC	Hb 11 g/dl
LFT	AST 60 u/l
	WCC 5 × 10⁹/l
	Bilirubin 11 μmol/l
	Platelets 160 × 10⁹/l
	Alkaline phosphatase 112 u/l
	MCV 105 fl
	Albumin 43 g/l
U&E	Normal
Chest X-ray	Kyphoscoliosis
	Clear lung fields
	Normal heart size
ECG	Normal
Gastroscopy	Gastro-oesophagitis

1. What is the diagnosis?
2. Give two explanations for the raised MCV.
3. How would you confirm the diagnosis?
4. How is the condition inherited, and where is the chromosomal defect?

Answer 110

1. Homocystinuria.
2. i. Phenytoin therapy. Phenytoin is thought to interfere with folate absorption. Other anticonvulsants causing folate deficiency include primidone and barbiturate therapy.
ii. The conversion of homocystine to methionine requires large amounts of the enzyme 5-methyl tetrahydrofolate methyltransferase, which utilises folate as a co-factor. During the enzyme reaction some of the folate is degraded, and folate deficiency can occur.
3. The urine gives a positive nitroprusside test. Raised levels of plasma methionine and homocystine are more reliable because the nitroprusside test is also positive in cystinuria.
4. Autosomal recessive inheritance. The gene is located on chromosome 21.

The chest pain due to oesophagitis has no connection with the underlying diagnosis. The examiner expects the reader to pick up on the skeletal, ocular and neurological abnormalities to come to a diagnosis of homocystinuria.

Homocystinuria is due to cystathionine deficiency. As a result, there is accumulation of homocysteine which in turn is oxidized to homocystine. There is no production of cystine. Plasma and urinary levels of homocystine are elevated. Homocystine is thought to affect cross-linking of collagen, leading to skeletal, ocular, neurological and vascular abnormalities.

Skeletal: The patients have the same skeletal abnormalities as in Marfan's syndrome. These include tallness, kyphoscoliosis, arachnodactyly, high-arched palate, pectus excavatum and flat feet. The ligaments are lax, and muscular development weak. Osteoporosis is a feature and classically affects the vertebrae. These patients need to be distinguished from Marfan patients, who have a strong family history, and often have evidence of cardiovascular involvement in the form of mitral valve prolapse and aortic root dilatation, but do not have associated neurological abnormalities. Osteoporosis is not a feature of Marfan's syndrome.

Ocular: The suspensory ligaments of the lens are weakened, causing lens dislocation which is usually downward. This is complicated by glaucoma, iridodonesis, myopia and cataracts. Optic atrophy and retinal detachment are also recognized ocular problems.

Neurological: Mental handicap occurs in approximately 50% of patients and 10–20% of patients have epilepsy. The degree of mental retardedness can be mild or severe. There is a form of homocystinuria which responds to pyridoxine. Patients with this form are less severely affected.

Vascular: Both venous and arterial thromboses occur and are thought to be due to the effects of methionine causing vascular damage, and increased platelet adherence. This has important therapeutic implications in patients undergoing surgery for correction of skeletal abnormalities, because there is a risk of deep-vein thrombus, and prophylactic heparin should be given following surgery. The oestrogen-containing oral contraceptive pill is contraindicated in women with homocystinuria. Recent studies have shown that homocystinuria is also associated with premature coronary artery disease.

Treatment is with dietary restriction of methionine and cystine supplements. Pyridoxine should be given immediately after the diagnosis has been made and is beneficial in some cases.

Question 111

A 59-year-old farmer was referred to a chest unit with an 18-month history of progressive breathlessness. Over the past four years, he had noticed a dry cough in the afternoons and evenings. His effort tolerance three years previously was very good, allowing him to work in the farm for almost 12 hours per day. Since then he had resolved to working only two days a week due to fatigue and breathlessness, and had asked both his sons to take over his farm.

His general practitioner diagnosed asthma, but his condition had continued to deteriorate despite the use of steroid and salbutamol inhalers. He was now breathless after walking just 200 metres. He was a non-smoker. There was no family history of lung disease. He had never worked with asbestos, and did not keep pets.

On examination, he was cyanosed and tachypnoeic. He had evidence of early clubbing. The JVP was not raised, and heart sounds were normal. On auscultation of the lung fields there were bilateral fine end-inspiratory crackles in both lungs.

Investigations are shown.

FBC	Hb 12 g/dl
	WCC 5 × 10^9/l
	Platelets 400 × 10^9/l
ESR	54 mm/h
Chest X-ray	Diffuse reticulonodular shadowing in both apices and midzones
FEV$_1$ (%)	50	Blood gases on air
FVC (%)	52	pH 7.45
FEV$_1$/FVC (%)	89	pCO$_2$ 3.5 kPa
TLC (%)	56	pO$_2$ 6.4 kPa
KCO (%)	60	Bicarbonate 22 mmol/l

1. What is the diagnosis?
2. List at least two tests which would help confirm the diagnosis.

Question 112

A 78-year-old male presented with a several weeks history of weakness, lethargy, weight loss and vomiting.

On examination, the blood pressure (standing) was 80/50 mmHg.

Blood results are shown.

Sodium	124 mmol/l
Potassium	4.9 mmol/l
Urea	15 mmol/l
Bicarbonate	15 mmol/l
Blood glucose	4.0 mmol/l

1. List three possible causes for this biochemical picture.

Question 113

A 51-year-old dentist presented to his general practitioner because he had difficulty lifting his right arm for over one week. For the past few days he could not holder the razor to the face with his right arm whilst shaving. About two weeks previously he received a hepatitis B booster vaccine which was associated with pain over his deltoid and shoulder region for almost 48 hours.

On examination there was wasting over the deltoid region. There was reduced power on abduction, flexion and internal rotation of the right arm and flexion of the right elbow. The right biceps and supinator reflexes were absent. All other examinations were normal.

Investigations are shown.

FBC	Hb 14.3 g/dl
	WCC 5 × 10^9/l
	Platelets 199 × 10^9/l
ESR	11 mm/h
Biochemistry	Normal
X-rays of chest and cervical spine	Normal

1. What is the diagnosis?
A. Polio.
B. Radiculopathy secondary to Lyme disease.
C. Neuralgic amyotrophy.
D. Syringomyelia.
E. Cervical rib.
F. Cervical myelopathy.
G. Motor neurone disease.

Answer 111

1. Extrinsic allergic alveolitis.
2. i. Precipitins from *Micropolyspora faenii*.
ii. High-resolution CT scan.
iii. Bronchoalveolar lavage.
iv. Bronchoscopy with transbronchial lung biopsy.

Extrinsic allergic alveolitis is a cell-mediated allergic reaction that occurs in response to inhalation of a variety of agents. It is characterized by interstitial inflammation and progressive lung fibrosis. Patients typically present with fever and dyspnoea several hours after inhaling the antigen. In this case, the farmer who has been working in the morning will not develop symptoms until late afternoon. During the reaction the patient will be tachypnoeic, febrile and have widespread coarse crackles throughout the lung. Continuing exposure and inflammation results in interstitial fibrosis, leading to progressive dyspnoea and functional limitation. The chest X-ray reveals nodular shadows in the upper zones that eventually involve the mid-zones. In severe cases the lung will have a honeycomb appearance on the X-ray due to severe fibrosis. Several antigens are recognized and several occupations are at risk. In farmers, the culprit antigen is commonly the spores of the fungus *M. faenii* that are inhaled while forking mouldy hay. Malt workers may be affected by inhalation of products of the fungus *Aspergillus clavatus* while turning germinating barley, and pigeon keepers may develop the condition after inhaling avian proteins from feathers of the birds.

The diagnosis relies on an abnormal chest X-ray, and the demonstration of antibodies to the culprit antigens. High-resolution CT scan of the thorax will reveal the extent of parenchymal involvement. Formal spirometry is useful in assessing lung reserve in patients with fibrosis. The KCO is reduced due to interstitial lung damage. Transbronchial lung biopsy is rarely required to make the diagnosis unless the cause of lung fibrosis is unclear. Bronchoalveolar lavage reveals increased cells that are predominantly lymphocytes.

Management is to remove the patient from the antigen. In the early stages of the disease, high-dose prednisolone will cause regression of the condition.

Answer 112

1. i. Addison's disease/primary hypoadrenalism.
ii. Diuretic therapy.
iii. Salt-losing nephritis.

The combination of lethargy, weight loss, vomiting, hypotension, hyponatraemia and hyperkalaemia are all suggestive of Addison's disease. Addison's disease is caused by destruction of the adrenal glands, resulting in deficiency of glucocorticoid and mineralocorticoid hormones. The most common cause of Addison's disease is autoimmune adrenalitis. Other causes are listed (*Table*). The condition has an insidious presentation in the majority of cases, but may present as a crisis. Lethargy, anorexia, nausea, vomiting, abdominal pain and symptoms of postural hypotension are common. Some patients are misdiagnosed as having depression. In the elderly, the condition may present as a confusional state. On examination, there may be evidence of pigmentation which is prominent in skin creases, scars and the buccal mucosa. The supine blood pressure may be normal, but there is a marked drop in systolic pressure on standing (>25 mmHg).

Acute Addisonian crisis is characterized by coma, profound hypotension, hypoglycaemia. The electrolytes are usually abnormal (as above) but may also be normal. Acute adrenal failure or Addisonian crisis is a medical emergency which should be aggressively treated with intravenous hydrocortisone and saline. Dextrose is used in hypoglycaemic cases.

Long-term treatment is with oral hydrocortisone, prednisolone or dexamethasone (glucocorticoids) and fludrocortisone (mineralocorticoid).

Addison's disease is diagnosed by performing the synacthen test. Serum cortisol is measured before and 30 min after intramuscular ACTH (synacthen). In normal individuals, the serum cortisol rises to above 600 nmol/l, or

---

Causes of Addison's disease (primary hypoadrenalism)

Autoimmune adrenalitis
TB
Carcinomatous infiltration of adrenal glands
(bronchial carcinoma)
Adrenal haemorrhage or infarction
(Waterhouse–Friedrichson syndrome)
Infiltration disorders:
haemochromatosis
amyloidosis
granulomatous disorders
Metyrapone therapy
Schilder's disease
Wolman's disease (hepatosplenomegaly and
steatorrhoea)

is increased by 300 from the basal level. Patients with Addison's disease will not demonstrate this level of rise. Adrenal antibodies are present in cases of autoimmune adrenalitis. In cases of tuberculous adrenal gland destruction there may be obvious calcification of the adrenal gland on the plain abdominal X-ray. Alternatively, the demonstration of an inappropriately raised serum ACTH and a low simultaneous serum cortisol level is diagnostic.

Diuretic therapy, with spironolactone (aldosterone antagonist) or combined loop diuretic and potassium-sparing diuretic preparations will produce the same biochemical picture. Dehydration from diuresis may lead to pre-renal failure, reflected by rising urea and a low bicarbonate. The serum aldosterone is elevated in dehydration due to diuretics. This is in direct contrast to Addison's disease, where the aldosterone level will be low. Salt-losing nephritis is characterized biochemically by hyponatraemia and impaired renal function.

Answer 113

1. C. Neuralgic amyotrophy.

The diagnosis is neuralgic amyotrophy. This is an inflammatory process affecting the roots of C5 and C6 and occasionally C7. It usually follows an infective illness or trauma to the deltoid region. It is preceeded by pain over the shoulder and arm followed by weakness and wasting of the muscles supplied by the affected roots.

Spontaneous recovery is usual but may take several months. The differential diagnosis of cervical cord compression but the absence of lower limb signs is against this. Lyme disease may produce a similar radiculopathy but in this case there is no history of a skin rash or tick bite. Furthermore, the history of imminization into the deltoid is more in keeping with amyotrophy. Syringomyelia is unlikely in the absence of sensory signs. Cervical rib is excluded by a normal chest X-ray.

Question 114

A 28-year-old obese female was admitted to the ward for further investigation after presenting with lethargy. She did not give any further history of significance. Her blood pressure in clinic was 128/85 mmHg. Blood results are shown.

After these blood results, the patient was questioned further about her bowel habit and medication. She denied having diarrhoea or taking any medication. She was observed on the ward for 48 hours, during which time her blood pressure did not fluctuate.

A repeat serum renin level was 1,600 pg/ml/h.

Biochemistry	Sodium 135 mmol/l
	Potassium 2.2 mmol/l
	Urea 7.3 mmol/l
	Creatinine 60 µmol/l
	Bicarbonate 36 mmol/l
Renin	1,500 pg/ml/h (normal range [lying supine] 300–1,300 pg/ml/h)
24-h urine output	500 ml
24-h urine potassium	10 mmol/l

1. Comment on the initial results.
2. Suggest a possible cause for the abnormalities, given the results of the tests performed while she was observed in hospital.

Answer 114

1. The patient has a hypokalaemic alkalosis and an appropriate hypokaluria. Patients with a serum potassium of <3.5 mmol/l conserve potassium and excrete less than 20 mmol/l of potassium in the urine. The urea is modestly elevated, as is her serum renin, both of which suggest hypoperfusion of the afferent glomerular vessels. This may occur in dehydration, shock, glomerular and renal parenchymal disease. However, in primary renal disease the serum creatinine is also elevated, and in this history the blood pressure is not suggestive of shock.

2. In the context of this history the most probable cause for the hypokalaemia is loss of potassium from the gastrointestinal tract. This is also causing dehydration and hence the elevated urea and renin. There is no history of diarrhoea or vomiting, but given her obesity there is a chance that she is abusing laxatives or has self-induced vomiting in order to try and lose weight (**114**).

Potassium may be lost via the gastrointestinal tract (diarrhoea, vomiting, intestinal fistulae, villous adenoma, nasogastric aspiration) or the kidneys (primary and secondary hyperaldosteronism, Cushing's syndrome, Liddle's syndrome, renal tubular disorders or drugs). Loss of potassium from the gastrointestinal tract is associated with conservation of potassium by the kidneys.

Hypokalaemia is generally associated with a metabolic alkalosis with the exception of RTA.

Many conditions associated with renal loss of potassium also cause hypertension. The most common cause of hypertension, hypokalaemia and alkalosis encountered in the MRCP and similar examinations is primary hyperaldosteronism (Conn's syndrome). However, other recognized causes include Cushing's, Liddle's syndrome (pseudohyperaldosteronism), accelerated hypertension, renal artery stenosis or hypertensive therapy with diuretics (*Table*). Liddle's syndrome is a tubular defect characterized by excessive sodium absorption and increased potassium excretion. The biochemistry is identical to that of Conn's syndrome, but there is no abnormality of the renin–angiotensin–aldosterone axis.

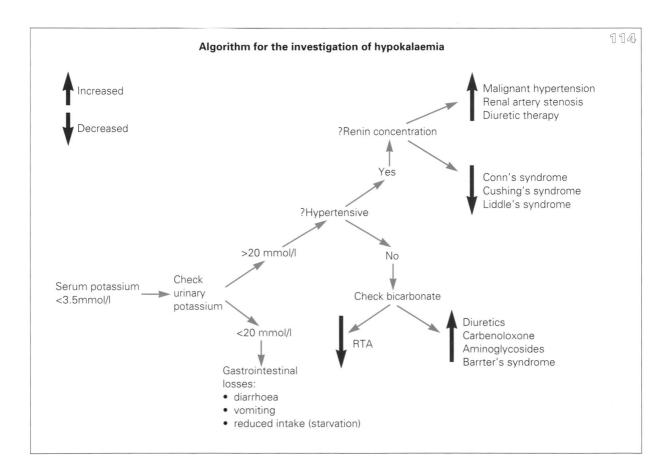

Algorithm for the investigation of hypokalaemia

Causes of hypokalaemic alkalosis and hypertension

Primary hyperaldosteronism (Conn's syndrome)
Cushing's syndrome
Liddle's syndrome
Accelerated hypertension
Hypertension treated with diuretics
Renal artery stenosis
Carbenoxolone therapy
Liquorice abuse
Congenital adrenal hyperplasia (11-β-hydroxylase deficiency)*

*In 11-β-hydroxylase deficiency, the aldosterone levels are low; however, there is excessive production of deoxycorticosterone which has strong mineralocorticoid effects and causes both hypertension and hypokalaemia

---

In the absence of hypertension, other causes of hypokalaemic alkalosis include carbenoxolone therapy, liquorice abuse, aminoglycosides, and Barrter's syndrome – which is due to hyperplasia of the juxtaglomerular apparatus. In Barrter's syndrome, affected children present with nocturia, muscle weakness and failure to thrive. It is important to note that carbenoxolone therapy and liquorice abuse may cause hypertension.

Question 115

A 17-year-old female was referred to the gynaecologist with primary amenorrhoea. She had been relatively well throughout her life. Her mother was concerned that she was not gaining any weight, despite eating well. She had been investigated for diabetes by the general practitioner and was found to have a normal blood glucose. Apart from complaining of intermittent headaches and feeling tired at the end of the day, there were no other symptoms. She was still at college. She had two brothers and a sister who were well. Her sister was aged 14 and had just started menstruating.

On examination, the patient measured 1.5 m and weighed 40 kg. She was pale, and had scanty axillary and pubic hair. Breast development had just begun.

Investigations are shown.

1. What is the cause of the patient's amenorrhoea?
2. What is the most probable underlying diagnosis?
3. Give two possible explanations for the alkaline phosphatase level.
4. Give two tests you would perform to confirm the diagnosis.

FBC	Hb 9.8 g/dl
	WCC 5 × 10⁹/l
	Platelets 190 × 10⁹/l
	MCV 104 fl
Blood film	Target cells, anisocytosis, macrocytes, poikilocytosis
Biochemistry	Sodium 137 mmol/l
	Potassium 4.1 mmol/l
	Urea 3 mmol/l
	Creatinine 78 μmol/l
	Calcium 2.0 mmol/l
	Phosphate 0.75 mmol/l
	Albumin 37 g/l
	AST 20 u/l
LFT	Alkaline phosphatase 300 u/l
	Bilirubin 11 μmol/l
Thyroid function	Thyroxine 100 nmol/l
	TSH 2.0 mu/l

Answer 115

1. Underweight due to malabsorption (malabsorption syndrome).
2. Coeliac disease.
3. i. Osteomalacia.
ii. Patient in a growth spurt.
4. i. Duodenal biopsy or jejunal biopsy.
ii Anti-endomyosium, anti-gliadin or anti-reticulin antibodies.

The patient is short for her age. She has a macrocytic anaemia. The blood film reveals hypochromasia, macrocytosis and target cells, suggesting either isolated folate (or possibly B_{12}) deficiency or combined iron and folate deficiency. The bone biochemistry is in keeping with vitamin D deficiency. The slightly low albumin level is indicative of poor nutritional status in this context. Failure to grow, or weight loss despite a normal appetite, plus a combination of nutritional deficiencies should always raise the question of a malabsorption syndrome. The lack of secondary sexual characteristics and delayed menstruation in this patient may be explained by the fact that she has yet to reach puberty, either due to a constitutional delay or that puberty has been delayed due to a malabsorption syndrome. Malabsorption syndromes are a recognized cause of primary and secondary amenorrhoea in girls and young women, predominantly as a result of poor malnutrition causing profound weight loss. Readers may fall into the trap of diagnosing hypopituitarism in this case, given the short stature and absent secondary sexual characteristics. However, the diagnosis of hypopituitarism fails to explain the normal thyroid function tests and the abnormal bone biochemistry. Anaemia is a recognized feature of hypopituitarism. It is usually normochromic normocytic, but may be macro- or microcytic.

A variety of conditions produce malabsorption syndromes (see *Table*), but the most common cause by far in the Western world is coeliac disease. This affects 1 in 2,000 patients in the UK, and is even more common in Ireland, affecting 1 in 300. The disorder is characterized by total villus atrophy in the small intestine as a result of ingestion of gluten-containing food. The majority (80%) of patients have the haplotype HLA A1, B8, DR7 or DQW2, suggesting a genetic basis. There is 30% disconcordance among identical twins, which suggests that non-genetic factors may also be involved. Small bowel injury occurs as a result of gluten ingestion. Gluten is a high-molecular weight compound which contains various gliadins. α-gliadin damages small bowel mucosa in these patients, probably through an immune-mediated mechanism. Anti-gliadin antibodies are strong evidence for this postulation. Small bowel damage produces malabsorption which manifests as weight loss, abdominal pain, diarrhoea and nutritional deficiencies. Diarrhoea may be absent in up to 20% of patients. The disease can present at any age. In children, it occurs soon after weaning and presents as failure to thrive. In adults, it presents with abdominal symptoms, weight loss and fatigue. Ankle oedema may complicate albumin deficiency. Mouth ulcers may occur as a result of iron deficiency. Osteomalacia, tetany and muscle weakness may be present due to vitamin D deficiency.

Anaemia is present in 50% of cases. Macrocytosis is invariably due to folate deficiency. Iron deficiency is common, but B_{12} deficiency is rare. Hypochromia and target cells may be present on the blood film.

Howell–Jolly bodies may be seen on the blood film in patients who develop splenic atrophy. The diagnosis is made by sampling small bowel from the second portion of the duodenum (D2 biopsy) via endoscopy or a jejunal biopsy (**115**). Anti-endomyosium antibodies are detected in almost 50% of all cases of coeliac disease, and are highly specific for the disorder. Anti-gliadin antibodies and anti-reticulin antibodies are found in the serum of the majority of patients.

Treatment is with a gluten-free diet. Gluten is present in the cereals wheat, rye, barley and oats. All of these should be excluded from the diet.

Associations of coeliac disease include autoimmune thyroid disorders, chronic liver disease, fibrosing alveolitis, ulcerative colitis and insulin-dependent diabetes mellitus. Complications include small bowel lymphoma and adenocarcinoma and splenic atrophy.

Small bowel malabsorption syndromes

Disorder	Additional comments
Coeliac disease	High anti-gliadin or anti-reticulin antibodies Anti-endomyosium antibodies highly specific
Dermatitis herpetiformis	Gluten-sensitive enteropathy. Associated subepidermal blistering rash
Bacterial overgrowth	Low B_{12} but normal or high serum folate. Previous gastric surgery (Billroth II), jejunal diverticuli
Giardiasis	May be detected on stool microscopy. Travel abroad or immunosuppressed
Whipple's disease	Associated locomotor /neurological/cardiac features HLA B27. PAS-positive macrophages which contain the bacillus, *Tropheryma whipelli* on small bowel biopsy
Tropical sprue	History of living in an endemic area for >3 months
Radiation enteritis	Previous history of abdominal irradiation
Crohn's disease	Abdominal pain/diarrhoea predominate. May have isolated B_{12} deficiency which is not corrected with intrinsic factor
Hypogammaglobulinacmia	Very similar to cystic fibrosis. Gut, respiratory and locomotor involvement. Low globulins. *Giardia* infections common
Zollinger–Ellison syndrome	History of recurrent peptic ulceration predominates
Intestinal lymphangiectasia	Hypoproteinaemia as a result of protein-losing enteropathy and steatorrhoea. Associated immunoglobulin deficiency. Congenital dilatation of small bowel lymphatics. May occur secondary to pericardial constriction or severe heart failure. Primary lymphatic abnormalities elsewhere may lead to chylous pleural effusions and chylous ascites

Question 116

A 30-year-old sailor was admitted to the navy hospital with a seven-day history of increasing confusion, malaise fever and reduced visual acuity in his left eye. Two weeks previously he had developed weakness affecting his left arm and left lower limb. He had a past history of Hodgkin's lymphoma which was successfully treated with chemotherapy five years ago.

On examination, he was confused. His temperature was 40°C (104°F). There was evidence of cervical lymphadenopathy on palpation of the neck. On examination of the fundi, there was widespread retinal scarring in both eyes, the right eye being more affected than the left. There was no obvious papilloedema. The left-sided limbs demonstrated marked weakness.

Investigations are shown.

FBC	Hb 11 g/dl
	WCC 6×10^9/l
	Platelets 190×10^9/l
ESR	80 mm/h
EEG	Diffuse slow wave activity

1. Suggest at least two possible diagnoses.
2. Give one investigation which would help make the diagnosis in each case.
3. What treatment would you institute for each of your diagnoses?

Answer 116

1. i. Cerebral toxoplasmosis.
ii. Tuberculous meningitis.
iii. Cryptococcal meningitis.
iv. Cerebral lymphoma.
2. i. CT scan brain (**116**). Multiple ring-enhancing lesions may suggest cerebral toxoplasmosis, TB abscesses, or lymphoma.
ii. CSF IgM levels or Sabin–Feldman dye test for *Toxoplasma gondii.*
iii CSF staining with auramine or Ziehl–Neelsen stain may detect TB and staining with Indian ink will identify cryptococcal meningitis.
iv. Brain biopsy.
3. i. Pyrimethamine and sulphadiazine for toxoplasmosis.
ii. Ansamycin and clofazimine for TB (particularly effective for atypical TB).
iii. Amphotericin for cryptococcal meningitis.
iv. Radiotherapy to the skull for cerebral lymphoma.

116

Cerebral manifestations of HIV

HIV dementia
Progressive multifocal leucoencephalopathy
Tuberculous meningitis/tuberculoma
Toxoplasmosis
Lymphoma
Herpes encephalitis
Peripheral neuropathy

The patient is a sailor. In MRCP and similar examinations questions, sailors are associated with a high level of promiscuity and high risk for HIV infection. This patient is confused, has focal neurological signs, and evidence of bilateral scarring of the retina. The confusion may be the manifestation of an encephalitis, meningitis, cerebral abscess or cerebral metastases in the context of the question.

Focal neurological signs may be caused by all of the above. The presence of chorioretinitis and focal neurological signs favours the diagnosis of cerebral toxoplasmosis, TB or cryptococcal meningitis. Cerebral lymphoma *per se* does not cause chorioretinitis, however, it is possible that the patient has both cerebral lymphoma and a CSF infection causing chorioretinitis. Other recognized causes of chorioretinitis in patients with HIV include CMV and syphilitic infection. The slow waves on the EEG are suggestive of an encephalitic process which may be part of the cerebral effect of the HIV itself, or as a result of opportunistic infections such as CMV, herpes virus, toxoplasmosis, atypical mycobacteria or lymphomatous infiltration.

The diagnosis and management for each condition are outlined above. It may be difficult to differentiate between cerebral lymphoma and toxoplasmosis in this case, and the best management policy would be to treat for cerebral toxoplasmosis in the first instance and repeat the CT scan in two weeks, which should reveal resolution of the ring-enhancing lesions if they are due to toxoplasmosis. If the lesions persist, then a tissue diagnosis using brain biopsy may become necessary.

The cerebral manifestations of HIV infection are listed (*Table*).

Question 117

A 60-year-old female presented with a two-month history of lethargy and dysphagia for solid food. Her appetite was slightly reduced, but there was no history of indigestion or weight loss.

The examination of her hands and tongue are shown (**117a, b**). There was no lymphadenopathy, or any other palpable masses in the neck. Examination of all the major systems was normal.

Investigations are shown.

FBC	Hb 8.8 g/dl
	WCC 6 × 10^9/l
	Platelets 170 × 10^9/l
Blood film (**117c**)	
Barium study (**117d**)	

1. What is the probable cause of the appearance of the hands and the tongue?
2. Comment on the blood film.
3. What is the abnormality on the barium study?
4. List two possible diagnoses.
5. Which single investigation would you perform?

Question 118

A 14-year-old female was referred to a specialist because she had difficulty in walking over the past eight months. She tripped easily. Her feet had adopted a strange shape and she had problems fitting her shoes. Her father had weakness affecting his legs and was under regular review by a neurologist.

On examination, she appeared well and a general examination was normal. There was wasting of the small muscles of the hand, but upper-limb tone was normal and the reflexes were preserved. On examination of the lower limbs she had bilateral pes cavus. The calf muscles were wasted and exhibited fasciculation. There was mild weakness of dorsiflexion, plantar flexion and eversion at the ankle joint. Examination of the thighs was normal. Both the ankle and knee reflexes were absent. Proprioception was impaired at the level of the first metatarsal joint. Two-point discrimination sense was also impaired in both feet but pain, temperature and pressure sense was normal.

1. What is the diagnosis?
2. Which three tests would you perform to confirm the diagnosis?

Answer 117

1. The female has koilonychia and glossitis which are features of iron-deficiency anaemia.
2. Anaemia with microcytosis, anisocytosis, poikilocytosis and hypochromia. The features are consistent with iron-deficiency anaemia.
3. Stricture in the upper oesophagus consistent with an oesophageal web (Paterson–Brown–Kelly or Plummer–Vinson syndrome).
4. The differential diagnosis is between oesophageal web and carcinoma of the upper oesophagus.
5. Oesophagoscopy and biopsy of stricture for histological analysis.

This woman has the features of oesophageal web, which is a rare condition characterized by submucosal inflammation, usually in the post-cricoid region, although any part of the oesophagus can be affected. The inflammation produces a 'web' or a concentric stenosis. The condition affects women in their fourth to sixth decade. The classic features are dysphagia, iron-deficiency anaemia, koilonychia and other stigmata of iron deficiency, such as glossitis. It is a pre-malignant condition, and can predispose to carcinoma of the oesophagus which needs to be excluded by endoscopy and biopsy of the stricture.

Answer 118

1. Charcot–Marie–Tooth disease (hereditary sensorimotor neuropathy (HSMN)/peroneal muscular atrophy).
2. i. Nerve conduction studies.
ii. Sural biopsy.
iii Family screening.

The patient presents with difficulty in walking. On physical examination, she has pes cavus, weakness of the distal aspects of the upper and lower limbs. The lower-limb reflexes are absent and proprioception and two-point discrimination sense are impaired. These are the features of HSMN. A family history is not given, but this should be an important part of the investigation.

HSMN is divided into Types I, II and III. Type I is the classic, familial type in which there is a diffuse demyelinating neuropathy which usually presents in the first two decades. Distal wasting of the lower limbs produces peroneal muscular atrophy and the characteristic 'inverted champagne bottle' appearance. Deformities of the feet and scoliosis are common. The sensory fibres of proprioception are affected, producing a sensory ataxia. Linkage studies on families with this neuropathy have localized the condition to a genetic defect on the long arm of chromosome 1. Nerve conduction is very reduced. Type II HSMN is similar, but much milder. In this condition, nerve conduction is only very slightly reduced or normal. HSMN III – also known as Dejerine–Sottas disease – is inherited as an autosomal recessive trait. It is a slow, progressive mixed sensory and motor neuropathy which starts in the first decade and is typically associated with enlargement of the peripheral nerves, which are easily palpable on examination. Differential diagnosis of thickened or enlarged peripheral nerves is listed below. Recently, the classification of the HSMN has been extended to include types IV and V. Descriptions of the latter are beyond the scope of this book.

Causes of thickened peripheral nerves

HSMN type III
Acromegaly
Tuberculoid leprosy
Neurofibromatosis
HIV syndrome

Question 119

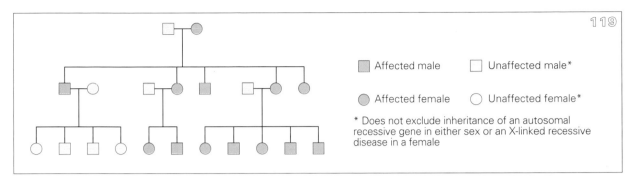

A family pedigree suffering from a very rare condition is shown (**119**).

1. What is the mode of inheritance?
2. Give one example of a condition inherited in this way.

Question 120

A 59-year-old female was referred to the out-patient clinic with lethargy and chest pain consistent with angina. She was on a gluten-free diet and on long-standing treatment for a skin rash (**120**). On examination, she was thin and had pale conjunctivae. She appeared cyanosed. The heart rate was 110 beats/min, with good volume; the blood pressure was 130/75 mmHg. The heart sounds were normal and the chest was clear.

Investigations are shown.

FBC	Hb 8 g/dl
	WCC 11×10^9/l
	Platelets 240×10^9/l
	MCV 110 fl
	PCV 0.34
	Reticulocytes 10%
Blood film	Polychromasia, macrocytosis, target cells, a few fragmented red cells
Serum B_{12}	470 ng/l
Red cell folate	65 µg/l
Serum folate	1.8 µg/l

1. Give two possible explanations for the folate levels.
2. What is the most likely cause for the blood picture?
3. What additional morphological feature in the blood film would be diagnostically helpful?
4. What test would you request to determine the cause of the cyanosis?
5. Give three reasons for the patient's chest pain.

Answer 119

1. Inheritance of maternal mitochondrial genetic abnormality.
2. Conditions inherited in this way are listed (*Table*).

During conception, all the mitochondria inherited by the zygote come from the ovum because the spermatozoon is relatively depleted of mitochondria by the time it reaches the ovum; therefore, abnormalities in mitochondrial DNA can only be transmitted by a female. An affected female will transfer the abnormal gene and the abnormal phenotype to all offspring; however, a male does not transfer the disease.

Mitochondrial DNA contains a limited number of genes which may be subject to point mutations, deletions or duplications. Abnormalities in mitochondrial DNA result in a variety of abnormalities include easy fatigue, myopathy, epilepsy, diabetes, optic atrophy, deafness, retinitis pigmentosa and cardiomyopathy. Calcification of basal ganglia is well recognized with mitochondrial disease. The most common mutation is an A to G mutation at nucleotide 3243. Most recognized mutations occur in transfer RNA or genes encoding the proteins involved in the oxidative phosphorylation pathway. The serum lactate/pyruvate ratio is elevated indicating impaired aerobic glycolysis. CSF lactate may be elevated even when serum lactate is normal.

> **Syndromes associated with mitochondrial gene mutations**
>
> MERRF: Myoclonic Epilepsy; Ragged Red Fibres (mutation in t-RNA Lys)
> MELAS: Mitochondrial Encephalomyopathy; Lactic Acidosis; Stroke (mutation in t-RNA Leu)
> NARP: Neuropathy, Ataxia, Retinitis Pigmentosa (mutation at nucleotide 8893; coding for ATPase 6)
> LHON: Leber's; Hereditary; Optic; Neuropathy (mutation in NADH dehydrogenase Subunit 4)
> Kearnes–Sayer syndrome: progressive external ophthalmoplegia, retinitis pigmentosa, heart block, myopathy, diabetes
> Usher's syndrome: deafness, retinitis pigmentosa, myopathy

Muscle biopsy may reveal red ragged fibres (increased fibre staining with stain for succinate dehydrogenase) representing abnormal mitochondria.

Answer 120

1. i. Malabsorption.
ii. Dapsone-induced haemolysis.
2. Dapsone-induced haemolytic anaemia.
3. The presence of Heinz bodies (oxidative haemolysis).
4. Serum methaemoglobin level.
5. i. Anaemia.
ii. Reduced delivery of oxygen to the heart due to leftward shift of the oxygen dissociation curve resulting from methaemoglobinaemia.
iii. Tachycardia.

The patient is on a gluten-free diet, suggesting that she has a gluten-sensitive enteropathy. She is on treatment for a long-standing rash (**120**) which is characteristic of dermatitis herpetiformis. The association between dermatitis herpetiformis and gluten-sensitive enteropathy is well recognized. Dermatitis herpetiformis is effectively treated with dapsone. An important side effect of dapsone is haemolytic anaemia because of its oxidant effect on Hb. This effect is severe in patients with glucose-6-phosphate dehydrogenase deficiency, but may also occur in some individuals as an idiosyncratic reaction, particularly with chronic use of the drug. Iron within the haem molecule of haemoglobin is oxidized from the ferrous state (Fe^{2+}) to the ferric state (Fe^{3+}), resulting in methaemoglobin (*Table*). This leads to depletion of the red cell NADPH (which is utilized to try and maintain iron in the ferrous form) and consequent reduction in the integrity of the red cell membrane. Patients with glucose-6- phosphate dehydrogenase deficiency have lower cellular levels of NADPH than normal individuals, and are more severely affected. Methaemoglobin has a very high affinity for oxygen molecules, resulting in a leftward shift in the oxygen dissociation curve and impaired unloading of oxygen to the tissues (*Table*). Methaemoglobinaemia causes a variable degree of cyanosis. Methaemoglobin levels exceeding 20% are associated with dyspnoea and headaches. Patients may develop angina, despite normal coronary arteries, due to reduced delivery of oxygen to myocardial cells. Collapse and sudden death may occur when levels exceed 60%. The blood film will demonstrate features of intravascular haemolysis (polychromasia, macrocytes, red cell fragmentation) and Heinz bodies, which are small red cell inclusions of denatured Hb.

Causes of methaemoglobinaemia	Causes of left-shift of O_2 dissociation curve
Genetic	Methaemoglobinaemia
NADPH diaphorase deficiency	Sulphaemoglobinaemia
Hb M	Carboxyhaemoglobinaemia
	Fetal Hb
Acquired	2,3 diphosphoglycerate deficiency
Drugs: Sulphonamides	Alkalosis
Primaquin	Hypocapnia
Phenacetin	Hypothermia
Toxins: Ferric cyanide	
Chlorate	
Aniline dyes	

These are scarce on the peripheral blood film unless the spleen has been removed. Other causes of methaemo-globinaemia are shown (*Table*). Dapsone-induced chronic haemolysis may lead to depletion of folate.

Question 121

A 76-year-old female was admitted to hospital with malaise, weakness, nausea and anorexia. She had been relatively well until two weeks previously when she developed a painful left calf for which she was prescribed 'some tablets' by her general practitioner. On examination, she appeared dehydrated and her blood pressure was 90/50 mmHg. She had clinical evidence of a deep-vein thrombosis in her left calf. All other physical examination was normal.

Investigations are shown.

1. What is the cause of this patient's low sodium?
A. Addison's disease.
B. Diuretic excess.
C. Acute tubulointerstitial nephritis secondary to NSAIDs.
D. Diabetic ketoacidosis.
E. Vomiting.

FBC	Hb 13 g/dl
	WCC 8×10^9/l
	Platelets 300×10^9/l
	MCV 88 fl
Biochemistry	Sodium 128 mmol/l
	Potassium 6.2 mmol/l
	Chloride 88 mmol/l
	Bicarbonate 13 mmol/l
	Urea 24 mmol/l
	Creatinine 297 µmol/l
	Blood glucose 10 mmol/l
U&E	24-hour urinary sodium
	68 mmol/l

Answer 121

1. C. Acute tubulointerstitial nephritis secondary to NSAIDs.

All five suggested answers can be responsible for hyponatraemia, but in a woman who has recently been treated for a painful calf it is most likely that she was prescribed some form of pain killer. She has subsequently presented with anorexia, malaise and vomiting and has deranged renal function. Urinalysis reveals a 24-hour urine of over 20 mmol/l sodium, which suggests a salt-losing state when one considers her low serum sodium. The most probable cause of her presentation is an acute nephritis secondary to prescription of a NSAID.

The biochemistry is partly consistent with Addison's disease; however, the diagnosis is less likely in the context of the history and the presence of a raised blood sugar. Diuretic excess is also possible. One could assume that she was prescribed a diuretic; this has resulted in dehydration and pre-renal failure, but the serum bicarbonate and the potassium suggest that this is unlikely. Diuretics used to treat ankle swelling alone comprise thiazides or loop diuretics which result in a hypokalaemic alkalosis. Potassium-sparing drugs such as amiloride alone or spironolactone are not the drugs of choice to treat ankle swelling. Vomiting is also a recognized cause of hyponatraemia, but there is no mention of it in the history and the raised potassium is unlikely to explain profuse vomiting which usually results in low sodium, potassium and chloride levels because gastric fluid contains high concentrations of all these ions.

Diabetic ketoacidosis would be lowest in the differential diagnosis because the blood sugar is relatively low. The hyponatraemia resulting from ketoacidosis is a result of osmotic diuresis from the very high blood sugar. A random blood sugar of 10 mmol/l could represent impaired glucose tolerance or mild non-insulin-dependent diabetes, but is against diabetic ketoacidosis.

NSAIDs may cause acute tubular necrosis or an acute tubulointerstitial nephritis (*Table*). Acute tubular necrosis is an increasing problem with NSAID prescription.

NSAIDs inhibit cyclo-oxygenase activity and decrease prostaglandin synthesis. Prostaglandins have a number of functions in the kidney, one of which is to stimulate renin production and thus activate the angiotensin–aldosterone system. With NSAIDs, there is a state of hyporenin-anaemic hypoaldosteronism causing hyperkalaemia, hyponatraemia, increased urinary sodium loss and dehydration. In patients with pre-existing renal disease, or in diabetics, this may be significant enough to produce acute renal failure. Such patients usually have a significant hyperkalaemia. Acute tubulointerstitial nephritis is often due to a hypersensitivity reaction to drugs (*Table*). NSAIDs and the penicillins are most commonly implicated in this country. Patients may present with malaise, arthralgia and/or acute renal failure. Many patients have eosinophilia or eosinophiluria. Treatment of both forms of renal failure involves withdrawal of the offending drug. The treatment of acute tubular necrosis is supportive, and involves careful fluid balance, correction of hyperkalaemia and hypovolaemia, and dialysis if necessary. Acute interstitial nephritis is treated in the same way, but in addition high-dose prednisolone is prescribed to reduce the acute inflammatory response in the kidney.

Causes of acute interstitial nephritis

Penicillins
NSAIDs
Sulphonamides
Allopurinol
Phenindione
Acute pyelonephritis
Sickle cell crisis
Lead poisoning

Renal manifestations of NSAIDs

Acute tubular necrosis
Acute interstitial nephritis
Minimal change glomerulonephritis

Question 122

The above (**122a, b**) are two rhythm strips from a 24-hour ECG in a 70-year-old male with dizziness and palpitation.

1. What is the diagnosis?
2. What is the management?

Question 123

A 40-year-old dentist presented with a five-month history of weight loss. He had recently become jaundiced.

Blood results are shown.

1. What is the diagnosis?
2. Which four tests would you perform next ?
3. What is the management?

LFT	AST 40 u/l
	Alkaline phosphatase 165 u/l
	Bilirubin 80 µmol/l
	Albumin 32 g/l
α-fetoprotein	40 ng/l
Serum ferritin	450 µg/l
Hepatitis serology	Hep B s Ag positive
	Hep B e Ag positive
	Hep B c Ab positive

Answer 122

1. Sick sinus syndrome. Rhythm strip A reveals sinus tachycardia followed by sinus arrest or sinus pause of 2.5 seconds. Rhythm strip B reveals atrial fibrillation with a rapid ventricular rate.
2. Symptomatic patients should be paced.

The diagnosis is consistent with sick sinus syndrome, which is a degenerative condition affecting the sino-atrial node and the atrial myocardium. It is characterized by long sinus pauses and paroxysmal atrial arrhythmias comprising atrial tachycardia, flutter and fibrillation. These patients are at increased risk of systemic emboli. Many go on to develop atrioventricular nodal disease.

Patients in sinus rhythm are implanted with an atrial pacemaker as they have effective atrial transport; however, those with atrial fibrillation are treated with ventricular pacing. Unlike atrioventricular block, pacing for sick sinus syndrome does not save lives.

Answer 123

1. Chronic active hepatitis B infection.
2. i. Hepatitis B e antibody (Hep B e Ab)/hepatitis s antibody (Hep B s Ab).
ii Liver ultrasound.
ii. Liver biopsy (if platelets and clotting not severely deranged).
iv. HIV antigen.
3. α-interferon.

The differential diagnosis of weight loss and jaundice is wide, but the presence of Hep B e Ag and Hep Bs Ag narrow this down to active hepatitis B infection. (Note: dentistry is a high-risk occupation for hepatitis B.)

The symptoms have been present for five months, suggesting that there is a chronic active infection. Investigations should be based on confirming the extent of hepatic damage and determining the patient's infectivity and immune status. The α-fetoprotein is modestly elevated in severe viral hepatitis and active cirrhosis. Levels exceeding 1,000 ng/l are strongly suggestive of hepatocellular carcinoma. Liver biopsy will reveal a ground-glass appearance of infected hepatocytes and evidence of balloon degeneration. Serological markers such as Hep B e Ab and Hep B s Ab will determine infectivity and immune response. Liver ultrasound may be useful in determining extent of liver damage when clotting and platelets are very abnormal. Hepatitis B-positive patients in high-risk occupations should also be offered HIV testing, because both conditions are acquired in the same manner from the same type of patients. There is evidence that treatment with α-interferon in patients with circulating Hep B s Ag and Hep B e Ag will reduce viral replication and infectivity.

Some 2% of patients with hepatitis B infection develop fulminant hepatitis, while 10% of patients become carriers after the initial infection. Some carriers are positive for Hep B s Ab, but have normal liver histology, while others have chronic active or chronic persistent hepatitis. Chronic active hepatitis may progress to cirrhosis of the liver. Patients with cirrhosis of the liver as a result of hepatitis B infection are more prone to hepatocellular carcinoma.

Hep B s Ag appears in the circulation 1–5 weeks before the onset of symptoms. It is no longer detectable when the infection has resolved, but its presence six months after infection indicates chronic infection.

Hep B e Ag appears in the circulation shortly before or 1–3 weeks after the onset of symptoms. Its presence indicates active viral replication, either in acute or in chronic infection, and high infectivity. Its disappearance is suggestive of resolution of infection. Hepatitis B virus DNA also appears at around the same time and its presence also indicates active viral replication. Disappearance of Hep B virus DNA correlates with resolution of infection. Hep B c Ag is only seen within hepatocytes, and does not circulate in the serum.

IgM anti-Hep B c Ab appears at the time of onset of symptoms. It is a marker of recent hepatitis B infection and may be the only marker of hepatitis B infection before the appearance of Hep B s Ag. IgG anti-Hep B c Ab is present lifelong after hepatitis B infection. It does not indicate immunity. Hep B e Ab appears after the c Ab. Its presence indicates reduced infectivity. Hep B s Ab is the last antibody to appear. Its presence indicates immunity.

Interferon therapy will reduce Hep B e and s Ag levels (40% and 10%, respectively). All patients with circulating e and sAg are offered treatment with interferon unless there is evidence of gross hepatic decompensation. Interferon has the effect of exacerbating coexisting autoimmune conditions, and is contraindicated in these situations.

Question 124

A 62-year-old female with rheumatoid arthritis was referred to an ophthalmologist with a three-day history of a painful left eye. The visual acuity was normal. She had a similar problem three years ago which required therapy with oral steroids. She was diagnosed with rheumatoid arthritis 21 years ago after presenting with pain in her hands, feet and elbows. Initial treatment comprised NSAIDs, then chloroquine, but over the past five years she was successfully managed on a combination of non-steroidals and penicillamine. On further questioning, she complained of a slightly reduced appetite, lethargy and breathlessness on trying to negotiate inclines, and swollen ankles. There was no other past medical history. She was a non-smoker. She was married and her husband worked as an architect.

On examination, the appearance of the eye was as shown (**124a**). The anterior chamber was clear and the pupils reacted normally to light. Visual acuity was 6/6 in the left eye, and 6/12 in the right eye. Examination of the fundi was normal. Examination of her hands and feet revealed evidence of a generalized, symmetrical deforming arthropathy. The heart rate was 90 beats/min and regular. The blood pressure was 140/90 mmHg. The jugular veins were not distended. The heart sounds were normal. Auscultation of the lung fields revealed fine inspiratory crackles at both bases, which persisted after coughing. On examination of the abdomen, there was a palpable spleen 3 cm below the costal margin. The liver was not palpable, and there was no ascites. Examination of the lower limbs revealed multiple bruises and pitting ankle oedema to the shins.

Investigations are shown.

1. What is the most probable cause of the painful eye?
2. Give two possible explanations for the FBC.
3. List two tests you would perform to ascertain the cause of the abnormal FBC.
4. List two possible causes for the ankle swelling?
5. What is the most likely cause of the breathlessness?
6. Which two investigations would you perform to ascertain the cause of the breathlessness?

FBC	Hb 7.4 g/dl
	WCC 3×10^9/l
	Platelets 45×10^9/l
	MCV 78 fl
ESR	56 mm/h
Biochemistry	Sodium 134 mmol/l
	Potassium 4.4 mmol/l
	Urea 13 mmol/l
	Creatinine 168 µmol/l
	Calcium 2.0 mmol/l
	Phosphate 1.2 mmol/l
	Alkaline phosphatase 200 u/l
	Albumin 29 g/l
Immunology	IgM 2.0 g/l
	IgG 19 g/l
	IgA 1.9 g/l
Immunoelectrophoresis	Increased gamma-globulin band
	No paraproteinaemia
	Rheumatoid factor positive 1 in 460
Chest X-ray	Normal
Urine dipstick	Protein ++
	Blood 0

Answer 124

1. Scleritis.
2. i. Penicillamine-induced marrow suppression.
ii. Hypersplenism (Felty's syndrome).
3. i. Bone marrow aspirate/trephine.
ii. Red cell sequestration study.
4. i. Penicillamine-induced membranous glomerulonephritis and secondary nephrotic syndrome.
ii. Renal amyloidosis.
5. Interstitial lung fibrosis or fibrotic lung disease.
6. Former spirometry and transfer factor.

This female with longstanding rheumatoid arthritis presents with a second attack of unilateral painful red eye which has previously required systemic steroids. The most probable diagnosis in scleritis. Other causes of a red eye in rheumatoid arthritis include episcleritis and keratitis secondary to Sjögren's syndrome. The former is painless, and the latter is bilateral. It is important to note that the only definitive method of differentiating scleritis from episcleritis without a history is by slit-lamp examination of the eye. Recurrent episodes of scleritis may result in perforation of the sclera (scleromalacia perforans) (**124b**).

In addition to the scleritis, she has other problems commonly seen in patients with rheumatoid arthritis which include anaemia, Felty's syndrome (which itself may be responsible for the anaemia), renal and respiratory involvement. Drugs used in the treatment for rheumatoid arthritis may themselves cause many of the complications seen in rheumatoid arthritis, and a knowledge of the drugs used – and their complications – is essential in the management of a patient with rheumatoid arthritis.

The anaemia is part of pancytopenia which, in the context of this question, is due to either penicillamine-induced marrow aplasia or hypersplenism resulting in Felty's syndrome. The former may be diagnosed by histological examination of the marrow, and the latter by demonstrating increased red cell uptake and destruction by the spleen.

The low albumin, swollen ankles and proteinuria are indicative of nephrotic syndrome, which may be due to a penicillamine-induced membranous glomerulonephritis or renal amyloid complicating chronic inflammation. Other causes of renal involvement in patients with rheumatoid arthritis are tabulated below. The fine inspiratory crackles at both lung bases probably represent interstitial lung disease, and require investigation with formal spirometry and KCO. Early interstitial fibrosis may not be identified on a chest X-ray, but respiratory function tests will reveal reduced lung volumes and reduced KCO. The haematological, ocular, renal, and respiratory complications of rheumatoid arthritis are tabulated (*Tables A–D*).

Table A. Causes of anaemia in rheumatoid arthritis

Iron deficiency secondary to NSAIDs
Marrow suppression from drugs such as penicillamine and gold
Hypersplenism seen as part of Felty's syndrome
Anaemia of chronic disease
Folate deficiency resulting from increased cell turnover in chronic inflammation
Autoimmune haemolysis
Associated pernicious anaemia

Table B. Causes of ocular involvement in rheumatoid arthritis

Episcleritis/scleritis/scleromalacia
Sjögren's syndrome
Cataracts secondary to steroid therapy
Retinopathy secondary to chloroquine
Extraocular muscle tendon synovitis
Extraocular muscle paralysis secondary to penicillamine-induced myaesthenia
Extraocular muscle paralysis secondary to a mononeuritis multiplex

Table C. Causes of renal involvement in rheumatoid arthritis

Acute tubulointerstitial nephritis secondary to NSAIDs
Renal papillary necrosis secondary to analgesic abuse
Renal amyloid
Membranous nephropathy secondary to gold or penicillamine
Minimal change glomerulonephritis complicating NSAIDs

Table D. Causes of respiratory involvement in rheumatoid arthritis

Cricoarytenitis
Pleural effusion
Pulmonary fibrosis
Bronchiolitis obliterans

Pneumonitis
Pulmonary nodules
Caplan's syndrome (nodules plus
progressive massive fibrosis in coal worker's disease

Question 125

An 11-year-old male was referred to the local paediatrician after his mother complained that he was unusually short for his age. His appetite was normal, and there was no history of recent diarrhoea or weight loss. He was performing well at school and enjoyed a relatively active life. His mother was short, measuring 1.48 m, but his father measured 1.81 m. There were no siblings.

On examination, the boy measured 0.97 m. There was no evidence of pallor, cyanosis or oedema. The heart sounds were normal and the chest was clear. The abdomen was soft, and there was no palpable organomegaly. The lower limbs appeared bowed. Neurological examination was normal.

Investigations are shown.

1. What is the abnormality on the X-ray?
2. What is the diagnosis?
3. Which tests would you perform to confirm the diagnosis?
4. What is the management?

FBC	Hb 11 g/dl
	WCC 5 × 10⁹/l
	Platelets 180 × 10⁹/l
Biochemistry	Sodium 135 mmol/l
	Potassium 4 mmol/l
	Urea 4 mmol/l
	Calcium 2.2 mmol/l
	Phosphate 0.3 mmol/l
	Albumin 39 g/l
	Alkaline phosphatase 500 u/l
X-ray of knees (**125**)	

Answer 125

1. Splaying of the metaphyses and widening of the epiphyseal plate, indicating rickets.
2. Hypophosphataemic rickets; X-linked dominant hypophophataemic rickets; Vitamin D-resistant rickets.
3. i. Urinary phosphate excretion (elevated).
ii. Renal tubular reabsorption rate of phosphate.
4. High-dose Vitamin D and oral phosphate supplements.

Both the boy and his mother are short. There is radiological evidence of rickets and a hypophosphataemia, but the serum calcium level is normal. The findings are consistent with the diagnosis of hypophosphataemic rickets or vitamin D-resistant rickets. The condition is inherited as an X-linked dominant condition. The fundamental abnormality is failure of phosphate reabsorption by the kidney. The diagnosis is confirmed by the demonstration of a high urinary phosphate excretion rate.

Unlike vitamin D-dependent rickets, myopathy does not occur. The main features of the condition are short stature and radiological evidence of rickets. Ossification of the ligamentum flavum is recognized and may cause paraplegia. The serum calcium and active metabolites of vitamin D are usually normal. Correction of the disorder is by a combination of high-dose vitamin D and oral phosphate supplements. Vitamin D alone aids resolution of biochemical rickets, but does not promote growth of height. Untreated patients are short and rarely measure more than 1.53 m.

Other causes of renal rickets are proximal RTA and Fanconi's syndrome (*Table A*). Vitamin D-dependent rickets is very rare. Two forms are recognized, the characteristics of which are listed (*Table B*).

Table A. Causes of rickets and osteomalacia

Vitamin D deficiency due to poor nutrition, malabsorption
Chronic renal failure (failure to synthesize 1α-hydroxycholecalciferol)
Renal tubular disorders (see above)
Anticonvulsants (rapid metabolism of 25-hydroxycholecalciferol to inactive derivatives)
Tumours (certain mesenchymal tumours; cause unknown; associated profound myopathy)
Vitamin D-dependent rickets (*Table B*)

Table B. Characteristics of Vitamin D-dependent rickets

	Type 1	*Type 2*
Mode of inheritance	Autosomal recessive	Autosomal recessive
Defect	Reduced 1α-hydroxycholecalciferol	Resistance to 1,25-dihydroxycholecalciferol
1,25-dihydroxycholecalciferol level	Reduced	Elevated
Myopathy	Present	Present
Associations		Alopecia
Treatment	Very high doses of 1,25-dihydroxycholecalciferol	Very high doses of 1,25-dihydroxycholecalciferol and i.v. calcium Spontaneous resolution with advancing age is recognized

Question 126

A 25-year-old homosexual male presented with an epileptic seizure.

Investigations were as follows:

1. List at least three possible diagnoses.
2. List three investigations you would perform on the CSF to help make the diagnosis.

CD4 count	300×10^6/l
Viral load	1,000 copies/ml
CT scan	Normal
CSF pressure	10 cm H_2O
CSF analysis	White cells 580/mm^3 (90% lymphocytes)
	Red cells 3/mm^3
	Protein 0.9 g/l
	Glucose 1.5 mmol/l
	Gram stain negative
	Ziehl–Neelsen stain negative
Blood glucose	5 mmol/l

Question 127

A 57-year-old male was admitted to the coronary care unit with a two-hour history of crushing central chest pain radiating to his jaw. On examination, he was sweating. His heart rate was 90 beats/min, and regular, and blood pressure 160/90 mmHg. He had a 12-lead ECG (**127**), after which he was given recombinant tissue plasminogen activator. Two hours later he complained of feeling dizzy and unwell. On examination, he was pale, but not cyanosed. His heart rate was 110 beats/min, and regular. His systolic blood pressure was 80 mmHg. The JVP was elevated 7 cm above the sternal angle. The heart sounds were normal and the chest was clear.

Investigations are shown.

Biochemistry	Sodium 136 mmol/l	FBC	Hb 13 g/dl
	Potassium 4.0 mmol/l		WCC 17 × 109/l
	Urea 8 mmol/l		Platelets 159 x 109/l
	Creatinine 90 μmol/l	Chest X-ray	Normal
	Glucose 6 mmol/l		

1. What is the ECG diagnosis?
A. Acute anterior myocardial infarction.
B. Acute inferior myocardial infarction.
C. Acute inferior myocardial infarction complicated by third degree atrioventricular block.
D. Acute posterior myocardial infarction.
E. Acute posterolateral myocardial infarction.
F. Acute lateral myocardial infarction.
G. Old inferior myocardial infarction.

2. What is the cause of his symptoms two hours after thrombolysis?
A. Haemorrhage complicating thrombolysis.
B. Complete heart block complicating myocardial infarction.
C. Allergic reaction to recombinant tissue plasminogen activator.
D. Acute pulmonary embolus.
E. Acute mitral regurgitation following papillary muscle rupture.
F. Acute VSD complicating myocardial infarction.
G. Right ventricular hypokinesia.
H. Pericardial tamponade.

Answer 126

1. i. Tuberculous meningitis.
ii. Cryptococcal meningitis.
iii. *Listeria* meningitis.
iv. Cerebral lymphoma or leukaemia.
v. Brucellosis.
2. i. Ziehl–Neelsen stain or PCR on the CSF for tuberculous meningitis.
ii. Indian ink stain on CSF to identify *Cryptococcus neoformans.*
iii. CSF analysis by the cytology department to look for malignant cells.

Causes of CSF lymphocytosis, raised CSF protein and CSF sugar less than half of blood sugar

Tuberculous meningitis
Brucellosis*
Fungal meningitis
Cerebral lymphoma
Leukaemic infiltration into the brain
Metastatic brain disease
Cerebral abscess

*This may be similar to that seen in viral meningitis.

This homosexual male with a low CD4 count presents with an epileptic seizure. The CD4 count suggests that he has advanced HIV infection. The CSF reveals a lymphocytosis, high protein, and a sugar concentration less than half of the blood sugar. The differential diagnosis of these CSF findings are listed above (*Table*). The normal CT scan is against the diagnosis of a cerebral abscess, and metastatic brain disease; however, all the other diagnoses listed are possible.

Answer 127

1. E. Acute posterolateral myocardial infarction.
2. G. Right ventricular hypokinesia.

The ECG on admission reveals ST-segment elevation of more than 2 mm in leads I and aVl. This is consistent with a limited lateral myocardial infarction. The J-point in leads II, and V3–V6 is elevated, but there is no pathological ST-segment elevation in these leads. There is also evidence of a dominant R-wave in leads V1–V3 which, in the context of the history, represents posterior extension of the infarct. Posterior infarction gives the opposite appearance of an acute anterior infarction; therefore instead of Q-waves (which would be seen in the case of an anterior infarction) there are prominent R-waves. The full diagnosis is acute posterolateral myocardial infarction.

There are several possible causes of hypotension in this man; however the only real possibility in this clinical scenario is right ventricular infarction and secondary right ventricular hypokinesia. This is a recognized complication of inferior and posterior myocardial infarction, and is characterized by a reduced cardiac output from the right heart causing hypotension and a raised JVP. Treatment is with a careful fluid challenge of 100 ml at a time to increase the PCWP to approximately 10 cm H_2O, which should be monitored using a Swan–Ganz catheter. Haemorrhage is unlikely with a raised JVP unless the patient has bled into his pericardial space. However, in this rare event one would expect an increased heart size on the chest X-ray. While allergic reactions are relatively common with non-human thrombolytic agents such as streptokinase, they are rare with recombinant human tissue plasminogen activator. In any case, allergic shock occurs during infusion of the drug rather than two hours afterwards. While pulmonary embolism is a recognized complication of myocardial infarction and could explain the raised JVP, low blood pressure and normal chest X-ray, it does not occur for at least three days after myocardial infarction. Both papillary muscle rupture and ventricular septal perforation, which usually occur 72 hours following myocardial infarction, are usually associated with an acute fall in cardiac output and pulmonary oedema. Complete heart block may cause hypotension, but is most unlikely in a patient with a heart rate of 110 beats/min.

Question 128

A 5-year-old male was admitted with a one-week history of fever, general malaise and pain in his hands and feet. Two weeks previously he had a bout of tonsillitis which required a course of antibiotics. On the day of admission he complained of intermittent chest pain radiating into his back and his arms. He was born at 41 weeks gestation and was a normal vaginal delivery. He had achieved his milestones normally. He was the only child. His father was a businessman, and his mother a teacher. He had been seen by the general practitioner two days earlier and diagnosed as having a viral illness for which he was prescribed paracetamol syrup.

On examination, he appeared unwell. He had a fever of 40°C (104°F). His heart rate was 140 beats/min and regular. His lips appeared oedematous, and examination of his mouth revealed a white-coated tongue with prominent papillae. On examination of the neck there was widespread, tender, cervical lymphadenopathy. Examination of the pharynx and tonsillar area was normal. The palms of his hands and feet were red, and there was evidence of early desquamation of the skin on the palmar surface of both hands. There was tenderness over the metacarpophalangeal joints of both hands. The interphalangeal joints in both feet were tender. Cardiovascular and respiratory examination was normal.

Investigations are shown.

FBC	Hb 10.5 g/dl
	WCC 15 × 10⁹/l
	Platelets 490 × 10⁹/l
ESR	90 mm/h
CRP	80 g/l
Biochemistry	Normal
Blood cultures	Normal
Chest X-ray	Normal
ECG	Sinus tachycardia
	Inverted T- waves V1–V6

1. What is the diagnosis?
2. What other important investigation would you perform?
3. List two important therapeutic steps in his management.

Question 129

A 33-year-old single male was admitted with a one-week history of fever, sore throat, a maculopapular rash on the trunk and cervical lymphadenopathy. His only past medical history comprised of treatment for urethritis one year ago following a trip abroad. His most recent sexual contact was eight weeks ago. Four months previously, he expressed the wish for HIV testing, which was negative.

Investigations are shown.

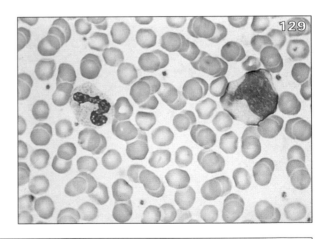

1. What is the cause of this patient's symptoms?
2. Which further definitive investigation is required?

FBC	Hb 11 g/dl	Toxoplasma titres	Negative
	WCC 6 × 10⁹/l	VDRL	Negative
	Platelets 180 × 10⁹/l	FTA IgG	Positive
Blood film (**129**)		Hep B s Ag	Absent
Paul Bunnell test	Negative	HCV Ab	Absent
CMV titre	Increased IgG at a titre of 1/16		

Answer 128

1. Kawasaki's disease.
2. Transthoracic echocardiography to visualize the coronary arteries on the short-axis views of the aorta.
3. i. Oral aspirin.
ii. Intravenous human immunoglobulin.

Key: 1 right coronary artery; 2 Aortic root; 3 left coronary artery.

The combination of mucocutaneous, rheumatological and dermatological involvement in a young boy shortly after a sore throat could be due to scarlet fever, Stevens–Johnson syndrome complicating streptococcal infection, an idiosyncratic reaction to antibiotics, or a systemic reaction to a general viral illness. The rash is not typical of Stevens–Johnson syndrome. The description of the tongue and the generalized erythema fits well with scarlet fever; however, the additional chest pain and abnormal ECG should raise the possibility of Kawasaki's disease.

Kawasaki's disease has been very topical, and it is only a matter of time before it appears in general examinations. It is an acute multisystem vasculitis which affects medium-sized arteries. It appears to be endemic in Japan, where there have been more than 100,000 cases since 1991. In contrast, the incidence in Britain is 35 per million. The disorder is thought to be due to a severe immune reaction following streptococcal or staphylococcal infections, although other organisms have also been implicated. The condition is almost confined to children below the age of six years.

Characteristic features include:
- Fever for more than five days.
- Erythematous palms and soles followed by desquamation of skin from these areas.
- Conjunctival congestion.
- Strawberry tongue and swollen lips.
- Polymorphous rash.
- Non-purulent cervical lymphadenopathy.

Vasculitis commonly affects the coronary arteries causing microaneurysms, coronary thrombosis and myocardial infarction. Death is usually from cardiac failure following infarction. Features of cardiac involvement include tachycardia, prolonged PR interval, ST segment elevation and T-wave inversion.

Other organs which may be affected include the lungs (pulmonary infiltrates), the brain (convulsions, cranial nerve palsies, deafness, CVA) and the gastrointestinal tract (abdominal pain from ischaemia). The small joints of the body may be affected in approximately 30% of cases.

The diagnosis is clinical. There are no specific tests, but inflammatory markers such as the ESR, CRP and platelets are elevated. The WCC is also elevated, as are the immunoglobulins. The haemoglobin may fall rapidly. Coronary involvement may be detected non-invasively by viewing the origins of the coronaries by echocardiography (**128**). This is not difficult in young children because they are thin.

The mainstay of treatment is oral aspirin and intravenous Sandoglobulin (c globulin). These reduce the mortality of the condition from more than 30% to less than 1%.

Differential diagnosis of Kawasaki's disease is streptococcal infection (scarlet fever), staphylococcal infection (scalded skin or toxic shock syndrome), Stevens–Johnson syndrome, juvenile chronic arthritis, leptospirosis, rickketsial infection and a generalized drug reaction.

Answer 129

1. The diagnosis is HIV seroconversion.
2. Repeat HIV antibody test.

HIV seroconversion occurs 2–6 weeks after HIV infection. The illness resembles infectious mononucleosis, comprising fever, pharyngitis, lymphadenopathy and a rash. The patient may have a mild anaemia, relative lymphopenia and thrombocytopenia. The blood film may reveal atypical lymphocytes (**129**). Other differential diagnoses include CMV infection, *Toxoplasma* infection and secondary syphilis.

Although secondary syphilis produces an identical syndrome to HIV seroconversion, the syphilis serology is suggestive of previous syphilis infection rather than secondary syphilis. In secondary syphilis, reagin antibodies become positive in almost 100% of cases, as do the more specific antibodies such as the FTA and the TPHA.

Positive syphilis serology in relation to the various stages of syphilis

Test	Primary syphilis (%)	Secondary syphilis (%)	Tertiary syphilis (%)
VDRL	70	99	77
FTA	55	100	96
TPHA	80	99	95

However, the VDRL test becomes negative in over one-third of patients following therapy or in tertiary and quaternary syphilis, whereas the more specific antibodies persist in almost every patient, even after successful treatment (*Table*). In this case, the negative VDRL in a patient with a pharyngitis and a rash is against secondary syphilis, the more likely diagnosis being HIV seroconversion. Persistent FTA suggests previous syphilis infection.

HIV IgG antibodies are detectable six weeks after infection with the virus. The detection of HIV antibody using a Western blot technique or ELISA is the most widely performed test if HIV infection is suspected. In the case of a negative HIV antibody test (usually in very early infection), the diagnosis may be confirmed by measuring HIV p24 antigen, a viral capsid protein which is detectable within 24 hours of the onset of illness. Alternatively, PCR methods may be used to detect viral RNA.

Question 130

A 39-year-old male presents with a three-month history of lower back pain. Over the past two years he has experienced three episodes of severe right lower quadrant pain.

Investigations are shown.

1. What is the diagnosis?
2. Which single investigation would you perform to confirm the diagnosis?
3. What is the cause of his back pain?
4. List two simple investigations which may help confirm the cause of his back pain.
5. What is the cause of his abdominal pain?
6. List two radiological tests which may help confirm the cause of his abdominal pain.

Biochemistry	
	Sodium 138 mmol/l
	Potassium 3.5 mmol/l
	Chloride 119 mmol/l
	Bicarbonate 13 mmol/l
	Urea 7 mmol/l
	Creatinine 112 µmol/l
	Calcium 2.1 mmol/l
	Phosphate 0.7 mmol/l

Answer 130

1. Distal (type I) RTA.
2. Early morning urinary pH measurement or measurement of urine pH after ammonium chloride infusion.
3. Osteomalacia.
4. i. X-ray of the lumbar spine may reveal osteopaenia or Looser's zones in osteomalacia.
ii. Serum alkaline phosphatase level which is characteristically raised in osteomalacia.
5. Renal colic.
6. i. Plain abdominal X-ray may identify a radio-opaque renal stone.
ii. Intravenous urography is the investigation of choice to identify stones in the renal tract.

The biochemical results reveal a hypokalaemic, hyperchloraemic acidosis. In addition, there are low calcium and phosphate levels. These are features of RTA, which is characterized by abnormalities in urinary acidification. RTA may be divided into type 1 (distal RTA) or type 2 (proximal RTA). The causes and associations or renal tubular acidosis are tabulated below. Distal RTA is due to defective excretion of H^+ in the distal convoluted tubule, and proximal RTA is due to failure of H^+ secretion by the proximal convoluted tubule. In both cases, there is hypokalaemia and hypercalcuria. Hypokalaemia can be explained as follows. In distal RTA the defective H^+ excretion means that the absorption of sodium requires increased potassium excretion. In proximal RTA, there is excessive bicarbonate loss, which in turn results in excessive sodium loss. The resulting hypotension activates the renin–angiotensin–aldosterone system to aid sodium and water retention, but at the expense of potassium loss. Hypercalcuria is more common in distal RTA. Osteomalacia is common to both, but nephrocalcinosis and nephrolithiasis is confined to distal RTA.

Patients with distal RTA may present at any age. In children, the condition presents with failure to thrive. In adults, it presents with renal colic or muscle weakness from hypokalaemia. Patients with proximal RTA present with symptomatic acidosis, polydipsia, polyuria, hypokalaemic myopathy and rickets or osteomalacia. The diagnosis should be suspected if an individual has a hyperchloraemic acidosis and can be confirmed by demonstrating an early morning urinary pH of >5.5. In some individuals in whom the diagnosis is suspected, but there is no evidence of systemic acidosis, an acid load test using ammonium chloride is required. This involves measuring urinary pH on samples collected hourly for 6 hours after intravenous ammonium chloride. Failure to acidify the urinary pH below 5.5 indicates RTA.

Treatment is with sodium bicarbonate and potassium citrate. The latter reduces calcium excretion and provides supplementary potassium.

Causes of RTA	
Distal (Type 1)	*Proximal (Type 2)*
Inherited	Inherited
	Part of Fanconi's syndrome
Acquired	Acquired
Primary biliary cirrhosis	Hyperparathyroidism
CAH	Heavy metal poisoning (lead, argon)
Obstructive nephropathy	Myeloma
Vitamin D intoxication	Acetazolamide
Tetracycline	

Question 131

A 64-year-old female was admitted to hospital with a three month history of increasing breathlessness and swollen ankles. She had been well until two-and-a-half years ago, when she was experienced a sudden onset of breathlessness while walking. She was observed in hospital overnight but was much improved the following day and allowed home. She had a further similar episode four months later, and then again a year later. On each occasion she improved within 24–48 hours. In between the two most recent episodes she had noticed that she was unable to exert herself as much without becoming breathless. There was no history of chest pain or a cough. Physical examination performed by the senior house officers during each hospital admission had been normal, with the exception of a sinus tachycardia of 110 beats/min. A chest X-ray performed on the admission one year ago is shown (131a). The patient had a past medical history of hysterectomy aged 43 years for menorrhagia due to uterine fibroids. Three years ago she had surgery for varicose veins of the lower limbs. She was a non-smoker. She was not taking any medication. She was a receptionist in a doctor's surgery for 20 years before retiring 20 years ago. She was married and lived with her husband. The couple had a dog and a parrot as pets.

On examination, she was breathless at rest and cyanosed. There was no clubbing. She had marked pitting lower-limb oedema up to her thighs. The heart rate was 102 beats/min and blood pressure 105/60 mmHg. The JVP was elevated to the level of the mastoid. Closer inspection revealed prominent c-v waves. On examination of the precordium, the apex was displaced to the anterior axillary line. There was a marked left parasternal heave. On auscultation of the precordium there was a soft systolic murmur and a loud fourth heart sound at the left lower sternal edge. The chest was clear. Abdominal examination demonstrated ascites and a pulsatile liver edge 5 cm below the costal margin.

The ECG performed on admission is shown (131b).

Respiratory function tests performed on this admission are shown.

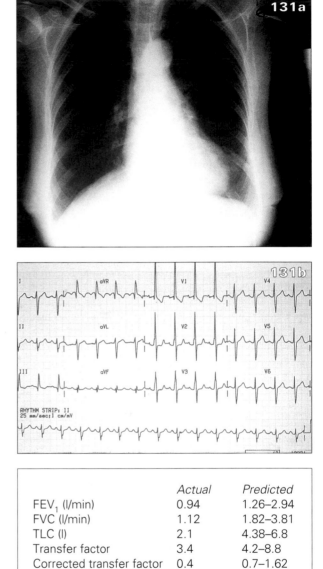

	Actual	Predicted
FEV$_1$ (l/min)	0.94	1.26–2.94
FVC (l/min)	1.12	1.82–3.81
TLC (l)	2.1	4.38–6.8
Transfer factor	3.4	4.2–8.8
Corrected transfer factor	0.4	0.7–1.62

1. List three abnormalities on the ECG.
2. What are the abnormalities on the respiratory function tests?
3. What is the most likely underlying diagnosis?
4. List three tests which would be useful in confirming the diagnosis.

Answer 131

1. i. Voltage criteria of right ventricular hypertrophy.
ii. Right axis deviation.
iii. Sinus tachycardia.
2. i. Restrictive lung defect.
ii. Reduced KCO.
3. Multiple pulmonary emboli or thromboembolic pulmonary disease.
4. i. Arterial blood gases.
ii. Ventilation/perfusion scan or spiral CT scan of the thorax.
iii. Right heart catheter plus pulmonary angiography.

The patient has a history of progressive breathlessness, and now presents with ECG evidence of right ventricular hypertrophy and a clinical picture of severe right heart failure. Lung function tests demonstrate a restrictive defect. She has cor pulmonale either complicating multiple pulmonary emboli, extrinsic allergic alveolitis, or CFA. The latter two diagnoses are unlikely in the absence of chest signs on three hospital admissions and the normal chest X-ray one year previously. In contrast the chest X-ray in multiple pulmonary emboli may appear relatively normal, the only evidence of pulmonary emboli being oligaemic lung fields. Another possible diagnosis is right heart failure due to chronic pulmonary hypertension from an ostium secundum ASD, however, the chest X-ray in this condition would reveal cardiomegaly. Investigations to confirm the diagnosis of multiple pulmonary emboli should include arterial blood gases (which will show low pO_2 and pCO_2 due to severe ventilation/perfusion mismatch) and a ventilation perfusion scan to demonstrate perfusion defects. A right heart catheter combined with pulmonary angiography would be diagnostic and would be useful in assessing the severity of pulmonary hypertension. Spiral CT scan of the thorax is an increasingly popular method of identifying peripheral pulmonary emboli, which may be difficult to detect with angiography. Echocardiography is useful in excluding an ASD with shunt reversal or tight mitral stenosis. Echo-Doppler may be useful in quantifying pulmonary artery pressure, however, it has no direct role in the diagnosis of multiple pulmonary emboli.

Question 132

A 42-year-old, insulin-dependent diabetic was investigated further after he was noted to have a positive dip stick for protein on urine analysis. He was diagnosed with diabetes at the age of 23 years after presenting with ketoacidosis. Initial management with porcine insulin was good; however, he was switched to human insulin 10 years ago because of severe lipoatrophy at sites of injection. Over the past three years blood glucose control had been suboptimal, and the dose of insulin had been increased on five occasions. He was married with two children. He owned a grocer's shop which was open seven days a week and was staffed by the patient and his wife at all times. He smoked five cigarettes per day. He did not consume alcohol.

On examination, he had bilateral corneal arcus. His heart rate was 80 beats/min and regular; blood pressure was 150/90 mmHg. There was no evidence of cardiac enlargement or cardiac failure. The peripheral pulses were all palpable, and there were no audible bruits over the carotid arteries or in the abdomen. Examination of his fundi is shown (**132a**).

Investigations are shown below.

FBC	Hb 12.8 g/dl	Glycosylated Hb	9% (normal range 3.8–6.4%)
	WCC 6 × 10⁹/l	Cholesterol	8.2 mmol/l
	Platelets 212 × 10⁹/l	Triglycerides	8 mmol/l
	MCV 89 fl	24-hour urine	Volume 2.7 l
Biochemistry	Sodium 136 mmol/l		Protein 0.7 g/l
	Potassium 3.4 mmol/l	Renal US	Two kidneys, 12 cm each
	Urea 6.8 mmol/l		Normal parenchymal
	Creatinine 117 µmol/l		texture
	Glucose 11 mmol/l	Renal biopsy (**132b** [haematoxylin and eosin stain])	

The patient was commenced on captopril, the dose of which was gradually increased to 50 mg, three times daily. Three months later, the patient was admitted with vague abdominal discomfort, nausea and anorexia. On examination, he appeared euvolaemic. The blood pressure was 120/65 mmHg.

Investigations are shown (right).

Another investigation was performed, which is shown (**132c**).

1. What is demonstrated on the examination of the fundi?
2. What is shown on the renal biopsy?
3. What is the cause of his proteinuria?
4. What was the cause of the marked deterioration in renal function?
5. List six management strategies to help ameliorate the renal function and the rate of future deterioration in renal function.

Biochemistry	
	Sodium 133 mmol/l
	Potassium 6.4 mmol/l
	Urea 32 mmol/l
	Creatinine 500 µmol/l
	Glucose 10 mmol/l

Question 133

A 16-year-old female was brought into the accident and emergency department with shortness of breath.

Blood gases on inspiring room air are shown.

1. What is the acid–base disturbance?
2. What is the underlying cause?
3. What is the management?

pH	7.49
pCO$_2$	2.4 kPa
pO$_2$	15.5 kPa
Bicarbonate	12 mmol/l
O$_2$ saturation	96%

Answer 132

1. Small retinal haemorrhages, and microaneurysms consistent with background diabetic retinopathy.
2. There is evidence of eosin staining (pink) fibrotic (hyaline) nodules characteristic of diabetic glomerulosclerosis, sometimes known as Kimmelsteil–Wilson nodules.
3. Diabetic nephropathy. Other causes of protein in the urine in diabetics include a urinary tract infection.
4. Angiotensin-converting enzyme (ACE) inhibitor-induced glomerular hypoperfusion in a patient with bilateral renal artery stenosis.
5. i. Stop ACE inhibitor.
ii. Bilateral renal angioplasty.
iii. Improve diabetic control.
iv. Control hyperlipidaemia.
v. Ensure blood pressure below 140/85 mmHg.
vi. Advise against smoking.

Overt diabetic nephropathy is based on the demonstration of over 0.5 mg of protein on a 24-hour urinary collection. A protein content of this level is easily detected on a urine dipstick. More recently, it has been noted that some patients pass small amounts of albumin in the urine (0.02–0.3 mg/24 h) before the development of a positive dipstick test. Such patients are said to have 'microalbuminuria' or incipient diabetic nephropathy.

The prevalence of diabetic nephropathy in the UK is 4–8%. The pathological basis for this is diabetic glomerulosclerosis, as shown in the renal biopsy (**132b**).

Patients with diabetic nephropathy have an increased mortality from cardiovascular and renal causes. Poor glycaemic control, raised blood pressure, and smoking expedite the development and progression of nephropathy. In patients with early nephropathy the GFR is increased, and the associated hyperinfiltration is thought to damage glomeruli by increasing the intraglomerular capillary blood pressure. Patients with nephropathy very often also have retinopathy, and vice versa.

The management includes good glycaemic control, maintaining blood pressure below 140/85 mmHg (this slows the rate of fall in the GFR rate by 60%). ACE inhibitors reduce albumin excretion in patients with microalbuminuria. In diabetic rats, ACE inhibitors reduce intraglomerular capillary pressure and prevent a decline in GFR. Whether they have the same effect in man is currently under investigation. Renal function should be observed carefully after the initiation of an ACE inhibitor because they may precipitate renal failure in patients with silent renal artery stenosis, as in this case. Renal failure is precipitated by reduction in the pressure within the afferent arteriole which causes a significant decrease in glomerular perfusion pressure in the presence of renal artery stenosis (**132c**).

Answer 133

1. There is a respiratory alkalosis and a metabolic acidosis.
2. Aspirin toxicity (see also Answer 90, page 118).
3. The management is dependent on the serum salicylate level. Levels below 500 mg/l are treated with intravenous saline to promote renal clearance. Levels between 500–750 mg/l may require forced alkaline diuresis on a high-dependency unit. Levels between 750–1,000 mg/l are best treated with haemodialysis.

There is a low pCO_2 and a high pH, suggesting a respiratory alkalosis. The serum bicarbonate is very low, indicating a coexistent metabolic acidosis. In chronic respiratory alkalosis there would be increased excretion of bicarbonate ions in an attempt to lower the arterial pH; however, the bicarbonate concentration is only modestly reduced. (See Acid-base Disturbance, page 228.)

Question 134

A 46-year-old garage mechanic was investigated in a medical clinic for weight loss. Six months previously he had commenced a voluntary diet to reduce weight. He lost 4 kg over two months, following which he stopped his diet. Despite a normal appetite he continued to lose another 4 kg in weight over the next four months. He had also noticed that he tired easily, and was finding it difficult to perform heavy manual work as part of his profession. His arms felt weak. He was breathless on strenuous effort and found heavy lifting increasingly difficult. More recently, he had developed lower back pain which was worse when he was sat upright and was associated with pain and numbness of his left calf and left foot. The pain was worsened by movement and he was forced to stop working. His appetite remained good. He had moved his bowels twice daily ever since he could remember. The stool was of normal consistency and did not contain blood. He was married with three children. He stopped smoking 15 years ago after an attack of bronchitis. He consumed 2–3 units of alcohol per week.

On examination, he was relatively well built. There was no evidence of pallor or clubbing. The heart rate was 102 beats/min and irregularly irregular. The blood pressure was 130/80 mmHg. The JVP was not raised. On examination of the upper limbs there was no muscle tenderness, but there was wasting of the proximal muscles of the upper limb with weakness of abduction and adduction. The upper limb reflexes were brisk. Sensory testing was normal. On examination of the lower limbs, there was wasting of the muscles of the thighs. Power testing demonstrated weakness of plantar flexion on the left side. Reflexes were brisk with the exception of the left ankle jerk which was absent. Plantar responses were normal. Sensory testing demonstrated reduced pin-prick sensation affecting the anterolateral aspect of the left foot.

Investigations were as follows:

FBC	Hb 14 g/dl
	WCC 6×10^9/l
	Platelets 210×10^9/l
ESR	10 mm/h
Chest X-ray	Normal
Biochemistry	Sodium 135 mmol/l
	Potassium 3.4 mmol/l
	Urea 5 mmol/l
	Calcium 2.4 mmol/l
	Phosphate 1 mmol/l
	Albumin 40 g/l

1. What is the cause of the absent ankle jerk?
A. Paraneoplastic syndrome.
B. Prolapsed intervertebral disc between L4/L5.
C. Prolapsed intervertebral disc between L5/S1.
D. Peripheral neuropathy.
E. Mononeuritis multiplex.
2. What is the diagnosis?
A. Polymyositis.
B. Polymyalgia rheumatica.
C. Thyrotoxic myopathy.
D. Eaton–Lambert syndrome.
E. Paraneoplastic syndrome.

Question 135

This ECG (**135**) is from a 35-year-old male with sudden onset of expressive dysphasia and right upper-limb weakness. On examination, he was apyrexial. The heart rate was 100 beats/min and regular; blood pressure was 110/80 mmHg. He had a soft systolic murmur. There were no carotid bruits He had been well and asympto-matic all his life, and was a non-smoker.

1. List three abnormalities.
2. What is the most likely cause for his murmur?
3. What is the most probable cause for his neurological signs?

Answer 134

1. C. Prolapsed intervertebral disc between L5/S1.
2. C. Thyrotoxic myopathy.

The patient has weight loss, despite a normal appetite. The differential diagnosis for this scenario is malabsorption, diabetes mellitus, phaechromocytoma and thyrotoxicosis. He has atrial fibrillation which is most consistent with thyrotoxicosis. He also has proximal muscle wasting of his limbs, a well-known feature of thyrotoxic myopathy. A paraneoplastic syndrome is unlikely because there is no immediate evidence of an underlying neoplastic process. For similar reasons, he is unlikely to have Eaton–Lambert syndrome, which is a myaesthenic syndrome associated with malignancy. Proximal myopathy is a feature, but reflexes are absent. In contrast to myaesthenia, weakness improves with repetitive muscular stimulation. Both polymyalgia rheumatica and polymyositis are associated with muscle tenderness and a raised ESR which are absent in this patient. Furthermore, polymyalgia rheumatica is a disorder which affects the elderly rather than young patients.

The chronic back pain worsened by movement and radiating to his left calf is consistent with a lumbar radiculopathy. A lateral disc protrusion is most likely. An absent ankle jerk (S1), weakness of dorsiflexion of the left side, and impaired sensation of the anterolateral aspect of the foot (L5 and S1) is consistent with a L5/S1 disc prolapse. In the case of an L4/L5 lesion the knee jerk would be absent. A peripheral neuropathy or mononeuritis multiplex cannot explain the root symptoms (back pain radiating to calf and made worse with movement) or the lack of neuropathy elsewhere (all other reflexes preserved).

Answer 135

1. i. Right axis deviation.
ii. RBBB.
iii. Voltage criteria for right ventricular hypertrophy.
2. Ostium secundum ASD.
3. Paradoxical embolus from the systemic veins.

The combination of right axis deviation and RBBB in a young, previously asymptomatic man with a soft systolic murmur is suggestive of an underlying ostium secundum ASD. Ostium primum defects are associated with left axis deviation and RBBB. Although both pulmonary stenosis and VSDs can produce similar ECG changes, a soft murmur in a patient with a VSD is suggestive of a large defect which would almost certainly cause symptoms of cardiovascular dysfunction before the third decade. Mild pulmonary stenosis is characterized by lack of symptoms and a soft systolic murmur, heard best in the left second intercostal space, but this is not usually enough to cause right ventricular hypertrophy. Moreover, it does not explain the neurological defect in this case, which has resulted from a paradoxical embolus of thrombus within the systemic veins to the brain via a defect in the interatrial septum. Paradoxical embolism is a rare but well-recognized complication of all septal defects. Thrombus from the systemic veins may result in emboli to the brain, limbs and gastrointestinal tract. Paradoxical embolus may be the presenting feature in a patient with a cardiac septal defect.

The differential diagnosis is a mycotic embolus complicating infective endocarditis involving an ASD; however, the patient is not febrile and infective endocarditis very rarely involves an ASD.

Question 136

A 22-year-old basketball player presented with sudden onset of severe left-sided chest pain radiating into his neck four hours before he was due to play in a large tournament. He had never experienced any previous chest pain, and was extremely fit, according to his team coach.

On examination, he was distressed with chest pain. His heart rate was 160 beats/min and blood pressure 190/110 mmHg. Examination of the precordium and the chest was normal. An ECG was performed immediately (**136**), and he was subsequently admitted to the coronary care unit. The following day he was asymptomatic and his blood pressure was normal. Examination of his fundi did not demonstrate any fundal changes of hypertension, and general examination did not reveal any peripheral stigmata of hyperlipidaemia. He denied any previous history of hypertension, diabetes mellitus or a family history of coronary artery disease. He had never smoked previously.

Investigations following admission are shown.

An echocardiogram performed three days later demonstrated minor apical hypokinesia, but satisfactory overall systolic function. Coronary angiography before discharge was entirely normal.

FBC	Hb 13 g/dl
	WCC 12×10^9/l
	Platelets 204×10^9/l
Biochemistry	Sodium 139 mmol/l
	Potassium 3.9 mmol/l
	Glucose 4.2 mmol/l
	Creatinine kinase 560 u/l

1. Which important piece of information should be elicited in the history to help ascertain the cause of his chest pain?
2. Which drug would you use in the management of his hypertension?

Question 137

A 66-year-old male with a long history of breathlessness presented with a three-day history of profound breathlessness and a cough productive of yellow sputum.

Arterial blood gases are shown.

1. What is the acid–base abnormality?

pH	7.33
pCO_2	8.8kPa
pO_2	6.5kPa
Bicarbonate	36 mmol/l
Base excess	+11

Answer 136

1. A history of amphetamine abuse.
2. A calcium channel blocker such as amlodipine or verapamil.

The clinical scenario is that of an elite athlete presenting with an acute myocardial infarction but subsequently has normal coronary arteries, although the echocardiogram is indicative of myocardial damage. While there are several causes of myocardial ischaemia despite normal coronary arteries (*Table A*), the possibility of cocaine abuse should be considered.

Cocaine abuse has reached epidemic proportions in some groups of elite athletes; however, the incidence of cardiac complications remains low. Cocaine inhibits reuptake of the catecholamine neurotransmitter nor-adrenaline, which is a potent vasoconstrictor. By this mechanism it may induce coronary artery spasm and myocardial infarction. The drug has also been implicated in causing myocarditis through direct effects on the heart. In addition, its local anaesthetic properties block the fast inward sodium and slow calcium currents within myocardial cells, thereby predisposing to lethal ventricular arrhythmias. Cocaine also prolongs the QT-interval and increases the risk of torsades de pointes-type polymorphic ventricular tachycardia. Arrhythmias are best treated by anti-arrhythmic agents which do not prolong the QT-interval. Beta blockers are contraindicated in the management of cocaine-induced cardiac problems because they would result in unopposed alpha activity, causing profound vasoconstriction. Cocaine is a relatively rare cause of sudden death in young elite athletes. Relatively more common causes are shown (*Table B*).

Non-cardiac causes of mortality from cocaine include CVA, status epilepticus and rhabdomyolysis.

Table A. Myocardial ischaemia/infarction with normal coronary arteries

HCM
Aortic stenosis
Hypertensive heart disease
Coronary arteritis, particularly polyarteritis nodosa
Coronary artery embolus secondary to intramural thrombus or vegetation
Severe anaemia
Thyrotoxicosis
Phaeochromocytoma
Cocaine
Amphetamines

Table B. Causes of sudden cardiac death in young elite athletes

HCM (almost 50% of all cases)
Coronary artery anomalies
Arrhythmogenic right ventricular cardiomyopathy
Myocarditis
Mitral valve prolapse
Wolff–Parkinson–White syndrome
LQTS
Drug abuse
Sarcoidosis
Rhabdomyolysis
Heatstroke

Answer 137

1. Partially compensated respiratory acidosis.

The high pCO_2 and low pH is diagnostic of respiratory acidosis. The arterial bicarbonate is high, indicating that there is increased absorption of bicarbonate ions by the kidney in an attempt to normalize the pH. As the pH is still slightly lower than normal, this is most accurately termed partial compensation. (See Acid–base Disturbance, page 228.)

Question 138

A 16-year-old Turkish female was referred to the gynaeco-logical outpatient clinic with a 14-month history of amenorrhoea. She started menstruating at the age of 13 years. She had almost regular periods until the age of 14 and after this had three scanty periods and none for the past year. She was born in Turkey and had only recently come to England. At the age of nine years she had been commenced on hydrocortisone 15 mg in the morning and 10 mg in the evening for an illness about which both parents were very vague. Apart from occasional dizziness on standing suddenly, and infrequent headaches, there was no other past history of note. She had an 18-year-old sister who was well. Her parents were first cousins. Her father worked as a tailor and her mother was a housewife. None of them spoke much English.

Examination was declined by the patient, but the height and weight were recorded (1.52 m (under 50th centile) and 42 kg (less than 3rd centile)), and the blood pressure measured (90/60 mmHg).

Investigations are shown.

FBC	Hb 13 g/dl	Endocrine tests	17-hydroxyprogesterone
	WCC 7×10^9/l	(continued)	23 nmol/l (normal
	Platelets 200×10^9/l		<5 nmol/l)
Biochemistry	Sodium 138 mmol/l		Androstenedione 16 nmol/l
	Potassium 4.0 mmol/l		(normal 5–12 nmol/l)
	Urea 4 mmol/l		Dihydroepiandrostenedione
	Creatinine 60 µmol/l		21 nmol/l
	Blood sugar 5 mmol/l		(normal <12 nmol/l)
	Calcium 2.4 mmol/l		Recumbent plasma renin
	Phosphate 1.0 mmol/l		9 pmol/l/ml/h (normal
	AST 22 u/l		0.2–2.2)
	Alkaline phosphatase 179 u/l		Ambulant plasma renin
Endocrine tests	Thyroxine 18 pmol/l		12 pmol/l (normal 1.2–4.4)
	TSH 3.1 mu/l		Prolactin 385 mu/l
	FSH 5 u/l (normal 1–7 u/l)		(normal <450 mu/l)
	LH 8 u/l (normal 2–20 u/l)		Urinary pregnantetriol
	Oestradiol 90 pmol/l		elevated +++
	(normal 40–92 pmol/l)	US ovaries	Normal-sized ovaries
	Testosterone 9 nmol/l		containing multiple cysts
	(normal 1–3 nmol/l)		Small uterus

1. What is the diagnosis?
2. Which other drug should this patient be given?
3. Suggest at least three possible causes for the amenorrhoea.

Question 139

A 75-year-old male was investigated for increasing dyspnoea.

Results of investigations are shown.

1. What sign would you ascertain on auscultation of the precordium?

Chamber	Pressure (cm H_2O)	Oxygen saturation (%)
Right atrium	6	65
Right ventricle	25/6	67
Pulmonary artery pressure	25/18	67
PCWP (mean)	16	
Left ventricle	210/18	98
Aorta	210/55	98

Answer 138

1. Congenital adrenal hyperplasia (21-hydroxylase deficiency).
2. Fludrocortisone.
3. i. Underweight.
ii. Inadequate treatment for congenital adrenal hyperplasia.
iii. Elevated testosterone.
iv. Coexistent polycystic ovary syndrome (PCOS).

The presenting complaint of amenorrhoea has a wide differential diagnosis (*Table A*); however, the endocrine tests are most compatible with the diagnosis of congenital adrenal hyperplasia. Congenital adrenal hyperplasia may be caused by a number of enzyme defects in the biosynthetic pathway for steroid hormone synthesis within the adrenal gland. The deficiencies are inherited as an autosomal recessive trait. The most common abnormality by far is 21-hydroxylase deficiency, the gene for which is on chromosome 6 (adjacent to the HLA B locus). The enzyme is responsible for the conversion of 17-hydroxyprogesterone to cortisol (**138**).

21-hydroxylase deficiency leads to elevated 17-hydroxyprogesterone, which is metabolized to adrenal androgens. These ketosteroids (particularly pregnanetriol) are found in high concentrations in the urine. The patients are cortisol-deficient, and some may also have aldosterone deficiency. Patients with severe 21-hydroxylase deficiency present in infancy with vomiting and failure to thrive. Ambiguous genitalia are common. Males may have hypospadias and females may have fusion of the labia. Males with mild deficiency may present with precocious puberty and females with primary amenorrhoea, hursutism and virilism. Hursutism occurring before menarche is suggestive of congenital adrenal hyperplasia. Lack of cortisol is responsi-

ble for high ACTH levels which continue to drive the biosynthetic pathway.

Laboratory investigations reveal an elevated plasma 17-hydroxyprogesterone and ACTH. Urinary pregnanetriol (ketosteroid) levels are also elevated. Treatment is with hydrocortisone replacement. The dose is similar to that used in Addison's disease. The therapeutic response is judged by suppression of the urinary pregnanetriol levels to the upper limit of normal. Considerable care should be taken not to give a very high dose of hydrocortisone, as this may stunt growth. Patients with aldosterone deficiency as judged by an elevated renin level and postural hypotension should receive fludrocortisone.

In this patient there are several potential causes of amenorrhoea. The most obvious cause is her very low weight (see also *Table A*). Another important cause is the raised testosterone levels caused by an inadequate dose of hydrocortisone. The dose should be enough to inhibit ACTH secretion and suppress androgen synthesis. In this case, the adrenal androgen levels (dihydroepiandrostenedione) are very high. The patient also has evidence of polycystic ovaries, which are themselves a cause of primary amenorrhoea but may coexist with hyperandrogenic states such as congenital adrenal hyperplasia and Cushing's syndrome. The differential diagnoses of congenital adrenal hyperplasia are shown (*Table B*).

Differentiating congenital adrenal hyperplasia from arrhenoblastoma is usually easy because in the former cortisol levels are low and dihydroepiandrosterone sulphate is high. Similarly, congenital adrenal hyperplasia can be easily distinguished from Cushing's by measuring

---

Table A. Causes of amenorrhoea

Physiological (pregnancy)
Systemic disease (e.g. coeliac disease)
Weight loss
Anorexia nervosa
Excessive stress
Hypopituitarism
Prolactinoma
Primary ovarian failure (see list of causes of primary hypogonadism)
Congenital adrenal hyperplasia
PCOS
Cushing's syndrome
Androgen-secreting adrenal tumour
Arrhenoblastoma

Table B. Differential diagnoses of mild 21-hydroxylase deficiency

Polycystic ovaries
Androgen-secreting adrenal tumour
Arrhenoblastoma
Cushing's syndrome

serum cortisol and ACTH.

Differentiation from an adrenal androgen-secreting tumour is possible by performing a low-dose dexamethasone suppression test which will reduce urinary pregnanetriol levels in congenital adrenal hyperplasia, but not in an adrenal androgen-secreting tumour.

The differentiation from PCOS is possible by measuring 17-hydroxyprogesterone levels and dihydroepiandrosterone sulphate, both of which are high in congenital adrenal hyperplasia. Alternatively, a synacthen test may be performed which is associated with a normal cortisol response in PCOS, but not in congenital adrenal hyperplasia.

Answer 139

1. A long early diastolic murmur at the left lower sternal edge and in the aortic area.

The only abnormality is the very wide pulse pressure in the ascending aorta, which would be consistent with the diagnosis of aortic regurgitation. (See Guidelines for the Interpretation of Cardiac Catheter Data, page 220.)

Question 140

A 58-year-old male presented with nausea and pain in his right upper quadrant. On examination he had tender hepatomegaly with an irregular edge.

Investigations are shown.

1. What is the cause of his anaemia?
2. What investigation would you perform to confirm the diagnosis?

FBC	Hb 8 g/dl
	WCC 18×10^9/l
	Platelets 100×10^9/l
Blood film	Neutrophils 68%
	Normoblasts 8%
	Myeloblasts 8%
	Myelocytes 4%
	Metamyelocytes 6%
	Lymphocytes 15%

Question 141

A 13-year-old male was admitted to hospital with complete loss of vision in his right eye. He had been placed in a juvenile offenders' residential home six months ago for stealing on several occasions. His parents had separated a few months previously, and before that he had been living with his father, who was an alcohol abuser, and three dogs. Two weeks before admission he had complained of reduced visual acuity in his right eye which had progressively become worse.

On examination, he appeared well. He had generalized lymphadenopathy, and was clinically blind in the right eye. Examination of the fundus in the right eye revealed two large, raised whites lesion situated adjacent to the optic disc and in the macular region. He was apyrexial and all other physical examinations were normal.

Investigations are shown.

FBC	Hb 11.4 g/dl
	WCC 6.6×10^9/l
	(differential below)
	Platelets 180×10^9/l
	Neutrophils 4.1×10^9/l
	Lymphocytes 1.2×10^9/l
	Eosinophils 1.1×10^9/l
	Monocytes 0.11×10^9/l
	Basophils 0.09×10^9/l
ESR	25 mm/h
Biochemistry	Normal

1. What is the diagnosis?
2. List two useful investigations in confirming the diagnosis.

Answer 140

1. Marrow infiltration by malignant cells.
2. Marrow aspirate for histological examination.

Causes of a leucoerythroblastic anaemia

Malignant infiltration of any type
Storage disorders, e.g. Gaucher's disease
Myelosclerosis
Marble bone disease (osteopetrosis)
Leukaemoid reaction secondary to severe infections

The patient has a leucoerythroblastic anaemia which is characterized by immature granulocytes and red cells (normoblasts) in the peripheral blood film. This characteristically occurs when the marrow is replaced by malignant cells, cells containing metabolic products of storage disorders, fibrous tissue and bone. Leukaemias, lymphoma, adenocarcinoma, myeloma and myeloproliferative disease are all capable of malignant infiltration. In this case, the patient has a 'knobbly' liver, suggesting liver metastases most probably from a primary lung carcinoma. Carcinoma of the lung also metastasizes to the bone and may result in marrow infiltration by malignant cells. Other causes of a leucoerythroblastic anaemia are tabulated above. In marble bone disease, bony replacement of the marrow causes the leucoerythroblastic anaemia. In myelosclerosis, the cause is extensive fibrosis within the marrow space, and in Gaucher's disease the cause is large white cells laden with glucocerebrosides.

Answer 141

1. i. Ocular *Toxocara* infection or ocular larva migrans.
2. i. IgM antibodies to *Toxocara* in the aqueous or vitreous humour of the eye.
ii. IgM antibodies to *Toxocara* in the blood.

The patient has contracted *Toxocara* infection from the dogs. Toxocariasis is due to migrating larvae of the parasite, *T. canis*. The disease occurs where there is a large dog or cat population. It is well-recognized in the Western world, and it is estimated that approximately 2–3% of the population carry antibodies to the parasite. The parasite is carried in dogs (*T. canis*) and cats (*T. catis*). Embryonated eggs are passed into faeces and may be ingested by humans, particularly children in close contact with cats and dogs (ingestion of contaminated fur or soil).

The larvae from the eggs hatch out into the small intestine and migrate to liver, lungs and brain where they stimulate local granuloma formation by the immune system. They do not mature into adult worms.

Toxocariasis can produce two distinct clinical patterns; the classical visceral larva migrans syndrome, and ocular toxocariasis. Most children who develop the classical larva migrans remain asymptomatic. The minority develop myalgia, cough and anorexia. An urticarial rash is not uncommon. Physical examination may reveal lymphadenopathy and hepatosplenomegaly. The blood picture comprises of a neutrophil leucocytosis and a significant eosinophilia. The acute illness is of 2–3 weeks' duration, following which complete recovery is usual. In some individuals complete recovery may take as long as two years. The diagnosis is made by demonstrating positive antibodies to the secretory or excretory products of *Toxocara*. Liver biopsy may demonstrate granulomas with eosinophilic infiltration.

Ocular toxocariasis is characterized by granuloma formation in the eye. If the macular area is involved, blindness may occur. The general manifestations of classical visceral larva migrans and accompanying eosinophilia may be absent. Physical examination reveals a round swelling near the optic disc. The diagnosis is made by the demonstration of IgM antibodies to *Toxocara* in the aqueous or vitreous humour.

Treatment of the classical visceral larva migrans is with thiabendazole or diethylcarbamazine. Ocular toxocariasis is treated with laser photocoagulation. Local or intra-ocular steroids may be used as adjunct therapy.

Question 142

142a

142b

FBC	Hb 9 g/dl
	WCC $10 \times 10^9/l$
	Platelets $180 \times 10^9/l$
	MCV 82 fl
Biochemistry	Sodium 136 mmol/l
	Potassium 6 mmol/l
	Urea 43 mmol/l
	Creatinine 500 µmol/l
	Calcium 2.0 mmol/l
	Phosphate 1.7 mmol/l
	Alkaline phosphatase 305 u/l
	Albumin 35 g/l
Chest X-ray	Slight increase in the cardiothoracic ratio
	Upper lobe venous distension
X-ray of hand (**142b**)	
Ultrasound of kidneys	Bilaterally shrunken kidneys

A 21-year-old male presented with headaches, drowsiness, nausea, lethargy and general malaise. His appetite was reduced, but he had not lost any weight. The only other positive feature in the history was that of troublesome back pain and cramps in the legs over the past 18 months. The past medical history comprised a long history of intermittent lower abdominal pains as a child which were associated with vomiting but had subsided by the age of 15 years. At the age of 17 he was seen by a paediatrician for short stature and delayed puberty, but was then lost to follow up. He had worked as an assistant in a florist's shop for eight years. He took very occasional analgesia for the back pain. He was single. He was a non-smoker, and did not consume alcohol.

On examination, he was 1.53 m tall and weighed 45 kg. Secondary sexual characteristics were present. The heart rate was 98 beats/min, and regular, and blood pressure was 210/110 mmHg. The jugular venous pulsation was just visible in the neck with the patient recumbent at 45°. On examination of the precordium, the apex was not displaced, but was heaving in nature. The second heart sound was loud. Examination of the respiratory system and the abdomen was normal. On examination of the central nervous system, the patient was slightly drowsy, and the Glasgow coma scale was 13/15. The pupils were both equal in size and reacted to light. The appearances on examination of a fundus is shown (**142a**).

Investigations are shown.

1. List four abnormalities on the fundi.
2. What is the cause of the hypertension?
3. Explain the low calcium.
4. Describe the abnormality on the hand X-ray, and with what is it consistent?
5. Explain the anaemia.
6. What is the best explanation for the tachypnoea?
7. What is the best management of the hypertension in the short term?
8. List five steps in the long-term management of this patient.

Answer 142

1. i. Arteriovenous nipping.
ii. Flame-shaped haemorrhages.
iii. Cotton wool spots or retinal infarcts.
iv. Blurred disc or papilloedema.
2. Chronic renal failure (*Table A*).
3. Failure of 1α-hydroxylation of vitamin D, causing low levels of 1,25-dihydroxycholecalciferol, which is an active vitamin D metabolite.
4. Subperiosteal bone resorption and severe demineralization of the third metacarpals bilaterally. There is also an expansion in the proximal phalanx of the left third digit. Such a cystic appearance is seen in severe hyperparathyroid-related bone disease.
5. Deficiency of erythropoietin.
6. Uraemic acidosis. Pulmonary oedema is less likely, given the relatively clear chest and absence of interstitial shadowing on the chest X-ray (*Table B*).
7. Haemodialysis.
8. i. Regular haemodialysis.
ii. Control hypertension.
iii. Erythropoietin for anaemia.
iv. α-1-calcidol for hypocalcaemia.
v. Calcium carbonate to bind phosphate and prevent osteodystrophy.

The patient presents with hypertension, grossly abnormal renal function, grade IV hypertensive retinopathy (*Table C*) and drowsiness. These features could be explained by primary accelerated hypertension; however, the anaemia, bone biochemistry and X-ray appearance of the hand indicate that the most likely cause for the hypertension is chronic renal failure. It is difficult to be certain about the aetiology of the renal impairment because the past history is vague and the kidneys are shrunken. Renal biopsy in these instances reveals extensive glomerular scarring and is rarely helpful in the management of the patient. The history of intermittent abdominal pain and vomiting and investigation for short stature suggest that the cause may be chronic pyelonephritis. Other causes of chronic renal failure and the complications are shown (*Tables A and B*). The long and short-term management of this patient is outlined in 7 and 8 above. It is important to be aware that erythropoietin itself may worsen hypertension; therefore, extra care is required in managing hypertension in an individual taking erythropoietin. Good hypertensive control will reduce the rate of decline in renal function; however, given his weight of just 45 kg, a serum creatinine of over 500 µmol/l almost certainly represents end-stage renal failure requiring dialysis. In some patients with chronic renal failure and hypertension, reducing intravascular volume with dialysis is all that is required to control blood pressure.

Table A. Causes of chronic renal failure

Chronic glomerulonephritis
Chronic pyelonephritis
APCKD
Diabetes mellitus
Chronic hypertension
Renal artery stenosis
Renal papillary necrosis secondary to chronic analgesia
Hyperuricaemic nephropathy
Chronic nephrolithiasis

Table B. Complications of renal failure

Anaemia secondary to erythropoietin deficiency
Osteomalacia/rickets secondary to deficiency of active vitamin D metabolites
Hypertension (secondary to salt and water retention) and its complications
Metabolic acidosis
Hyperkalaemia
Osteodystrophy secondary to hyperparathyroidism resulting from chronic hyperphosphataemia
Fluid overload causing pulmonary and peripheral oedema
Pruritis secondary to hyperphosphataemia
Skin pigmentation
Hyperlipidaemia
Premature coronary artery disease (combination of hypertension and hyperlipidaemia)
Neuropathy

Table C. Wegener's classification of hypertensive retinopathy

I   Silver wiring of the arterioles
II Arteriovenous nipping
III Flame-shaped haemorrhages and cotton wool spots
IV Papilloedema

Question 143

A 42-year-old male was investigated for a three-year history of intermittent abdominal pain. He had suffered four episodes of pyelonephritis in the past four years which were treated by his general practitioner. There was a long history of migraines, for which he took mefenamic acid and paracetamol. Over the past few months he complained of increasing lethargy. There was no history of diarrhoea, weight loss, urinary hesitancy, nocturia or post micturition dribble. Four months ago he was noted to have a blood pressure of 180/110 mmHg which was under review. He was a florist by occupation. He was a non-smoker and consumed very occasional alcohol. His father died suddenly from a subarachnoid haemorrhage at the age of 40 years, but his mother was still alive and well. He had three brothers aged 44, 45 and 46 years respectively; the eldest brother had hypertension.

On examination, he appeared well at rest. There was no clubbing or peripheral oedema. The blood pressure was 180/105 mmHg. Examination of the abdomen revealed tenderness in both loins. Deep palpation of the loins was difficult due to tenderness. The percussion note throughout the abdomen was resonant and auscultation demonstrated normal bowel sounds. Examination of the cardiovascular and respiratory system was normal. Fundoscopy demonstrated silver wiring and arteriovenous nipping.

Investigations are shown.

FBC	Hb 15 g/dl
	WCC 5×10^9/l
	Platelets 240×10^9/l
ESR	15 mm/h
Biochemistry	Sodium 128 mmol/l
	Potassium 3.8 mmol/l
	Urea 20 mmol/l
	Creatinine 400 µmol/l
	Calcium 2.1 mmol/l
	Phosphate 1.9 mmol/l
	Albumin 39 g/l
Serum renin	Elevated
Urinalysis	Protein ++
	Blood ++
	24-hour urinary sodium 89 mmol/l

1. What is the most likely diagnosis?
A. Bilateral renal artery stenosis.
B. Chronic pyelonephritis.
C. Hypernephroma.
D. APCKD.
E. Analgesic nephropathy.

Question 144

A 16-year-old East African female was admitted with a two-week history of intermittent, sharp, right upper quadrant pain which is worse on inspiration. The pain radiated to the umbilicus and right loin and was most severe on the night of admission. There were no other symptoms. She had just finished menstruating. Her family had very recently immigrated to Britain from Kenya.

On examination, she had shallow respiration. The temperature was 37.5°C (99.5°F). There was tenderness and guarding in the right hypochondrium. The liver was palpable 6 cm below the costal margin, and there was tenderness in the 9th intercostal space in the mid axillary line. The right lung base was dull to percussion with reduced air entry on auscultation.

Investigations are shown.

FBC	Hb 13 g/dl
	WCC 16×10^9/l (neutrophil leucocytosis)
	Platelets 590×10^9/l
ESR	70 mm/h
U&E	Normal
Chest X-ray	Raised right hemidiaphragm
	Clear lung fields
Urinalysis	Normal

1. What is the most likely diagnosis?
2. List at least three investigations you would perform to confirm the diagnosis.

Answer 143

1. D. APCKD.

This middle-aged patient presents with abdominal pain and advanced renal failure. All of the options given may cause abdominal pain and renal failure (*Table*). The episodes of pyelonephritis in a middle-aged male should raise suspicion of obstructive uropathy or an anatomical abnormality in the renal tract. In the context of the possibility of the latter, the family history of subarachnoid haemorrhage and hypertension should arouse the suspicion of APCKD. The normal Hb in the presence of chronic renal failure should clinch the diagnosis because APCKD is one of the few causes of chronic renal failure where the Hb is preserved. This is due to inappropriate erythropoietin secretion in some patients with the condition. Hypernephroma may also cause polycythaemia for the same reason but does not cause a salt-losing nephropathy as seen in this case.

APCKD is inherited as an autosomal dominant trait. It is characterized by multiple thin-walled cysts in the kidney which become progressively larger over the years and cause renal failure by compression of the nephrons. In 90% of patients, the abnormal gene is on the short arm of chromosome 16 which encodes a transmembrane protein termed polycystin. The exact function of it is unclear but it is thought to be involved in mediating cell-matrix interactions. Of the other 10% of patients, some

Abdominal pain and renal failure
Henoch–Schönlein purpura
Haemolytic uraemic syndrome
Polyarteritis nodosa
APCKD
Nephrolithiasis
Analgesic nephropathy
Retroperitoneal fibrosis
Dissecting aortic aneurysm
Legionnaire's disease
Acute pancreatitis
Ethylene glycol poisoning

have abnormalities linked to a locus on chromosome 4. Clinical symptoms comprise flank pain, haematuria, nocturia and recurrent urinary tract infections. Hypertension develops in 75% of cases. End-stage renal failure may occur at any age. The patients may be anaemic due to haematuria and uraemia; however, polycythaemia secondary to increased erythropoietin is recognized. Malignant transformation within cysts is also recognized. Associations include berry aneurysms causing intracranial haemorrhage and mitral valve prolapse. Management includes family screening of first-degree relatives, early treatment of urinary tract infections, and meticulous blood pressure control.

Answer 144

1. Hepatic abscess secondary to *Entamoeba histolytica* (amoebic liver abscess).
2. i. Ultrasound of the liver.
ii. Microscopy from liver aspirates.
iii. Indirect haemagglutination tests (over 95% with liver abscess are positive, but the test cannot distinguish between past and current infection).

The patient presents with hepatomegaly, a raised right hemidiaphragm, and localized tenderness in the 9th intercostal space. These features are consistent with a hepatic abscess. She has been in East Africa, which makes an amoebic abscess the most probable cause of her signs and symptoms. Some 50% of patients with amoebic abscess have no history of dysentery. Symptoms include right hypochondrial pain, fever, sweating, intermittent fever and rigors. Hepatic enlargement and localized

tenderness in the right hypochondrium or intercostal spaces. Enlargement of the liver abscess is usually upwards, and may cause compression of the right hemidiaphragm and atelectasis of the overlying lung. Jaundice and abnormality of LFT are rare. US or CT scan will demonstrate the abscess or abscesses. Aspiration of the pus may demonstrate the organism. Sigmoidoscopy and biopsy for microscopy and stool microscopy have a low yield, but indirect haemagglutination tests have high titres in the presence of a hepatic abscess. The lesions may be as large as 10 cm. Rupture of the abscess into the lung and development of a hepatobronchial fistula is a recognized complication (anchovy-sauce sputum). Peritonitis, pericarditis and cutaneous sinus formation are rare complications.

Treatment is with metronidazole or tinidazole. Diloxanide is also given to eliminate any on-going gastrointestinal infection.

Question 145

A 14-year-old male was admitted to hospital with a 12-hour history of colicky right-sided abdominal pain and vomiting. He had a past history of recurrent chest infections which had been treated by his general practitioner. He was also thought to be asthmatic, and took a regular bronchodilating inhaler. He had intermittent loose, bulky stool but had

FBC	Hb 10 g/dl
	WCC 14 × 10⁹/l
	Platelets 480 × 10⁹/l
	MCV 80 fl
Biochemistry	Sodium 135 mmol/l
	Potassium 3.2 mmol/l
	Urea 9 mmol/l
	Total protein 70 g/l
	Albumin 34 g/l
	Calcium 2.2 mmol/l
	Phosphate 0.7 mmol/l
Chest X-ray (**145c**)	
Abdominal X-ray (**145d**)	

never experienced abdominal pain. He had a younger brother and sister who were well. His father was a shop assistant and his mother was a part time general practitioner's receptionist.

On examination, he did not appear acutely unwell. He had mild clubbing. The abdomen was distended. There was generalized tenderness on palpation, as well as a firm mass in the right iliac fossa. Bowel sounds were tinkling. The rectum was empty. Auscultation of the lung fields revealed coarse crackles throughout the lung fields.

Growth charts for height and weight are shown (**145a**, **145b**). Investigations are shown.

1. What is the abnormality on the growth chart?
2. Comment on the chest X-ray.
3. Comment on the abdominal X-ray.
4. What is the cause of his presentation problem?
5. What is the management of his current problem?
6. What is the full diagnosis?
7. Which test would you request to confirm the diagnosis?

Answer 145

1. This patient has fallen off the third centile for height at the age of 10 years and for weight at the age of 14 years.

2. The chest X-ray is grossly abnormal. There is widespread fibrotic change, patchy consolidation, and bronchiectasis. In the context of this history the findings are consistent with cystic fibrosis.

3. The erect abdominal X-ray reveals dilated loops of small bowel and multiple fluid levels consistent with small bowel obstruction.

4. Meconium ileus equivalent. This is bowel obstruction resulting from a combination of steatorrhoea and viscid intestinal secretions causing faecal impaction in the ascending colon or the ileocaecal junction.

5. The management steps are as follows:
- Rest the bowel; the patient should be completely restricted from oral solids and fluids and should have intravenous fluid supplements. A nasogastric tube should be placed in situ to prevent gastric dilatation and vomiting.
- Diagnostic and therapeutic manoeuvres: a gastrograffin enema should be performed which is both diagnostic and therapeutic. Patients with any form of obstruction should not have barium studies.
- Other therapeutic steps: acetylcysteine given intravenously or through the nasogastric tube has been shown to be very useful in resolving bowel obstruction.
- In the long term, the plan is to reduce steatorrhoea, which can be done by increasing pancreatic supplements. There have been recent reports of fibrous colonopathy in association with a high dose of *Pancrease* pancreatic supplements. The risk of the condition with *Creon* pancreatic supplements is very small.

6. The full diagnosis is cystic fibrosis. The diagnosis should be suspected in any young child who presents with chronic gastrointestinal and respiratory complaints.

7. The diagnosis of cystic fibrosis can be confirmed by demonstrating a sweat sodium concentration exceeding 60 mmol/l.

Cystic fibrosis is an autosomal recessive condition with a prevalence of 1/2,500 which is characterized by viscid respiratory and gastrointestinal secretions. The abnormality is in the gene encoding a chloride ion channel in the nasal epithelium, lungs, salivary glands, pancreas, intestine and bile ducts. This chloride ion channel has been

---

Table A. The clinical manifestations of cystic fibrosis

Respiratory
Nasal polyps
Otitis media
Asthma

Bronchiolitis	Recurrent pneumonia	*Staphylococcus aureus, Haemophilus influenzae, Pseudomonas aeruginosa*
Bronchiectasis	Lung abscess/empyema	
	Haemoptysis	
	Aspergillus infection	
	Lung fibrosis	
	Pneumothorax	
	Cor pulmonale	

Gastrointestinal
Meconium ileus (birth)
Rectal prolapse (neonate)
Steatorrhoea (pancreatic insufficiency)
Meconium ileus equivalent (infancy onwards)
Malabsorption (fat-soluble vitamins due to pancreatic insufficiency usually, or biliary obstruction)
Gall stones
Secondary biliary cirrhosis

Miscellaneous
Non-erosive arthropathy
Infertility in males

Table B. Causes of a false-positive sweat sodium test
Hypothyroidism
Familial hypoparathyroidism
Mucopolysaccharidoses
α-1 antitrypsin deficiency
Addison's disease

mutation which results in the deletion of the amino acid phenylalanine on position 508. This mutation accounts for 70–80% of all cases. The clinical manifestations are listed (*Table A*). The differential diagnoses are other causes of recurrent respiratory infections and diarrhoea in young children which include hypogammaglobulinaemia and intestinal lymphangiectasia. The genetic heterogeneity of the condition means that the diagnosis continues to rely on the demonstration of a sweat sodium >60 mmol/l. However, there are conditions associated with a false-positive sweat sodium test (*Table B*). It is also worth noting that a small proportion of patients with cystic fibrosis do not have a positive sweat sodium test.

termed the CFTR. The gene is located on chromosome 7. Over 200 different mutations have been described within the gene, but by far the most common is a point

---

Question 146

A 6-year-old female was seen in the accident and emergency department with a two-year history of a painful swollen right knee which developed after she fell at school. Two years previously she had a similar episode affecting the left knee, following which she had persistent swelling and discomfort for several weeks. At that stage she had a FBC which was normal and an X-ray of the left knee which revealed soft tissue swelling. In the interim she had recurrent episodes of painful swelling of the left knee for no obvious reason which would subside after a few days. At the age of two years she sustained a large haematoma on her forehead after a fall at home. The only other past history of note was a recent review by the ophthalmologist for a left convergent squint.

She had achieved her milestones normally, but had problems with reading which were attributed to her squint. She was one of three siblings. All three were adopted and had come from different families. Her parents appeared very caring. The father was a businessman who spent many days away from home and the mother was a housewife.

On examination, she was below the third centile for height and was on the 50th centile for weight. There was a painful swelling over the left knee consistent with a synovial effusion. The right knee was not swollen, but movement of the knee demonstrated crepitus. There was an obvious convergent squint. The neck was short and the hands, particularly the fourth and fifth digits appeared small.

Investigations are shown.

FBC	Hb 11 g/dl
	WCC 6×10^9/l
	Platelets 112×10^9/l
Blood film	Normal
Clotting	PT 12 s
	APTT 94 s
	BT 8 min
Biochemistry	Sodium 136 mmol/l
	Potassium 3.8 mmol/l
	Urea 6 mmol/l
	Creatinine 80 μmol/l
	Calcium 2.3 mmol/l
	Phosphate 1.0 mmol/l
	Albumin 40 g/l
X-ray of left knee	Soft-tissue swelling
	No bony deformity
X-ray of right knee	Chondrocalcinosis

1. List two different diagnoses.
2. What is the mechanism for the swollen knee?
3. Give two possible underlying causes for the swollen knee.
4. Which two investigations would you request to confirm your answer to 1?

Answer 146

1. i. Turner's syndrome.
ii. Haemophilia A or Haemophilia B.
2. Haemarthrosis; bleeding into the knee joint.
3. i. Haemophilia A.
ii. Haemophilia B.
4. i. Buccal smear for karyotyping to confirm Turner's syndrome.
ii. Factor VIII assay or Factor IX assay to confirm haemophilia A or B respectively.

The patient has several morphological features of Turner's syndrome (see *Table C* in Answer **158**, page 209). All of these morphological features, particularly short metacarpals may also occur in pseudohypoparathyroidism; however, the normal bone biochemistry is against the diagnosis. Short metacarpals may occur in other conditions (*Table A*).

The patient also has an important clotting abnormality, suggested by the elevated APTT. The swollen knee is most probably due to haemorrhage into the joint. The right knee has features of chondrocalcinosis possibly due to recurrent haemarthroses. The PT is normal, suggesting that the defect is in the intrinsic pathway of the clotting cascade.

Causes of a raised APTT include deficiency in any one of the clotting factors in the intrinsic pathway, DIC, or heparin therapy. The normal PT and fibrinogen level makes DIC very unlikely. The normal BT excludes Von Willebrand's disease. The most likely clotting abnormality here is either factor VIII (haemophilia A) or factor IX (haemophilia B; Christmas disease) deficiency. Both are X-linked recessive; thus normal females with two X chromosomes will not exhibit the disease phenotype, even if they have inherited the abnormal gene. However, patients with Turner's syndrome have just one X chromosome and effectively have the same chance of being affected by an X-linked recessive genetic condition as males.

Table A. Causes of short metacarpals

Turner's syndrome
Noonan's syndrome
Pseudohypoparathyroidism
Sickle cell dactylitis
Juvenile chronic arthritis
Recurrent hand trauma

Table B. Differentiation between haemophilia A, B and Von Willebrand's disease

	HA	*HB*	*Von Willebrand's*
PT	Normal	Normal	Normal
APTT	↑	↑	↑
BT	Normal	Normal	↑
Factor VIII$_c$	↓↓	Normal	↓
Factor VIII$_{VWB}$	Normal	Normal	↓
Ristocetin platelet aggregation	Normal	Normal	↓

Question 147

A 48-year-old clerical worker in a large insurance company was admitted with malaise, increasing shortness of breath and confusion. One week before admission he had a dry cough, chills, headaches and generalized aches throughout his body. He saw his general practitioner, who prescribed amoxycillin 500 mg, three times daily. Two days later, the patient developed generalized abdominal pain and loose motion. Over the next 24 hours, he had become increasingly confused, and started to hallucinate. His wife became concerned, and brought him to the accident and emergency department. He had been in Spain six weeks before his illness. He smoked 20 cigarettes a day, and consumed 4 units of alcohol a night.

On examination, he appeared unwell and dehydrated. His temperature was 38.7°C (101.7°F). The heart rate was 110 beats/min, and regular, and the blood pressure was 120/70 mmHg. On examination of the respiratory system he was noted to have a respiratory rate of 35/min. On auscultation, there were coarse crackles at the right lung base. Examination of the precordium was normal. Abdominal examination revealed generalized abdominal tenderness, but no guarding or rigidity. Central nervous system examination revealed a Glasgow coma score of 9/15. The patient was disorientated in time and space, but there was no focal neurological abnormality.

Investigations are shown.

FBC	Hb 13.5 g/dl	Arterial blood	pH 7.37
	WCC 12.1 × 10^9/l (neutrophils	gases	pO$_2$ 7.3 kPa
	10.2 × 10^9/l; lymphocytes		pCO$_2$ 4 kPa
	1.5 × 10^9/l)		Bicarbonate 18 mmol/l
	Platelets 140 × 10^9/l		Oxygen saturation 83%
Biochemistry	Sodium 128 mmol/l	Chest X-ray	Right lower lobe
	Potassium 4 mmol/l		consolidation, and a small
	Urea 10 mmol/l		associated pleural effusion
	Creatinine 160 μmol/l	ECG	Sinus tachycardia
	Bilirubin 22 μmol/l	Urinalysis	Trace of blood
	ALT 75 u/l		Protein ++
	Alkaline phosphatase 102 u/l		
	Gamma GT 102 u/l		
	Albumin 29 g/l		

1. What is the most probable diagnosis?
2. List three possible causes for the low sodium.
3. List three further investigations you would perform to make a rapid diagnosis.
4. Which antibiotic therapy would you institute whilst awaiting the definitive diagnosis?
5. List three therapeutic interventions you would initiate to manage this condition assuming a definitive diagnosis has already been made.

Question 148

A 34-year-old West African female presented with a three-month history of increasing ankle oedema and abdominal distension. There was no history of cough, exertional dyspnoea or orthopnoea. She was married with a five-year-old daughter. She was a non-smoker, and drank alcohol very occasionally. She had worked as a fish farm administrator in Nigeria before moving to England three years ago.

On examination, there was no evidence of pallor, jaundice or lymphadenopathy. She had considerable, pitting, lower-limb oedema. The heart rate was 100 beats/min, and irregularly irregular. The blood pressure was 95/75 mmHg. The JVP was elevated to the level of the ear lobes. On examination of the precordium the apex beat was not palpable. The heart sounds were soft. There were no cardiac murmurs. Auscultation of the lung fields was normal. Abdominal examination revealed firm hepatomegaly palpable 6 cm below the costal margin and shifting dullness. The spleen was not palpable. Neurological examination and examination of the skin was normal.

Investigations are shown.

FBC	Hb 12 g/dl
	WCC 7 × 10^9/l
	(normal differential)
	Platelets 300 × 10^9/l
Urinalysis	Protein +
Chest X-ray	Normal cardiac size and clear lung fields
ECG	Low QRS voltage and non-specific lateral T-wave changes

1. Which investigations would be most useful in making the diagnosis?
2. What is the most probable diagnosis?

Answer 147

1. Legionnaire's disease.
2. i. Syndrome of inappropriate ADH secretion.
ii. Diarrhoea and vomiting.
iii. Salt-losing nephritis/acute tubulointerstitial nephritis.
3. i. Urine for *Legionella* antigen.
ii. Direct immunofluorescent antibody test on sputum, bronchial washings, pleural effusion or blood.
iii. IgM RMAT for *Legionella*.
4. Intravenous cefotaxime and oral erythromycin.
5. i. Oxygen.
ii. Intravenous erythromycin or azithromycin and oral rifampicin.
iii. Intravenous rehydration with CVP monitoring.

Conditions simultaneously involving the lower respiratory tract and central nervous system

Infections
HIV
TB
Legionnaire's disease
Mycoplasma pneumonia
Streptococcal/staphylococcal pneumonia
Malaria
Cystercercosis

Malignancy
Primary or secondary bronchial carcinoma

Granulomatous disease
Sarcoidosis
Histiocytosis X

Vasculitides
Polyarteritis nodosa
Wegener's granulomatosis
SLE

Neuroectodermal syndromes
Neurofibromatosis
Tuberose sclerosis

Sickle cell syndromes

This previously fit middle-aged man presents with respiratory problems, abdominal symptoms and confusion. Biochemical tests reveal a low sodium and evidence of renal dysfunction. The full blood count reveals a mildly raised WCC with a relative lymphopenia. The most probable diagnosis which ties all of this together is Legionnaire's disease. The condition is caused by the organism *Legionella pneumophilia*. Epidemic outbreaks can occur among previously fit individuals staying in hotels, institutions or hospitals where the cooling systems have been contaminated with the organism. It can also occur in sporadic cases and in the immunocompromised where the source of infection is unknown. It is spread via the aerosol route. Incubation period is between 2–10 days. Males are affected more than females.

Legionnaire's disease is preceded by a prodromal illness similar to a viral infection with headaches, myalgia, anorexia and pyrexia. Approximately 50% have abdominal symptoms (nausea, vomiting and diarrhoea). Neurological symptoms such as confusion, hallucinations, peripheral neuropathy, myelitis and, rarely, a cerebellar syndrome can occur. Patients may develop renal failure, usually secondary to an acute tubulointerstitial nephritis. Liver involvement is usually mild and characterized by abnormal LFT.

Hyponatraemia is common and is usually due to inappropriate ADH secretion; however, loss of sodium from the kidneys (acute tubulointerstitial nephritis) and gastrointestinal tract (diarrhoea and vomiting) may also contribute. Other biochemical features include hypocalcaemia, hypophosphataemia, and raised creatinine kinase (myositis). On the blood film there is a normal or mildly raised WCC with a moderate neutrophilia and relative lymphopenia. A mild coagulopathy can occur. Chest X-ray usually shows a unilateral lobar and then multilobar shadowing, with or without an associated pleural effusion.

A rapid diagnosis can be made using the tests mentioned above. Urinary *Legionella* antigen has a yield of 90% within the first week of the illness. Serology relies on measuring antibody titres in acute and convalescent serum samples separated by 10–14 days; therefore a reader would not score marks if asked specifically for tests to make a rapid diagnosis. Similarly, culturing this fastidious organism (using buffered charcoal yeast media) may take up to three weeks and has a low yield, and therefore would not score marks.

Treatment involves high-concentration oxygen and antibiotic therapy with intravenous erythromycin or azithromycin plus oral rifampicin. Before the diagnosis of Legionnaire's disease is confirmed, the patient should also receive a cephalosporin to cover the possibility of pneumonia due to *Streptococcus pneumoniae* which may present similarly. Rehydration would have to be performed with CVP monitoring as the patient has evidence of renal involvement and the plasma electrolytes should be monitored daily.

Conditions causing lung and brain involvement simultaneously are common in postgraduate examinations in which Legionnaire's disease is commonly tested. Other causes of simultaneous lung and cerebral involvement are tabulated.

Answer 148

1. i. Echocardiography.
ii. Cardiac MRI.
iii. Left and right cardiac catheter.
2. i. Pericardial constriction.
ii. Restrictive cardiomyopathy.

The patient has signs of severe right heart failure, but the chest X-ray reveals a normal-sized heart. The differential diagnosis of severe heart failure in the absence of significant cardiac enlargement is between pericardial constriction and a restrictive cardiomyopathy.

If we consider the possibility of restrictive cardiomyopathy (*Table A*), then there is little information in the history to suggest systemic sclerosis, haemochromatosis, carcinoid syndrome or anthracycline therapy. We are left with the possibility of malignancy, amyloidosis, EMF or idiopathic restrictive cardiomyopathy; however, the latter is extremely rare and some cardiologists are unsure if it even exists. There is no real evidence of malignancy. Cardiac amyloidosis is usually associated with myeloma of which there is no real evidence in this case. Moreover, it is more common in the 6th and 7th decade and more common in males. It is often associated with macroglossia and neuropathy, which appears to be absent here. EMF has two variants; the tropical and temperate form (*Table B*). The findings in favour of the tropical form of EMF is its insidious presentation and normal eosinophil count. However, tropical EMF is confined to young malnourished, poverty-stricken individuals with a high parasite load, and it is highly unlikely whether any of these factors would apply to a fish-farm administrator.

The most probable diagnosis is pericardial constriction. This is usually insidious and presents with signs of severe right heart failure, but little in the way of left heart failure. Contrary to popular belief, most cases of pericardial constriction are idiopathic. Other causes of pericardial constriction are listed in *Table C*.

In a tropical country, tuberculous pericarditis would be a possible aetiological candidate; however, there is complete absence of radiological evidence of previous pulmonary TB.

Echocardiography is useful in differentiating peri

Table A. Causes of restrictive cardiomyopathy

Idiopathic (extremely rare)
EMF: temperate
         tropical
Systemic sclerosis
Amyloidosis
Haemochromatosis
Carcinoid syndrome
Malignancy
Anthracycline

Table B. Differences between temperate and tropical EMF

	Temperate	*Tropical*
Presentation	Acute	Insidious
Fever	Common	Unusual
Multisystem involvement	Common	Unusual
Previous ill health or malnourishment	Uncommon	Very common
Eosinophil count	High	Normal

Table C. Causes of pericardial constriction

Idiopathic	Bacterial pericarditis
TB	Radiotherapy

Table D. Echocardiographic features of pericardial constriction and restrictive cardiomyopathy

	Pericardial constriction	Restrictive cardiomyopathy
Left and right atria	Enlarged/normal	Enlarged
Left and right ventricles	Normal	Usually normal/enlarged
Endocardium	Normal	Bright
Myocardial texture	Normal	Normal/bright
Valves	Normal	Affected (mitral and tricuspid regurgitation)
Doppler	Low E/A inspiration High E/A expiration	Large E*, small A**
Pericardium	May be thickened	Normal

* Early or passive left ventricular filling
** Late or active ventricular filling

cardial constriction from a restrictive cardiomyopathy (*Table D*). Restrictive cardiomyopathy has classic echo-cardiographic features. In pericardial constriction, the pericardium may seem to be thickened. Cardiac MRI may be more useful than echocardiography in demonstrating pericardial thickness.

An unequivocal method of differentiating the two condition is by performing a left- and right-heart cardiac catheterization. Pericardial constriction encases the whole heart, therefore the right and left end-diastolic pressures are equal, as are the atrial pressures. In contrast, restrictive cardiomyopathy is patchy; thus LVEDP is slightly higher than right ventricular end-diastolic pressure (**148**). In addition, there is evidence of mitral and/or tricuspid regurgitation, which is generally absent in pericardial constriction.

Pericardial constriction | Restrictive cardiomyopathy

Question 149

A 23-year-old homosexual requested an HIV test after his partner had been diagnosed as having the condition. Apart from a febrile illness eight weeks previously, he had been relatively well. Physical examination was entirely normal.

Investigations performed in clinic are shown.

1. Does this patient require treatment?
2. Which medication(s) should be considered?

FBC	Hb 13 g/dl
	WCC 6×10^9/l
	Platelets 310×10^9/l
HIV serology	IgG HIV antibody-positive
CD4 count	510×10^6/l (normal range $500–1,300 \times 10^6$/l)
Viral RNA	20,000 copies/ml
Chest X-ray	Normal

Question 150

A 57-year-old male was admitted with a seven-month history of increasing breathlessness and swollen ankles. Just before admission he had developed paroxysmal nocturnal dyspnoea. He had seen his general practitioner who had prescribed 80 mg of frusemide, with very slight effect. He had no past medical history of note, and there was no family history of cardiovascular disease. He was a non-smoker and consumed about 7 units of alcohol per week. He had been a patron for a large charity organization for several years.

On examination, he appeared pale and was breathless on very slight exertion. The heart rate was 100 beats/min, and regular; blood pressure was 90/60 mmHg. The JVP was raised 6 cm above the sternal angle and revealed prominent a- and c–v waves. The apex was not palpable, but on auscultation of the precordium there was a loud third heart sound. On examination of the lungs there was reduced air entry bilaterally at both lung bases. Abdominal examination revealed hepatomegaly palpable 7 cm below the costal margin, and some ascites.

Investigations are shown.

FBC	Hb 11 g/dl
	WCC 6 × 10⁹/l
	Platelets 100 × 10⁹/l
	MCV 88 fl
ESR	70 mm/h
Biochemistry	Sodium 135 mmol/l
	Potassium 3.9 mmol/l
	Urea 15 mmol/l
	Creatinine 110 µmol/l
	Bilirubin 33 µmol/l
	AST 64 u/l
	Alkaline phosphatase 200 u/l
	Albumin 18 g/l
ECG (**150a**)	
Chest X-ray (**150b**)	
Renal US	Renal size enlarged slightly bilaterally, but no ureteric obstruction
Echocardiogram (**150c**)	
Renal biopsy (**150d**)	

1. Comment on the chest X-ray.
2. Comment on the ECG.
3. What is the renal diagnosis?
4. What is the cause of cardiac failure?

5. What is the overall diagnosis?
6. List two important investigations which you would perform.

Answer 149

1. The patient is HIV-positive. His CD4 count is within normal limits, but he has a very heavy viral load which is generally a poor prognostic marker of disease progression and an indicator for treatment.
2. Combination of two nucleoside analogues and a protease inhibitor.

AIDS-defining conditions

Pneumocystis carinii pneumonia
TB (*Mycobacterium avium intracellulare*)
Cryptococcus neoformans
Cryptosporidium
Isospora belli
Oesophageal or disseminated *Candida* (but not oral)
Herpes infection
CMV retinitis, colitis, oesophagitis and encephalitis
Oral leukoplakia
Toxoplasmosis
Kaposi's sarcoma

Patients infected with HIV may present following the seroconversion syndrome, with generalized lymphadenopathy or with AIDS-defining opportunistic illnesses (*Table*). The management of HIV infection is dependent on the CD4 count and the viral RNA load. Recommendations for initiating therapy in patients infected with HIV include all patients with a CD4 count of $<500 \times 10^6/l$, as well as asymptomatic patients who have a CD4 count $>500 \times 10^6/l$ but evidence of active viral RNA ($>10,000$ viral copies per ml). Some experts will initiate treatment in patients with a CD4 count $>500 \times 10^6/l$ in the presence of any detectable level of virus. Patients with AIDS-defining illnesses usually have a CD4 $<200 \times 10^6/l$. Treatment is in the form of triple therapy, comprising combinations of nucleoside analogues which inhibit the viral reverse transcriptase enzyme and a protease inhibitor which inhibits viral protein synthesis.

Examples of nucleoside analogue combinations include AZT and didanosine (AZT/ddI), AZT and zalcitabine (AZT/ddC) or AZT and lamivudine (AZT/3TC). Commonly used protease inhibitors include ritonavir, indinavir and saquinavir.

Answer 150

1. i. Bilateral pleural effusions; the right effusion being larger than the left.
ii. Prominent pulmonary arteries.
2. Small voltage complexes with T-wave inversion in the lateral leads.
3. Nephrotic syndrome due to renal amyloidosis.
4. Restrictive cardiomyopathy secondary to cardiac amyloid.
5. Primary amyloidosis.
6. i. Serum immunoglobulins/immunoelectrophoresis.
ii. Urinalysis for Bence–Jones protein estimation.

The combination of nephrotic syndrome and cardiac failure should always raise the suspicion of primary amyloidosis or AL amyloid. Primary amyloid affects approximately 10–15% of all patients with myeloma. In primary amyloidosis, the amyloid is made up of immunoglobulin light chains and glycoprotein. Clinical features include restrictive cardiomyopathy, macroglossia, peripheral neuropathy, nephrotic syndrome, purpura, and isolated clotting factor X deficiency. Cardiac amyloid has a poor prognosis as it results in a stiff ventricle with poor systolic and diastolic function. It responds poorly to diuretics. Arrhythmias and conduction tissue disease are common. The ECG commonly reveals small complexes, pathological Q-waves and non-specific T-wave changes. Echocardiography demonstrates thickened left and right ventricular walls, which have a ground-glass appearance. The ventricular cavities are small, but the atria are enlarged (as in this case). The interatrial septum is often bright. The definitive diagnosis of amyloidosis rests on tissue diagnosis. Rectal or gingival biopsy are useful; however, the former has a lower yield. Serum amyloid protein (SAP) scans are useful in identifying tissues infiltrated with amyloid; however, an important exception is cardiac infiltration, which is best identified with cardiac biopsy.

The other important type of amyloidosis for the candidate doing higher specialist examinations in internal medicine includes systemic amyloidosis. In this case, the protein comprising amyloid is protein AA. This occurs in chronic inflammatory conditions or infections. Examples include rheumatoid arthritis, bronchiectasis, inflammatory bowel disease and familial Mediterranean fever. This type of amyloid has a predilection for the kidneys, causing nephrotic syndrome, haematuria and renal failure. Hepatosplenomegaly is present in over 20% of cases.

Question 151

A 28-year-old female presented with a four-week history of progressive difficulty with walking, clumsiness of her hands, and slurring of the speech. Before this she had been relatively well, with the exception of occasional episodes of central chest pain and breathlessness when she was stressed, or on rushing suddenly. In the past four weeks she had fallen twice because she was 'not in control of her lower limbs'. Her hands were clumsy and she was having difficulty washing dishes or holding cups. There was no history of headaches or any family history of neurological disease. She was a non-smoker and consumed 1–2 glasses of wine per week.

On examination, she appeared well at rest. She measured 1.81 m. She had a high-arched palate, kypho-scoliosis and mild bilateral pes cavus. Her speech was mildly dysarthric. On examination of her upper limbs the power was normal. The tone was slightly increased in both forearms. There was clinical evidence of an intention tremor, past pointing, finger nose ataxia and dysdiado-chokinesia. The reflexes were brisk bilaterally. On examination of the lower limbs the power was slightly reduced bilaterally. The tone was increased and heel–shin ataxia was present. The knee reflexes were brisk, but the ankle jerks were absent. The plantar response was upgoing bilaterally. On examination of the cardiovascular system the heart rate was 90 beats/min, and regular; blood pressure was 100/70 mmHg. The apex was not displaced, but was heaving in nature. On auscultation there was a harsh ejection systolic murmur at the left lower sternal edge which was louder on standing suddenly and softer on squatting. The remainder of the physical examination was normal.

1. What is the diagnosis?
2. What is the cause of the cardiac murmur?
3. List two other associations of the condition.

Question 152

A 44-year-old Nigerian male was investigated for right upper quadrant pain, abdominal distension and ankle swelling:

Chamber	Pressure (mmHg)	Oxygen saturation (%)
Right atrium	17	68
Right ventricle	48/30	68
Pulmonary artery	40/22	68
PCWP	18	
Left ventricle	90/30	96
Aorta	85/65	96

A lateral view chest X-ray is shown (152a).

1. What are the abnormalities in the cardiac catheter data?
2. What is the abnormality on the chest X-ray?
3. What is the diagnosis?

152a

Answer 151

1. Friedreich's ataxia.
2. i. Hypertrophic cardiomyopathy (hypertrophic obstructive cardiomyopathy).
3. i. Diabetes mellitus.
ii. Optic atrophy.

The patient has pes cavus, signs of cerebellar and pyramidal tract disease. In addition, there is a history of chest pains and breathlessness suggesting cardiovascular disease and a cardiac murmur which is compatible with dynamic left ventricular outflow tract obstruction characteristic of hypertrophic obstructive cardiomyopathy. The complete diagnosis is Friedreich's ataxia.

Friedreich's ataxia is an autosomal recessive condition due to a mutation in a gene encoding the protein frataxin on chromosome 9. The mutation comprises of unstable expansions of the GAA repeat of variable size (120–1,700) in the first intron. The exact function of frataxin is unknown but early reports suggest that it is a mitochondrial iron transport protein. The prevalence is 1/50,000. It is the most common example of the hereditary ataxias. There is degeneration of the dorsal spinal columns, the spinocerebellar tracts, the pyramidal tracts, and the dorsal root ganglion cells. The syndrome is dominated by progressive ataxia. The usual age of onset is the second decade, but the disease may not appear until as late as the fourth decade. The lower limbs are generally affected before the upper limbs. Difficulty in walking and stumbling regularly are early signs. Cerebellar signs may proceed rapidly and include a coarse intention tremor, ataxia affecting the limbs and the trunk, nystagmus (25%) and dysarthria which may become severe. Involvement of the pyramidal tracts causes weakness of the lower limbs. The tone may be only slightly increased because of the accompanying disturbance affecting the afferent fibres from the muscle spindles. The plantar response is extensor. Dorsal column involvement causes loss of joint position, vibration and two-point discrimination sense. There is a peripheral neuropathy associated with muscle wasting, and depressed or absent reflexes. Optic atrophy is present in approximately 30% of patients. Associated skeletal deformities include kyphoscoliosis, pes cavus, pes equinovarus and high arched palate. Kyphoscoliosis and high arched palates are also present in Marfan's syndrome and homocystinuria, but neither of these conditions is associated with spinocerebellar degeneration.

The condition is associated with HCM in between 50–70% of patients. The frequency of HCM increases with the size of the GAA expansion in the first intron. The ECG is abnormal in over 70% of patients and demonstrates widespread T-wave inversion. Diabetes mellitus is present in approximately 10%. A very small proportion of patients may also have sensorineuronal deafness. Death usually occurs in the fourth decade, and is due to cardiac failure.

Answer 152

1. i. Elevated and equal right and left atrial pressures.
ii. Elevated and equal left and right ventricular end-diastolic pressures.
2. Calcification of the pericardium (**152b**, arrowed).
3. The findings are consistent with the diagnosis of pericardial constriction.

(See Guidelines for the Interpretation of Cardiac Catheter Data, page 220.)

152b

Question 153

A 52-year-old male presented with night sweats and lethargy. On examination, he was pale and had a palpable spleen 7 cm below the costal margin.

Investigations are shown.

1. Suggest two possible diagnoses.
2. Apart from the bone marrow, which two investigations would help differentiate between the two diagnoses?

FBC	Hb 9 g/dl
	WCC 52 × 10⁹/l
	Platelets 680 × 10⁹/l
	MCV 88 fl
Blood film	Neutrophils 67%
	Myoblasts 8%
	Myelocytes 10%
	Metamyelocytes 8 %
	Lymphocytes 2%
	Eosinophils 1%
	Basophils 2%
	Nucleated red cell 2%

Question 154

A 59-year-old female presented to the accident and emergency department with sudden onset of retrosternal pain on bending down to get into her car. On examination, she was jaundiced. Her blood pressure was 140/80 mmHg. She was extremely tender over the midsternal area, particularly when she attempted deep inspiration. The heart sounds were normal and her chest was entirely clear. Abdominal examination revealed hepatomegaly which was palpable 4 cm below the costal margin and a palpable tip of the spleen. Only three days earlier she had seen her general practitioner with a six-week history of malaise and was noted have jaundice which was under preliminary investigation. There was no history of abdominal pain or weight loss. She also complained of increasing weakness, with particular difficulty in rising from a sitting position. She had never had any previous hospital admissions, but had seen the general practitioner for troublesome pruritis over the past four years for which she took chlorpheniramine. She was noted to have a serum cholesterol level of 10.5 mmol/l during a routine health check one year ago, for which she had been taking simvastatin. She was widowed two years ago and now lived alone. There was no recent history of travel abroad.

Investigations are shown.

FBC	Hb 11 g/dl
	WCC 10 × 10⁹/l
	Platelets 108 × 10⁹/l
	MCV 90 fl
Biochemistry	Sodium 135 mmol/l
	Potassium 4.7 mmol/l
	Urea 9 mmol/l
	Creatinine 125 μmol/l
	Bilirubin 90 μmol/l
	AST 70 u/l
	Alkaline phosphatase 400 u/l
	Albumin 33 g/l
	Protein 80 g/l
	Calcium 2.0 mmol/l
	Phosphate 0.9 mmol/l.
	Cholesterol 7 mmol/l
	Creatinine kinase 900 u/l
Chest X-ray	Normal-sized heart
	(PA view)
	Clear lung fields
	Looser's zone right clavicle
ECG	Sinus rhythm
	Partial RBBB

1. What is the most probable explanation for the chest pain?
2. Which investigation would you perform to confirm the diagnosis?
3. What is the cause of the failure to rise from a sitting position?
4. Why is the serum cholesterol elevated?
5. How would you account for the raised creatinine kinase?
6. List two steps in the management of her hypercholesterolaemia.
7. What is the cause for her jaundice?
8. List two investigations you would perform to confirm the cause of her jaundice.

Answer 153

1. i. Chronic myeloid leukaemia.
ii. Myelofibrosis.
2. i. Neutrophil leucocyte alkaline phosphatase.
ii. Karyotype for Philadelphia chromosome.

Both chronic myeloid leukaemia and myelofibrosis are myeloproliferative disorders characterized by a high (usually $>50 \times 10^9$/l) WCC consisting of the granulocyte series. Both may be associated with a large spleen, and therefore the differentiation between the two on clinical grounds alone is difficult. Myclofibrosis is characterized by fibrous replacement of the marrow, and although the white cell and platelet count may be very high, a leucoerthyroblastic blood picture is more characteristic. A list of features which may help distinguish chronic myeloid leukaemia from myelofibrosis is shown (*Table*).

Features which may help distinguish chronic myeloid leukaemia from myelofibrosis		
Parameter	*Chronic myeloid leukaemia*	*Myelofibrosis*
WCC	$>50 \times 10^9$/l	$>50 \times 10^9$/l
Large spleen	Present	Present
Blood film	Numerous granulocytes at varying stages of maturation. May be leucoerythroblastic (**153**)	Leucoerythroblastic Tear drop cells.
Neutrophil leucocyte alkaline phosphatase	Low	Normal/high
Philadelphia chromosome	Present in 90%	Absent
Marrow	Numerous granulocytes at varying stages of maturation	Myelofibrosis; stains black with reticulin.

Answer 154

1. Fractured sternum due to osteomalacia.
2. Lateral chest X-ray.
3. Proximal myopathy due to osteomalacia.
4. Reduced excretion of cholesterol due to biliary stasis.
5. Simvastatin-induced myositis/rhabdomyolysis.
6. i. Dietary measures, low-fat diet.
ii. Cholestyramine.
7. PBC.
8. i. Anti-mitochondrial antibodies (IgM2).
ii. Liver biopsy, provided that clotting was not abnormal.

The patient has PBC. There is the classic history of pruritis preceding the onset of jaundice by a few years. The raised serum cholesterol and biochemical and radiological evidence of osteomalacia are suggestive of chronic cholestasis in a jaundiced patient. Hypercholesterolaemia is the result of reduced biliary excretion because bile is the only means of the human body to dispose of cholesterol; thus, many patients with PBC have xanthelasma and palmar xanthomas which are stigmata of hypercholesterolaemia. Osteomalacia is due to vitamin D deficiency resulting from fat malabsorption. Bile excretion into the small intestine is necessary for fat digestion and absorption. Failure to absorb fats results in failure to absorb fat-soluble vitamins, notably vitamins A, D, E and K. Vitamin D deficiency leads to osteomalacia and pathological fractures. This patient's presentation is almost certainly due to a sternal fracture, which may be detected on a lateral chest X-ray. The raised creatinine kinase is unlikely to represent an acute myocardial infarction, given the chest tenderness. The most likely explanation for the high creatinine kinase level is simvastatin-induced myositis. In liver and/or renal failure, simvastatin may cause frank rhabdomyolysis. Patients also taking fibrates and cyclosporin with the statins are at risk of this complication. In this case, the best method of managing the hypercholesterolaemia is by a low-fat diet and by therapy with cholestyramine, a resin which binds bile and promotes its excretion.

The diagnosis of PBC is confirmed by the demonstration of IgM anti-mitochondrial antibodies (subtype M2) which are present in over 90% of the patients. A liver biopsy shows a dense infiltration of the portal tract with lymphocytes and plasma cells. There is periportal fibrosis and cholestasis, and granulomas are present around the small bile ducts.

ANF antibodies and rheumatoid factor are present in up to one-third of cases. Associations include CREST (Calcinosis, Raynaud's syndrome, Esophageal problems, Scleroderma and Telangiectasia) syndrome, membranous glomerulonephritis, RTA and Sjögren's syndrome.

There is no specific proven therapy. Liver transplantation should be considered when the serum bilirubin exceeds 100 µmol/l.

Question 155

A 35-year-old female with Crohn's disease since the age of 15 years presented with a six-month history of foul-smelling diarrhoea and weight loss.

Investigations are shown.

1. List two possible causes for this patient's symptoms.
2. Which investigation would you perform next?

FBC	Hb 10 g/dl
	WCC 7×10^9/l
	Platelets 199×10^9/l
	MCV 106 fl
Serum folate	22 µg/l
Serum B$_{12}$	65 ng/l
Faecal fat	50 mmol/l
	(normal range <20 mmol/l)
Schilling test	Pre-intrinsic factor 2% B$_{12}$
	isotope excreted
	Post-intrinsic factor 2% B$_{12}$
	isotope excreted

Answer 155

1. i. Primary B_{12} malabsorption.
ii. Bacterial overgrowth.
2. Repeat Schilling test after a two-week course of antibiotics.

Table A. The Schilling test

Part 1
- Give 1 mg ^{58}Co-B_{12} orally to a patient who has fasted overnight, and also give 1 mg of non-radioactive B_{12} by intramuscular injection to saturate B_{12} binding proteins. Collect urine for 24 hours.
- Normal subjects excrete >10% of the radioactive dose.

If part 1 is abnormal:

Part 2
- Repeat Schilling with oral intrinsic factor.
- If excretion becomes normal, the primary abnormality is intrinsic factor deficiency.
- If excretion remains abnormal, then the differential is between primary B_{12} malabsorption and bacterial overgrowth.

Table B. Differentiation of primary B_{12} malabsorption from bacterial overgrowth

	1° B_{12} malabsorption	*Bacterial overgrowth*
1. Schilling test after antibiotics	Abnormal	Normal
2. Small bowel meal	Terminal ileal stricture	Fistulae, jejunal strictures
3. Jejunal aspirate	Normal bacteria	High concentration of *Escherichia coli/Bacteroides*
4. ^{14}C-glycocholate breath test	Positive	Positive

The patient has a history of Crohn's disease and now presents with steatorrhoea, B_{12} deficiency and an abnormal Schilling test (*Table A*), with and without intrinsic factor. The two most likely causes for the B_{12} deficiency in Crohn's disease are primary B_{12} malabsorption due to terminal ileal disease, or intestinal destruction of dietary B_{12} by bacterial overgrowth within small bowel strictures. Both conditions also cause steatorrhoea by impairing fat absorption due to disturbances in bile salt absorption; the former by preventing absorption of bile salts which are required for micelle formation, and the latter by deconjugation and dehydroxylation of bile salts. Repeating the Schilling test after a two-week course of metronidazole and tetracycline may help to differentiate between terminal ileal disease and bacterial overgrowth (*Table B*). Antibiotics destroy the large concentrations of *Escherichia coli* and/or *Bacteroides* which are responsible for bacterial overgrowth, and following this the Schilling test (without intrinsic factor) becomes abnormal. In terminal ileal disease, the test will remain abnormal. A small-bowel enema may also help in the differentiation by demonstrating a terminal stricture responsible for primary B_{12} malabsorption, and any structural defects which will predispose to bacterial overgrowth. Another method of

Table C. Causes of B_{12} deficiency

Low dietary intake (vegans)

Intrinsic factor deficiency
Congenital
Pernicious anaemia
Gastrectomy
Chronic atrophic gastritis

Primary B_{12} malabsorption
Terminal ileal disease
Bacterial overgrowth
Coeliac and tropical sprue (longstanding)
Pancreatic insufficiency

Miscellaneous
Fish tapeworm (*Diphyllobothrium latum*)
Drug, e.g. colchicine, neomycin

differentiation is by jejunal aspiration and culture. Although *E. coli* and *Bacteroides* are found in the jejunum, it is unusual to find concentrations exceeding 10^6/ml unless there is overgrowth. A ^{14}C-glycocholate breath test

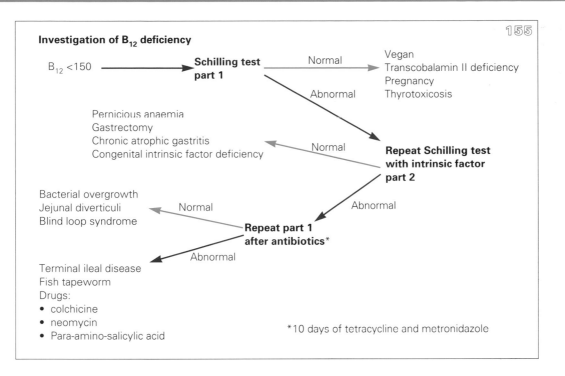

Investigation of B$_{12}$ deficiency

B$_{12}$ <150 → **Schilling test part 1**

Normal → Vegan / Transcobalamin II deficiency / Pregnancy / Thyrotoxicosis

Abnormal → **Repeat Schilling test with intrinsic factor part 2**

Normal → Pernicious anaemia / Gastrectomy / Chronic atrophic gastritis / Congenital intrinsic factor deficiency

Abnormal → **Repeat part 1 after antibiotics***

Normal → Bacterial overgrowth / Jejunal diverticuli / Blind loop syndrome

Abnormal → Terminal ileal disease / Fish tapeworm / Drugs:
- colchicine
- neomycin
- Para-amino-salicylic acid

*10 days of tetracycline and metronidazole

is characteristically positive in bacterial overgrowth, as bacteria deconjugate bile salts to release ^{14}C-glycine, which is metabolized to $^{14}CO_2$. The radioactivity in the breath is easy to measure; however, it is important to realize that the test may also be positive in terminal ileal disease because unabsorbed radiolabelled bile salts pass into the colon where the concentration of *E. coli* is very high, leading to deconjugation of bile salts and liberation of ^{14}C-glycine. In terminal ileal disease, faecal radioactivity is also high, whereas in bacterial overgrowth the radioactivity level is relatively low.

Question 156

A 65-year-old male was seen in the out-patient's clinic with a one-year history of dizziness which was worse on getting out of bed, and occasionally associated with collapse. The patient also complained of weakness affecting both legs. On further questioning, he admitted to urinary incontinence and his wife noted that he was generally slow and had an intermittent tremor affecting his right hand.

On examination, he appeared slightly withdrawn. His pulse was 84 beats/min, and blood pressure 155/85 mmHg. The heart sounds were normal. Examination of the respiratory and gastrointestinal systems was normal. On examination of the central nervous system he had sluggish pupillary reflexes and nystagmus. Examination of the fundi was normal. There was a pin-rolling tremor affecting the right hand. There was increased tone in both legs, with the right leg being affected more than the left. Power was slightly reduced (grade 4/5) in all limbs. The reflexes were generally brisk. The plantar response in the left foot was extensor, but was equivocal in the right foot. Sensation was normal. His gait was ataxic.

1. What is the most likely diagnosis?
2. List two further investigations you would pursue to confirm your diagnosis.

Answer 156

1. Multisystems atrophy or Shy–Drager syndrome.
2. i. Lying and standing blood pressure.
ii. Autonomic nervous system testing (loss of sinus arrhythmias on ECG, loss of reflex bradycardia on carotid sinus massage, absence of a reflex tachycardia after the Valsalva manoeuvre).

Causes of autonomic failure

1. Central (primary)
Progressive autonomic failure (no obvious cause)
Progressive autonomic failure with multisystem
  atrophy (Shy–Drager syndrome)
Progressive autonomic failure with Parkinson's
  disease

2. Central (secondary)
Central brain lesions: craniopharyngioma, vascular
  disease
Encephalitis, tabes dorsalis, Chaga's disease
Spinal cord lesions
Familial dysautonomia

3. Distal autonomic neuropathies
Guillain–Barré syndrome, diabetes mellitus,
  amyloid, porphyria, rheumatoid arthritis,
  myaesthenia gravis, Fabry's disease

*4. Tricyclic antidepressants, MAOIs, ganglion-
  blocking drugs*

The patient has a pill-rolling tremor and increased muscular tone, indicating an extrapyramidal syndrome such as Parkinson's disease. The presence of additional neurological findings suggests that he has a Parkinson-plus syndrome. There are several Parkinson-plus syndromes in the literature, but the ones which are most commonly tested include multisystem atrophy and the SROS. Multisystem atrophy is the name given to a sporadically occurring condition which begins in adult life, usually in the sixth decade. It is characterized by neuronal cell loss and gliosis changes in:

- The substantia nigra pathways which causes parkinsonism.
- The olivopontocerebellar tract causing ataxia, dysarthria, nystagmus and pyramidal signs.
- The intermediolateral cell column (preganglionic sympathetic neurones in the lateral horns of the spinal cord) causing autonomic nervous system failure. Other causes of autonomic failure are shown (*Table*).

These changes often overlap and may present as a mixture of neurological abnormalities. When features of Parkinson's disease predominate, the disorder is called striatonigral degeneration. When features of the autonomic failure predominate, the disorder is commonly known as Shy–Drager syndrome, and when cerebellar features predominate it is called olivopontocerebellar atrophy. When all three systems are involved the disorder is known as multisystem atrophy. Unlike Parkinson's disease, there is a shortened life expectancy, with a median survival of 9.3 years.

In Shy–Drager syndrome, impotence is often the first symptom. Incontinence is common in both sexes. Speech differs from the hypophonic monotony of Parkinson's disease, incorporating quivering, straining, slurring, and dysarthric components. Patients may develop aphonia, anarthria and dysphagia, which are the same as in Parkinson's disease. Respiratory stridor can occur in about 30% of patients. There is no specific treatment for multisystem atrophy and the associated disorders. The use of compression stockings, fludrocortisone, and pressor agents such as ephedrine have been used for the postural symptoms. The response to L-dopa is usually absent or poor.

Steele–Richardson–Olszewski syndrome (SROS)
This is another multisystem degeneration syndrome. It is characterized by cell loss and neurofibrillary tangles in the brainstem, globus pallidus, subthalamic and dentate nuclei and causes the syndrome of progressive supranuclear palsy. It begins in the seventh decade. Patients present with imbalance, particularly falling backwards, a coarse dysarthria, involuntary groans, and dysphagia. Perseverance may be obvious in speech with repetition of syllables and words (palilalia) or even of whole phrases (palilogia). Involuntary eye closure is often seen. The brow may be furrowed and the eyebrows raised from frontalis hyperactivity in an attempt to keep the eyes open, resulting in a surprised expression. The characteristic feature in SROS is a supranuclear palsy of voluntary gaze. Voluntary downgaze is slow and incomplete, but when the patient's neck is passively extended while fixing his gaze on the examiner's nose, a downward gaze is obtained. Patients may therefore have problems with reading and eating. Patients with SROS can masquerade as having Parkinson's disease because of axial rigidity and gait disturbances, but lack features of distal parkinsonism (distal limb akinesia or rigidity). Resting tremor is almost never seen. There is no effective treatment. Median survival is about 6–7 years.

Question 157

A 31-year-old male was admitted to hospital with a two-week history of progressive dyspnoea on exertion and wheeze. He complained of aches and pains in his arms and legs. He had suffered from ulcerative colitis for four years, and required several courses of high-dose prednisolone until the last two months when his colitis was relatively quiescent. He also had a past history of hyperthyroidism which was medically treated with carbimazole. He was currently maintained on sulphasalazine 1 g twice daily for the ulcerative colitis.

On examination, he was dyspnoeic, had mild cervical and axillary lymphadenopathy, and a generalized maculopapular rash. He had a fever of 38.5°C (101.3°F). The heart rate was 110 beats/min and regular. The blood pressure was 140/80 mmHg. Heart sounds were normal. Auscultation of the lung fields demonstrated widespread wheeze. His abdomen was very muscular and difficult to examine. All other examinations were essentially normal.

Investigations are shown.

FBC	Hb 13 g/dl
	WCC 15.3 × 10^9/l (neutrophils
	10.1 × 10^9/l, lymphocytes
	1.0 × 10^9/l, eosinophils
	4.2 × 10^9/l)
	Platelets 308 × 10^9/l
U&E	Sodium 126 mmol/l
	Potassium 4.3 mmol/l
	Urea 7 mmol/l
	Creatinine 100 µmol/l
ESR	98 mm/h
Blood and sputum cultures	Negative
Arterial blood gases (on air)	pH 7.4
	pCO$_2$ 3.3 kPa
	pO$_2$ 8.7 kPa
	Bicarbonate 21 mmol/l
	O$_2$ saturation 92%
Chest X-ray (**157a**)	

1. Give two possible diagnoses.
2. List three investigations you would perform.
3. Give two steps in the management of this patient.

Answer 157

1. i. Eosinophilic pneumonia secondary to sulphasalazine.
ii. Churgg–Strauss syndrome.
2. i. Transbronchial lung biopsy (would detect eosinophilic infiltration and vasculitis).
ii. Bronchoalveolar lavage.
iii. Serum ANCA.
3. i. Stop sulphasalazine.
ii. Start prednisolone.

The patient has a generalized illness comprising of a widespread macular rash, generalized lymphadenopathy, and a very high eosinophil count. He has a wheeze, and his chest X-ray reveals patchy consolidation which is worse in the right lung. He had been on prednisolone for ulcerative colitis but has recently commenced sulphasalazine. The symptoms and signs have appeared after the drug was commenced, and the most likely diagnosis for his respiratory problem is an eosinophilic pneumonia. This question tests the reader's knowledge of causes of eosinophilia (**157b**) of which there are many; however, the most common cause is allergy. An allergic reaction to drugs may precipitate a profound eosinophilia with multi-system involvement, including eosinophilic infiltration into the lungs. Sulphonamides are a well-recognized cause of eosinophilia and subsequent eosinophilic consolidation. Other drugs include erythromycin, nitrofurantoin and imipramine. The most obvious management of a drug-related eosinophilia is to stop the culprit agent. Pulmonary involvement responds well to high-dose steroids, which may be tailed off over a few weeks. However, relapse is not uncommon and some patients require a maintenance dose of 5 mg prednisolone for several months to prevent recurrence.

The differential diagnosis here is the Churgg–Strauss syndrome, which is a small-vessel granulomatous vasculitis characterized by skin rash, respiratory involvement giving asthmatic symptoms, neuropathy and eosinophilia. It is a variant of Wegener's granulomatosis, but is a much milder disease and does not usually involve the kidneys. Lymphoma is also associated with eosinophilia, however, it is would have to be fairly extensive to involve the cervical and axillary lymph nodes as well as the chest. The normal Hb and lymphocyte count are not consistent with extensive lymphoma.

Although the patient had been on steroids and is currently taking carbimazole, his normal neutrophil count is highly against the development of an opportunistic infection such as TB or *Pneumocystis carinii* pneumonia.

Ulcerative colitis itself is a recognized cause of a mild eosinophilia; however, an eosinophilia as high as in this case and pulmonary involvement cannot be explained by the disease.

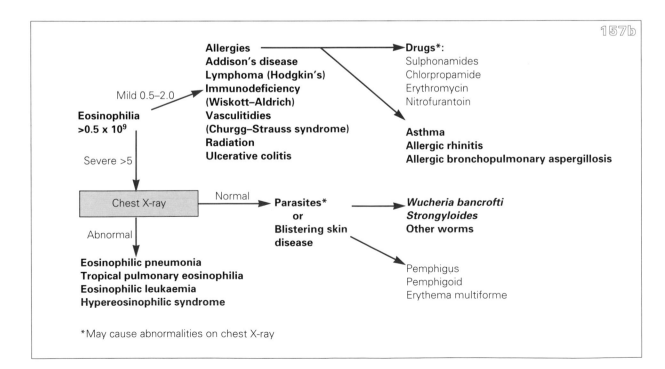

Question 158

A 16-year-old female is investigated for short stature. The results of a dynamic pituitary function tests following 0.15 u/kg of insulin, 100 μg of LHRH, and 200 μg of TRH are as follows:

Time (min)	Glucose (mmol/l)	GH mu/l	Cortisol (nmol/l)	TSH mu/l	LH u/l	FSH u/l	Oestradiol pmol/l
0	4.0	1.4	400	2.0	29	16	4
20	2.8	12.0	860	5.2	40	24	5
30	1.6	28	1270	-	-	-	–
40	1.5	32	1450	-	-	-	–
60	2.2	20	1120	8	34	20	6

1. The following statements are true with respect to the pituitary function tests above:
A. There was an inadequate stimulus for GH secretion.
B. The GH response was abnormal.
C. The findings are consistent with pituitary Cushing's syndrome.
D. The patient is hypothyroid.
E. There is evidence of primary hypogonadism.
2. The following investigations would be useful in confirming the diagnosis:
A. Buccal smear for karyotyping.
B. CT scan of the pituitary gland.
C. Dexamethasone suppression test.
D. Investigation of other family members.
E. Thyroid antibodies.
3. The following diagnoses are possible in this patient:
A. Hypothyroidism.
B. Turner's syndrome.
C. PCOS.
D. Testicular feminization syndrome.
E. Coeliac disease.

Question 159

A 70-year-old male on treatment for congestive cardiac failure with an angiotensin converting enzyme inhibitor, spironolactone, digoxin and frusemide was admitted with nausea. An ECG taken on admission is shown (**159**).

1. What is the abnormality?
2. Which investigation would you perform next?

Answer 158

1. E. There is evidence of primary hypogonadism.
2. A. Buccal smear for karyotyping.
3. B. Turner's syndrome.

In order to answer this question correctly the reader requires knowledge of the normal results of a dynamic pituitary function test and gonadotrophin and sex hormone levels (*Tables A* and *B*).

In this case, there is an adequate stimulus to GH and cortisol secretion. The GH response is normal, and there is no evidence of hypothyroidism. The basal oestradiol is low and the basal LH and FSH are high, suggesting primary hypogonadism. The LHRH test is normal (as is the case) in primary hypogonadism. The most probable diagnosis is Turner's syndrome. Turner's syndrome is characterized by a single X chromosome (karyotype 45 XO). It has an incidence of approximately 1 in 2,500. The main abnormality is gonadal dysgenesis, the consequences of which are primary amenorrhoea and infertility. Oestradiol levels are low, resulting in elevated gonadotrophin levels via the positive feedback on the pituitary. The patients are typically short and have a number of other morphological abnormalities (*Table C*). The diagnosis is confirmed by a Buccal smear which reveals an absent Barr body. There are several other causes of hypogonadism in females (*Table D*).

Polycystic ovary syndrome may also cause partial hypogonadism, but in contrast with the other causes of hypogonadism given in *Table D*, the oestradiol levels are only slightly reduced and the FSH level is low (*Table E*). Although coeliac disease is a recognized cause of short stature (and also delayed puberty), the gonadotrophin response to LHRH is entirely normal. The commonly examined causes of short stature in the MRCP and similar examinations are listed (*Table F*).

Testicular feminization syndrome is due to the absence of testosterone receptors on end organs. The patient has male karyotype, but is phenotypically female due to the absence of the effect of testosterone in the normal development of male gonads. Testicles are present but are usually intra-abdominal or in the hernial orifices. Serum testosterone levels are very high. Lack of testosterone receptors on the pituitary means that there is no negative feedback system to inhibit gonadotrophin secretion, therefore both LH and FSH are very high. Excess stimulation of the testicular remnants leads to excess oestrogen production by the testes which is comparable with levels found in females. The oestrogen initiates breast development and maintains breasts. Lack of the testosterone effect means that pubic hair may be absent or scanty. These patients are not particularly short. They present with amenorrhoea. The diagnosis can be confirmed by karyotyping.

Pituitary Cushing's is unusual in this age group. It is due to a basophil adenoma within the pituitary which secretes ACTH causing adrenal hyperplasia and excess cortisol production. The serum cortisol is >900 nmol/l and there is loss of diurnal variation i.e the midnight cortisol is also >900 nmol/l (normally 150–750 nmol/l). In the majority of cases high dose dexamethasone (8 mg per day) suppresses cortisol production (see also Answer 70, page 94). In some cases the cortisol response to dexamthasone is unaffected and in these instances the main definitive method of diagnosing pituitary Cushing's is to perform inferior petrosal sinus sampling for ACTH.

Table A. Normal responses to dynamic pituitary function tests

- Following an insulin tolerance test, the GH level rises to >20 mu/l and the serum cortisol level should rise to ≥550 nmol/l and increase by 180 nmol/l from the basal level. The blood sugar should fall below 2.2 mmol/l to ensure adequate metabolic stress for GH and cortisol secretion. Note: An insulin tolerance test should not be performed if the basal cortisol level is below 180 nmol/l.
- Following a TRH test, the TSH should increase by >2 mu/l from the basal level. Basal TSH levels are between 0.5–5 mu/l.
- Following an LHRH test, the LH and FSH should double from the basal level.

Table B. Normal gonadotrophin and sex hormone levels in males and females

Females
Follicular phase, FSH 1–10 u/l and LH 2–20 u/l
Oestradiol <110 pmol/l
Testosterone 0.5–3 nmol/l

Males
FSH 1–7 u/l and LH 1–10 u/l
Testosterone 10–35 nmol/l

Table C. Morphological features of Turner's syndrome

Skeletal
Short stature
Cubitus valgus
Short fourth metacarpals
High-arched palate*
Shield chest with widely spaced nipples

Cardiac anomalies
Septal defects
Coarctation of the aorta

Renal anomalies
Horse-shoe kidneys

Miscellaneous abnormalities
Webbed neck (fused cervical vertebrae)
Lymphoedema
Low hair line
Multiple naevi
Increased incidence of autoimmune thyroiditis
  and diabetes

* Also present in Marfan's syndrome, homocystinuria and Friedreich's ataxia

---

Table D. Causes of primary hypogonadism in females

Turner's syndrome
Pure ovarian dysgenesis*
Swyer's syndrome**
Autoimmune oophoritis

Ovariectomy
Chemotherapy
Steroid biosynthetic defect
  (17-α-hydroxylase deficiency)

* The pathology is the same as Turner's, but differs in that there is a normal complement of chromosomes and the other morphological features of Turner's syndrome are absent. Some patients may have sensorineuronal deafness.
** Swyer's syndrome is characterized by the XY karyotype and gonadal dysgenesis. Affected individuals are phenotypically female. It is associated with a high incidence of gonadoblastomas.

Table E. Characteristics of PCOS (Stein–Levental syndrome)

Irregular menstruation
Impaired fertility
Hursutism
Acne
Obesity
Low oestradiol levels

Testosterone level slightly higher than 3.0 nmol/l
High oestrone levels
Slightly elevated LH level
Slightly depressed FSH level
LH/FSH ratio generally exceeds 2

Table F. Causes of short stature

Constitutional delay*
Familial
Systemic disorder, e.g. coeliac disease
Endocrine causes e.g. hypothyroidism or GH deficiency

Drugs, particularly steroids
Emotional deprivation
Skeletal abnormalities (achondroplasia,
  vitamin D-resistant rickets)

* Slow growth from the beginning, spontaneous puberty, slight delay in bone maturity, normal LHRH test.

Answer 159

1. Tall T-waves (>12 mm).
2. Serum potassium.

Tall tented T-waves is an ECG feature of hyperkalaemia. In this case, the cause of hyperkalaemia is a combination of potassium sparing drugs and obstructive uropathy. (See *Table B* in Answer **96**, page 125.)

Question 160

A 65-year-old female was referred to a neurologist with a six-month history of progressive weakness and clumsiness of her left hand. She mentioned having particular difficulty in washing the dishes and using the gear stick whilst driving her car. Her husband noticed that her gait had been unsteady and she had suffered a few falls in the past year. On systemic enquiry there was no history of headaches, visual disturbance or weight loss, but she had experienced dizziness on turning her head suddenly.

On examination she was thin and had marked kyphoscoliosis. There was evidence of wasting of the small muscles of the hands which was more prominent on the left side than the right. There was reduced power on flexion and abduction of the arms. The supinator and biceps reflexes on the left side were absent but present on the right. The triceps reflexes were brisk bilaterally. The power in both lower limbs was grade 4 out of 5 in all muscle groups. The tone was increased. The ankle and knee reflexes were brisk bilaterally. The left plantar response was upgoing but the right one was equivocal. Sensation was normal with the exception of vibration sense at both ankle joints.

1. What is the diagnosis?
A. Motor neurone disease.
B. Syringomyelia.
C. Multiple sclerosis.
D. Cervical myelopathy.
E. Subacute combined degeneration of the spinal cord.
F. Cervical cord tumour.
2. Which investigation would you perform to perform to confirm the diagnosis?
A. Myelography.
B. X-ray cervical spine in extension and flexion.
C. MRI cervical spine.
D. Nerve conduction studies and electromyography.
E. CSF analysis for ologoclonal bands.
F. Serum B_{12} level.
G. VDRL.
H. Muscle biopsy.

Question 161

A young alcoholic who is well known to the local accident and emergency department was admitted to hospital after being found collapsed. On examination, he was unrousable. His temperature was 36.5°C (97.7°F). His heart rate was 120 beats/min, and regular, with a weak pulse volume. The blood pressure was 80/40 mmHg. The heart sounds were normal. Auscultation of the lung fields revealed a few crackles at both lung bases. The abdomen was rigid and bowel sounds were absent. Rectal examination demonstrated soft brown stool. Examination of the fundi was normal.

Investigations are shown.

1. What is the diagnosis?
A. Diabetic ketoacidosis.
B. Rhabdomyolysis.
C. Perforated duodenal ulcer.
D. Gastrointestinal haemorrhage secondary to oesophageal varices.
E. Acute alcohol intoxication.
F. Acute pancreatitis.
G. Dissecting aortic anuerysm.
H. Methanol poisoning.
I. Ethylene glycol poisoning.
2. List five investigations which you would perform on this patient immediately.

FBC	Hb 7 g/dl
	WCC 23 × 10⁹/l
	Platelets 50 × 10⁹/l
	MCV 102 fl
INR	1.9
Biochemistry	Sodium 131 mmol/l
	Potassium 5.6 mmol/l
	Urea 17 mmol/l
	Creatinine 200 µmol/l
	Bicarbonate 16 mmol/l
	Calcium 1.9 mmol/l
	Phosphate 1.0 mmol/l
	Albumin 30 g/l
	AST 64 u/l
	Bilirubin 53 µmol/l
	Alkaline phosphatase 204 u/l
	Gamma GT 190 u/l
	Glucose 21 mmol/l
Urine	Protein +1
	Blood 0
	Ketones +1

Question 162

162a

162b

A 44-year-old West Indian male presented with a three-week history of polydipsia, polyuria and nocturia. He was passing copious amounts of urine several times per day, and felt excessively thirsty. According to his wife he was consuming up to five 2-litre bottles of cola per day, and several large 1-litre flasks of water. His appetite and weight had been normal. He was not taking any medication. For four years he had been intermittently unwell, firstly with chest problems, and then with arthritis affecting his hands and feet. The respiratory problems were of relatively sudden onset which were characterized by a dry cough and accompanied by night sweats, pains in his ankles and tender, raised lesions on his shins. The joint pains responded to pain killers prescribed by a doctor who he saw in the West Indies, but the chest symptoms persisted for several months despite four long courses of antibiotics. The skin lesions on the shins resolved about three months after the onset of his illness. He was eventually referred to a chest physician with breathlessness on exertion, and after respiratory function tests (top panel of results) and a chest X-ray was told he had scarring on the lung, possibly due to several previous chest infections, and was prescribed a steroid inhaler.

The patient's breathing remained stable. He was able to walk for over two miles on the flat, but experienced breathlessness on negotiating inclines. After two years, he developed pain and swelling in his hands and feet which was controlled to some extent with co-proxamol. His only other complaint was of a gritty feeling in the eyes as the day progressed, and dryness of the mouth for several months before he developed polyuria. He worked as a bus conductor. His brother, aged 58 had rheumatoid arthritis which was complicated with lung fibrosis.

On examination, the patient appeared well at rest, but had mild bilateral parotid gland enlargement. The appearance of the eyes is shown (162a). His eyes were red, but the visual acuity, visual fields, pupils and fundi were normal. There was no focal neurological deficit. There was no evidence of a previous BCG scar. There was bone swelling affecting several phalanges in the hand and feet. There was no joint swelling. Cardiovascular examination was normal. Auscultation of the lung fields revealed fine inspiratory crackles in the anterior chest, but auscultation of the posterior aspect of the chest was normal.

Investigations are shown (second panel of results).

	Actual	Predicted
FEV$_1$ (l)	2.2	4.1
FVC (l)	2.5	5.4
TLC (l)	3.3	6.3
KCO (mmol/min/kPa)	0.9	1.40

Biochemistry	Sodium 143 mmol/l
	Potassium 4.5 mmol/l
	Urea 6 mmol/l
	Creatinine 90 μmol
	Calcium 2.3 mmol/l
	Phosphate 1.1 mmol/l
	Alkaline phosphatase 120 u/l
Blood glucose	4.2 mmol/l
X-ray of hand (162b)	

Fluid deprivation test:

Time (min)	$P_{mOsm/l}$	$U_{mOsm/l}$
0	303	120
60	310	120
120	318	120
180	328	120
240	335	120
8 h after desmopressin		800

1. What were the painful lesions on the shins?
2. What do the patient's respiratory function tests demonstrate?
3. What does the X-ray of his hand reveal?
4. Why does he have gritty eyes?
5. What is the interpretation of the water deprivation test?
6. What is the overall or underlying diagnosis?
7. Which three investigations would you perform to confirm your diagnosis?
8. Give three therapeutic steps in his management.

Answer 160

1. D. Cervical myelopathy
2. C. MRI scan cervical spine

The patient presents with progressive weakness affecting her arms and hands. She has a combination of upper and lower motor neurone signs in the upper limbs and purely upper motor neurone signs in the lower limbs. There is loss of vibration sense in at the level of the ankle. This may be a normal finding in patients in their seventh decade but may indicate pathology in the dorsal columns.

The differential diagnosis is between motor neurone disease, cervical cord tumour and cervical myelopathy, and subacute combined degeneration of the spinal cord.

Features against motor neurone disease include her gender (more common in males), the mid-cervical reflex pattern (absent supinator and biceps reflex but exaggerated triceps reflex) which is more suggestive of cervical myelopathy, the association of her symptoms with rigidity in the neck and dizziness on turning suddenly which again suggests pathology in the cervical cord, and the absence of weight loss which is usually marked in motor neurone disease.

Subacute combined degeneration of the spinal cord is a remote possibility, but one would want more evidence of a sensory neuropathy in this condition, for example, absence of light touch and proprioception and absent knee or ankle jerks.

Both cervical myelopathy and a cervical cord tumour may present with predominantly upper limb signs, which characteristically produce lower motor neurone disturbances at the level of the lesion and upper motor signs below it. The best investigation to differentiate between the two is an MRI scan of the spinal cord which has superseded myelography. In this case, the lesion appears to affect the C5 and C6 segments of the cervical cord, hence the absent biceps and supinator reflexes on the left side. This would not explain the weakness and wasting of the muscles of the hand as they are supplied by C8 and T1; however, small muscle wasting in cervical myelopathy appears to be due to reduced blood flow to the lower segments of the cord rather than to direct compression of the C8 and T1 spinal nerves. It is worth noting that sensory disturbance in the upper limbs may be absent or very mild in cervical myelopathy.

Cervical myelopathy is due to bulging or extrusion of the disc material into the cervical canal, which results in pressure atrophy and ischaemia. The main cause is osteoarthritis of the cervical spine. The posterior columns (dorsal tracts carrying proprioception, vibration sense and light-touch fibres) and the lateral columns (pyramidal tracts carrying upper motor neurones) are affected. The 5th–7th cervical segments are most commonly affected. The symptoms are those of lower motor neurone signs at these levels and upper motor neurone signs below. Neck stiffness and upper limb pain may be present. Spasticity of the lower limbs is common and more pronounced than physical examination would suggest. Ataxia may occur due to dorsal column involvement (senosry ataxia). L'hermitte's sign (electrical shock feeling down the spinal cord and into the legs) is recognized, but may also occur with cervical cord tumours, multiple sclerosis and subacute combined degeneration of the spinal cord.

The presence of lower motor neurone signs and the absence of cerbellar signs is against multiple sclerosis.

The absence of dissociated sensory loss is against syringomyelia.

Answer 161

1. F. Acute pancreatitis.
2. i. Serum amylase.
ii. Arterial blood gases.
iii. Full clotting screen.
iv. Chest X-ray.
v. Ultrasound of the abdomen.

The clinical scenario is of an alcohol abuser who presents with unconsciousness and a rigid abdomen. The differential diagnosis is between a perforated duodenal ulcer, acute pancreatitis, ethylene glycol poisoning and methanol poisoning, as all four are recognized causes of abdominal pain in alcoholism. The raised gamma GT supports alcohol abuse. The low calcium favours either acute pancreatitis or ethylene glycol poisoning (oxidation of ethylene glycol to

Diagnoses to consider in an unconscious alcoholic
Hepatic encephalopathy
Wenicke's encephalopathy
Methanol poisoning
Ethylene glycol poisoning
Alcohol intoxication
Subdural haemorrhage
Haemorrhage from peptic ulcer or varices
Acute haemorrhagic pancreatitis
Tuberculous meningitis
Alcohol-induced hypoglycaemia

oxalic acid results in chelation of calcium). However, the diabetic state is more in keeping with acute pancreatitis, which results in damage to the islets of Langerhans that produce insulin. Methanol poisoning may also cause hyperglycaemia, but hypocalcaemia is unusual. Furthermore, the acidosis is more severe in methanol poisoning and there is usually evidence of optic atrophy. The anaemia is quite severe, suggesting that there may be ongoing peritoneal bleeding from the pancreatitis. The MCV is high, indicating either alcohol-related marrow toxicity or alcohol-related liver damage. The low platelets indicate either hypersplenism secondary to portal hypertension or a DIC process complicating acute pancreatitis. The raised INR may be due to hepatocellular dysfunction or part of the DIC. Diabetic ketoacidosis would not explain the unconsciousness in this patient given the fact that the bicarbonate is not very low and the ketonuria is mild. The mild ketonuria in this case is due to reduced dietary intake. Rhabdomyolysis is unlikely because the creatinine is not very high, and there is no evidence of blood in the urine on dipstick testing (remember that myoglobin gives a positive dipstick test for blood).

A very high serum amylase would confirm acute pancreatitis in this case. The most common causes of death in acute pancreatitis are haemorrhage, renal failure and respiratory failure; therefore a FBC, blood gases, chest X-ray and clotting would give important prognostic information.

Answer 162

1. Erythema nodosum. Causes of erythema nodosum are shown (*Table A*).
2. A restrictive lung defect with a low KCO. The differential diagnosis for conditions causing this picture is discussed in Answer 93, page 120.
3. The X-ray of the hand demonstrates several lucent lesions at the ends of most phalanges.
4. Bilateral keratoconjunctivitis.
5. The fluid-deprivation test reveals an inability to concentrate urine until the administration of exogenous desmopressin (an ADH analogue), which is indicative of cranial diabetes insipidus. Interpretation of a fluid-deprivation test is discussed below. Conditions causing cranial diabetes insipidus and an abnormal chest X-ray include sarcoidosis, TB, and histiocytosis X. In rare situations, bronchial carcinoma may metastasize to the hypothalamus or pituitary and cause diabetes insipidus. Other causes of diabetes insipidus are shown (*Table B*).
6. The combination of erythema nodosum, ocular, lung, bone, parotid and lachrymal gland involvement strongly suggest the diagnosis of sarcoidosis.
7. i. Transbronchial lung biopsy to demonstrate non-caseating granulomas.
ii. MRI scan of the pituitary to demonstrate high-intensity lesions in the mid brain.
iii. Serum ACE level. This is not specific for the diagnosis of sarcoidosis and may be elevated in TB, histoplasmosis, berylliosis, silicosis, lymphoma, diabetes mellitus, chronic liver disease, hyperthyroidism and Gaucher's disease.
8. i. High-dose steroids.
ii. Desmopressin.
iii. Artificial tears.
Indications for high-dose steroids in sarcoidosis include cerebral involvement, acute diffuse lung disease, uveitis, and hypercalcaemia.

Sarcoidosis is a multisystem granulomatous disease of unknown aetiology which usually affects females more commonly than males. It is much more common in the Negroid race, and may present acutely with the Lofgren's syndrome which is characterized by erythema nodosum,

---

Table A. Causes of erythema nodosum

Common conditions	Other conditions
Streptococcal infections, including rheumatic fever	Behçet's syndrome
	TB
	Leprosy
Sarcoidosis	Histoplasmosis
Oral contraceptive pill and pregnancy	*Yersinia*
	Neisseria meningitidis and gonococcal infections
Inflammatory bowel disease	
Sulphonamide drugs	*Pasteurella pestis*

Table B. Causes of diabetes insipidus

Cranial	Nephrogenic
Familial	X-linked (vasopressin receptor-2 gene)
Autosomal dominant	
DIDMOAD syndrome	Autosomal recessive (aquaporin receptor gene)
Cerebral tumour	
Sarcoidosis	
TB	Hypokalaemia
Histiocytosis X	Hypercalcaemia
Trauma	Lithium
Pituitary haemorrhage	Post-obstructive uropathy
	Sickle cell anaemia
	Glibenclamide
	Aminoglycosides
	Amphotericin

arthralgia, dry cough, bilateral hilar lymphadenopathy on the chest X-ray, and anterior uveitis. Patients with sarcoidosis may have lachrymal and parotid gland involvement which is characterized by gland enlargement and sometimes referred to as Mikulicz syndrome (causes of parotid gland enlargement are listed in *Table C)*. Affected patients may complain of xerostomia and gritty eyes respectively, the latter being due to keratoconjunctivitis resulting from impaired lachrymation. Mikulicz syndrome may also complicate TB, lymphoma and leukaemia. Mikulicz syndrome is relatively common and when it is associated with acute uveitis and facial nerve palsy it is referred to as Heerfordt's syndrome. In most patients the acute illness will resolve, although some will continue to have respiratory symptoms for up to two years, and a small percentage develop a chronic illness characterized by relapses and remissions.

In chronic cases, lung parenchyma becomes involved, leading to fibrosis commonly affecting the apices. Ocular involvement is well recognised. Manifestations include anterior and posterior uveitis, which are characteristically associated with visual symptoms and pupillary abnormalities, and episcleritis, scleritis, choroiditis, cataracts and glaucoma. Corneal calcification complicating hypercalcaemia may also occur in sarcoidosis.

Skin infiltration occurs in the chronic form of the illness and comprises papules on the eyelids and around the mouth. Papules affecting the nose may be disfiguring and are referred to as lupus pernio. Arthralgia affecting the hands and feet is common; X-rays demonstrate small lucent cysts in multiple phalanges. Cerebral involvement is rare, but features include cranial nerve lesions, aseptic meningitis, psychosis and a multiple sclerosis-type syndrome. Mononeuritis multiplex is a recognized manifestation of the peripheral nervous system. Hypercalcaemia occurs due to the presence of excessive production of 1,25-DHCC by granulomatous cells. Other conditions where a similar phenomenon occurs include TB and *Candida* infection.

Water deprivation test
In patients with polyuria and polydipsia and a normal blood glucose, the differential diagnosis is between cranial diabetes insipidus, nephrogenic diabetes insipidus and compulsive water deprivation. The water deprivation test will help differentiate compulsive water drinking from both types of diabetes insipidus (*Table D*). However, the differentiation of cranial diabetes insipidus from nephrogenic diabetes insipidus involves measurement of plasma and urine osmolality following administration of desmopressin. Patients with cranial diabetes insipidus are deficient of ADH and respond dramatically to desmopressin with an increase in urine osmolality, whereas patients with nephrogenic diabetes insipidus are resistant to the effects of ADH and therefore the urine osmolality is not affected by desmopressin.

Table C. Causes of parotid gland enlargement

Mumps	Haemochromatosis
Sarcoidosis	Amyloidosis
Lymphoma	Acromegaly
Leukaemia	Malabsorption syndromes
Sjögren's syndrome	Drugs; propylthiouracil
Alcohol abuse	Toxins; lead
Bulimia	Hyperlipidaemia
Cystic fibrosis	

Table D. After a water deprivation test

	P mOsm/l	U mOsm/l
Normal	300	Over 720 or double the plasma osmolality
Compulsive water drinking	300	Incomplete response, i.e. the U mOsm/l is not quite 720 and does not exceed twice the value of the P mOsm/l. Typical value 600–700 mOsm/l
Cranial diabetes inspidus	>300	<150; over 720 mOsm/l after desmopressin
Nephrogenic diabetes insipidus	>300	<150; remains <150 mOsm/l after desmopressin

Question 163

A 26-year-old female presented with a six-month history of light headedness on hanging the washing. She was seen by her general practitioner at the onset of her illness who noted a blood pressure of 80/50 mmHg in both arms but no other abnormality. Over six months she had on episode of weakness and numbness of the right arm and face for almost an hour and two near syncopal episodes. She developed increasing lethargy, night sweats, and aches and pains in her upper limbs. Her appetite had reduced and she had lost almost 3 kg in weight. There was no other past medical history of note. She smoked 10 cigarettes per day for three years from the age of 17.

On examination she was had flushed cheeks but there was no skin rash. The heart rate was 90 beats/min and regular. The systolic blood pressure was 80 mmHg in both upper limbs, but the diastolic blood pressure could not be ascertained. On examination of the precordium, the apex was heaving in nature but not displaced. On auscultation there was an audible fourth heart sound. The radial pulses were absent bilaterally, the brachial pulses were weak bilaterally, the right carotid pulse was absent. The left carotid pulse was prominent. Both femoral pulses were easily palpable. Neurological examination was normal.

Investigations are shown.

FBC	Hb 9.4 g/dl
	WCC 8 × 10⁹/l
	Platelets 430 × 10⁹/l
ESR	112 mm/h
Biochemistry	Sodium 135 mmol/l
	Potassium 4.5 mmol/l
	Urea 6 × 10 mmol/l
	Creatinine 84 µmol/l
	Glucose 4.5 mmol/l
	Cholesterol 5.3 mmol/l
Autoantibody screen	Rheumatoid factor absent
	Anti-nuclear antibodies present in a titre of 1in 16
Syphilis serology	VDRL and TPHA absent
Chest X-ray	Normal sized heart
	Clear lung fields
ECG	Voltage criteria for left ventricular hypertrophy
CT scan brain	Normal

1. What is the diagnosis?
A. Giant cell arteritis.
B. Polyarteritis nodosa.
C. Buerger's disease.
D. Takayasu's arteritis.
E. Relapsing polychondritis.

2. Which investigation would you request to confirm the diagnosis?
A. Aortrography.
B. Invasive blood pressure monitoring.
C. Serum anti-neutrophil cytoplasmic antibody.
D. Fluorescent treponemal antibody.
E. Cardiac biopsy.

3. Which of the three below would best explain the reason for left ventricular hypertrophy on the ECG?
A. Cardiac amyloid.
B. Essential hypertension.
C. Hypertension secondary to renal artery stenosis.
D. Chronic renal failure.
E. Fibromuscular dysplasia.
F. Renal vasculitis.
G. Acquired co-arctation of the aorta.
H. Reduced distensibility of the ascending aorta.

Answer 163

1. D. Takayasu's arteritis.
2. A. Aortrography.
3. C. Hypertension secondary to renal artery stenosis.
    G. Acquired co-arctation of the aorta.
    H. Reduced distensibility of the ascending aorta.

The absence of pulses in the arms and neck and the associated with a high ESR in a young woman should raise the diagnosis of Takayasu's arteritis. Takayasu's arteritis is a rare disorder with prevalence of 1.5–2 per million. It has a strong female predisposition and is more common in parts of Africa and Asia. The mean age of onset is 29 years, but it can occur from any age between infancy and middle age. It is very uncommon after middle age. The condition is caused by granulomatous vasculitis of large vessels, particularly the aortic arch, which results in obliterative changes in the lumnia of the vessels affected. Inflammation may be multisegmental, interspersed with normal segments. Symptoms comprise of a systemic illness (sweats, weight loss, amorexia and myagia) as well as vascular insufficiency in the limbs affected. Physical signs include pulseless vessels. Hypertension is present in 50% of cases, but was not detected in this case because of disease in both subclavian arteries. The cause of hypertension inlcudes renal artery stenosis, acquired co-arctation and reduced distensibility of the aortic arch. Complications are those of long-standing hypertension, aortic regurgitation and congestive cardiac failure. Inflammatory markers are usually raised and there may be an anaemia of chronic disease, but the diagnosis is a clinical one and can be confirmed with aortography. In this case, the patient had an occluded brachiocephalic and left subclavian artery. The differential diagnosis is between other conditions which may produce an aortic arch syndrome, such as syphilitic aortitis and relapsing polychondritis; however, in this case syphilis serology is negative and there are no clinical features of relapsing polychondritis. Treatment is with steroids and vascular stents.

Aortography in this patient demonstrated occluded innominate and left subclavian arteries (**163**). Only the left common carotid artery is patent.

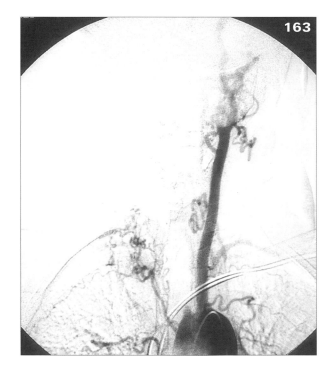

Data Interpretation

Calcium Biochemistry

Condition	Ca	PO$_4$	Alkaline phosphatase	Additional
1° and 3° hyperparathyroidism	↑	↓	↑	
2° hyperparathyroidism/CRF	↓/N	↑	↑	
Hypoparathyroidism	↓	↑	N	PTH absent
Pseudohypoparathyroidism	↓	↑	N	PTH elevated
Magnesium deficiency	↓	↑	↑	PTH normal
Pseudopseudohypoparathyroidism	N	N	N	
Osteomalacia/rickets	↓	↓	↑	
Osteoporosis	N	N	N	
Myeloma	↑	N	N*	
Paget's disease	N**	N	↑	↑ urinary hydroxyproline
Malignancy (bony metastases)	↑	N/↑	↑	
Sarcoidosis	N/↑	N	N	
Vitamin D intoxication	↑	↑	N	

* Increased with pathological fractures.   ** Increased after prolonged immobilization.

Genetics

Patterns of inheritance

Autosomal dominant inheritance
- Males and females are equally affected.
- All individuals inheriting the abnormal gene are affected.
- Offspring of affected parents (irrespective of the parental sex) have a 50% chance of inheriting the disease.
- This is in contrast to X-linked conditions where male-to-male transmission of disease does not occur.

Autosomal recessive inheritance
- Males and females are equally affected, but are fewer in number than in autosomal dominant conditions.
- Not all generations will be affected.
- If both parents are carriers for the recessive gene 25% of the offspring will be affected, 50% will become carriers, but will not have the disease and 25% will not have the abnormal gene.
- If an affected individual marries a carrier, then 50% offspring will be affected and 50% offspring will be carriers.
- If an affected individual marries another affected, then all offspring will be affected.

X-linked dominant inheritance
- Males and females are both affected.
- No male-to-male transmission.
- Affected males transmit the disease to 100% of their daughters.
- An affected female will transmit the disease to 50% of all offspring.

X-linked recessive inheritance
- Males are affected.
- Females are carriers.
- No male-to-male transmission.
- Daughters of affected males will be carriers.
- Female carrier will have 50% affected sons and 50% daughters who are carriers.

Inheritance of maternal mitochondrial genetic abnormalities
- During conception, only mitochondria from the ovum are passed on to the zygote.
- Affected females will pass the disease to 100% offspring.
- Affected males will not transmit disease to offspring.
- Examples include Leber's optic atrophy, Kearnes–Sayer syndrome, MELAS (mitochondrial encephalopathy, lactic acidosis and stroke-like syndrome), MERF (mitochondrial encephalopathy and red ragged fibres).

Audiograms

An audiogram of both ears may be presented on the same graph, or there may be a separate audiogram for each ear. A separate suffix will be given to differentiate between air conduction (AC) and bone conduction (BC).

In senosineuronal deafness, both air and bone conduction are diminished. The air–bone gap is usually narrow, i.e. there is not much difference between air and bone conduction. In conduction deafness, bone conduction is superior to air conduction on the affected side.

Normal hearing can detect sounds of a frequency between 250–8,000 Hz at a sound intensity of 0–10 dB (1). The following audiograms are most commonly tested in higher post-graduate examinations.

Senosorinuronal deafness at progressively higher frequencies. In degenerative senorineuronal loss (presbycusis), deafness is usually bilateral most profound at sounds with high frequencies (2). Other causes of bilateral senorineuronal deafness include congenital rubella infection, mumps infection and drugs, such as high dose loop diuretics and aminoglycosides.

Fluctuating low tone deafness (below 4,000 Hz) suggests Ménière's disease. This is bilateral in 10% of cases (3) and may progress to senorineuroanl deafness in 25% of patients (2).

Sudden and profound hearing loss at a frequency of 4,000 Hz is suggestive of noise-induced hearing loss (4).

Unilateral senorineuronal hearing loss (5) may be degenerative or due to unilateral auditory nerve damage as a result of a neuropathic process. It should also raise the suspicion of lesion in the cerebello-pontine angle on the affected side, for example, an acoustic neuroma.

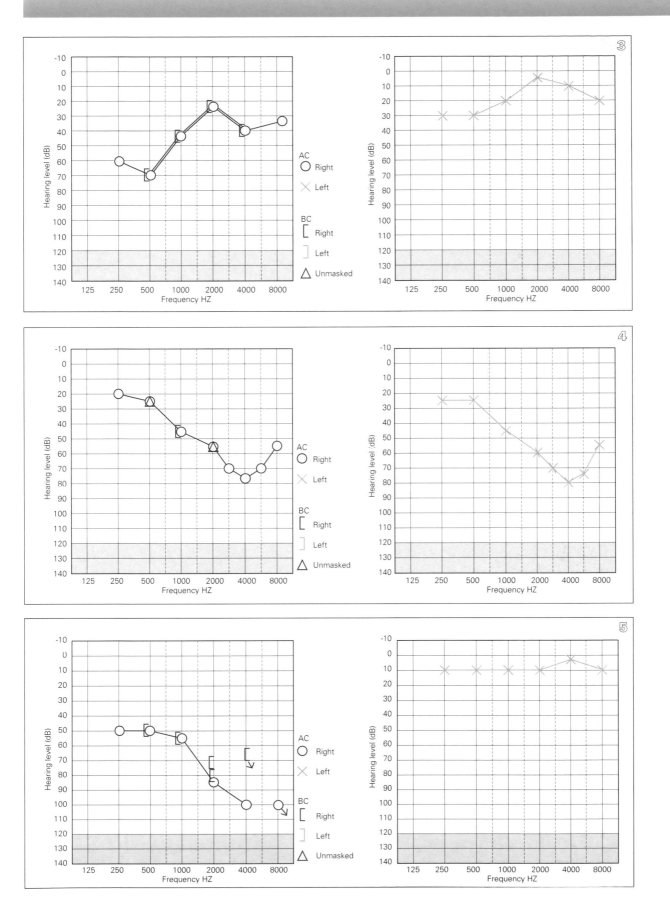

In the example below, bone conduction is superior to air conduction suggesting conduction deafness (**6**). Causes of conduction deafness are shown (*Table*).

> **Causes of conduction deafness**
>
> Ear wax
> Chronic suppurative otitis media
> Middle ear granuloma
> Otosclerosis

Guidelines for the Interpretation of Cardiac Catheter Data

- Right-heart saturations do not exceed 75%. Saturations more than this are suggestive of a left-to-right shunt.

- Left-heart saturations vary from 96–98%. Saturations less than this are suggestive of a right-to-left shunt.

- In right-to-left shunts, the arterial saturations do not change with inspired high-concentration oxygen.

- A VSD with a right-to-left shunt and pulmonary stenosis can be differentiated from Fallot's tetralogy by examining the oxygen saturation in the left ventricle and the ascending aorta. In the case of a VSD, the saturations in the left ventricle and the aorta will both be low and very similar. In the case of Fallot's tetralogy, the aortic oxygen saturation will be much lower than the oxygen saturation in the left ventricle because the right ventricle pumps most of the deoxygenated blood into the overriding aorta.

- A pulmonary artery pressure exceeding 35 mmHg is suggestive of pulmonary hypertension.

- A pressure drop of more than 10 mmHg across the aortic or pulmonary valve is suggestive of aortic or pulmonary stenosis, respectively.

- The PCWP is equal to the LVEDP. When the PCWP exceeds the LVEDP, the diagnosis of mitral stenosis should be considered.

- The diagnosis of mitral regurgitation cannot be made unless you are given the PCWP 'v-wave'. A v-wave higher than 20 mmHg is highly suggestive of mitral regurgitation.

- Aortic regurgitation is diagnosed by a wide pulse pressure in the aortic pressure.

- The right and LVEDP and the left and right atrial pressures are roughly equal in pericardial constriction.

Respiratory Function Tests

Obstructive lung defect

Examples:
- Chronic bronchitis.
- Emphysema.
- Asthma.
- Bronchiectasis.

Spirometry	
FEV_1 (l)	↓↓
FVC (l)	↓
FEV_1/FVC	<70% (normal 70–80%)
TLC (l)	↑ (gas trapping)
RV	↑
TLCO (l)	↓
KCO (mmol/min/kPa)	↓*

*The KCO is always low in obstructive airways disease, with the very rare exception of a limited number of patients with asthma who may have a high KCO during an attack. The exact mechanism for this is not understood. The KCO is significantly reduced in emphysema, and if a young patient or a non-smoker has a low KCO in the context of an obstructive lung defect, always consider the possibility of α-1 antitrypsin deficiency

Restrictive lung defect

Examples:
- Interstitial lung disease:
  sarcoidosis,
  fibrotic lung disease.
- Pulmonary emboli.
- Pulmonary oedema.
- Neuromuscular disease affecting respiratory muscles.
- Pulmonary haemorrhage.
- Lymphangitis carcinomatosa.
- Thoracic cage defects.

Spirometry	
FEV_1 (l)	↓
FVC (l)	↓↓
FEV_1/FVC	>80%
TLC (l)	↓
RV	↓
TLCO (l)	↓
KCO** (mmol/l/kPa)	↓

** KCO is charcteristically reduced in most cases of restrictive defect, with the exception of pulmonary haemorrhage, where it is increased, and thoracic cage deformities/neuromuscular defects and pneumonectomy where it is unchanged or increased

KCO

Increased KCO:
- Polycythaemia.
- Left-to-right shunts.
- Pulmonary haemorrhage.
- Asthma (exceptionally rare).
- Thoracic cage deformities (may be normal).

Reduced KCO:
- Interstitial lung disease.
- Primary pulmonary hypertension.
- Multiple pulmonary emboli.
- Pulmonary oedema.
- Lymphangitis carcinomatosa.
- Arteriovenous malformation.
- Anaemia (spirometry normal).
- Obstructive airways disease (rare exception is asthma).

Interpretation of Respiratory Flow Loop Curves

The normal flow loop curve has a triangular expiratory flow limb and a semi-circular inspiratory flow limb (**7**). The explanation for this is as follows: Following a full inspiration, the lung's recoil is maximal, as is pleural pressure. The onset of expiratory flow is therefore explosive and reaches its peak within 0.01 s. The expiratory curve decreases its flow gradually as the lung volume drops from TLC to RV. This reflects the gradual drop in the lung's elastic recoil as the lung gets smaller. In contrast to expiration, inspiration does not reach an instant maximal flow. As the respiratory muscles contract, the power increases progressively from the start of the inspiration to achieve a maximal flow. This takes a relatively long time, and the maximal inspiratory flow is only achieved by the mid-point of the vital capacity. The flow then slows again as the maximum inspired volume is reached, giving the inspiratory limb a semi-circular appearance.

Flow loops tested in the examination are those of obstructive airways disease, extrathoracic airways obstruction, intrathoracic airways obstruction, and a restrictive lung defect.

Obstructive airways disease

In obstructive airways disease the amount of elastic recoil in the lung is reduced; therefore the onset of the expiratory limb is not as explosive as in a normal individual and reaches its peak later than usual. As expiration continues the small airways collapse rapidly to produce a very early decline in flow which results in a 'flat' expiratory flow loop curve after the initial peak (**8**).

Extrathoracic airways disease obstruction

Extrathoracic airways may be variable or fixed. In extrathoracic obstruction, the inspiratory loop is reduced significantly compared with the expiratory flow. Normally, during inspiration, the negative intrathoracic pressure pulls the intrathoracic airways open and promotes inspiratory flow. In extrathoracic obstruction this does not happen; therefore the inspiratory flow rate is reduced. In variable extrathoracic obstruction the expiratory flow limb is preserved (**9**). Examples of variable obstruction include tumour in the upper airways, fat, pharyngeal muscle weakness, vocal cord paralysis or enlarged lymph nodes. In fixed extrathoracic obstruction, such as tracheal stenosis, both expiratory flow and inspiratory flow limbs are 'blunted'; however, the inspiratory limb is affected much more than the expiratory limb (**10**).

Intrathoracic airways obstruction

When obstruction is intrathoracic, inspiration is preserved because the large extrathoracic airways are patent; however, the expiratory flow is diminished because an increased intrathoracic pressure is required to overcome the obstruction, which results in closure of the small airways (**11**).

Restrictive lung disease

The flow loop curve has the same shape as the normal curve (**7**), but the lung volume is much smaller.

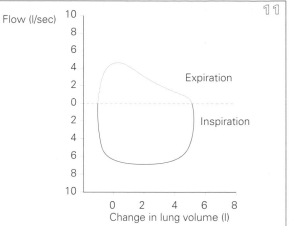

Echocardiography

Echocardiography has featured, and will continue to feature, in postgraduate examinations because it is widely requested, and pictures from 'still frames' are relatively easy to interpret. Both M-mode and two-dimensional (2D) echocardiography are tested, although the latter is being shown with an increasing frequency because it allows the reader to have a better appreciation of cardiac chambers.

Normal values for cardiac dimensions are shown in the table.

Normal values for cardiac dimensions	
Chamber/structure	*Measurement*
Left atrium	<4.5 cm
Left ventricular diastolic size	<5.5 cm
Interventricular septum	<1.2 cm
Posterior wall	<1.2 cm

2D echocardiography

The view which is shown most often is the parasternal long-axis view (**12**). In this view it is not always easy to study the right ventricle in detail, and therefore it is unusual to be shown right-sided pathology in the examination. Four-chamber views resemble what the reader envisages the heart to look like, except that the ventricles are at the top and the atria are at the bottom (**13**). Most echocardiograms are accompanied by a scale where each square represents 1 cm.

Key:
1 Interventricular septum
2 Left ventricle
3 Mitral valve
4 Left atrium
5 Left ventricular posterior wall
6 Aorta
7 Right ventricle
8 Right atrium

Figures **14** and **15** are diagrammatic representations of a common parasternal long axis and an apical four-chamber view respectively.

Common examples of conditions shown in examinations using 2D echocardiography:
- Pericardial effusion (**16**, effusion is arrowed).
- Left atrial myxoma (**17**, myxoma is arrowed).
- Mitral stenosis (**18**, stenosed mitral valve is arrowed).
- Vegetation on mitral valve (**19**, vegetation on the anterior mitral valve leaflet is arrowed).

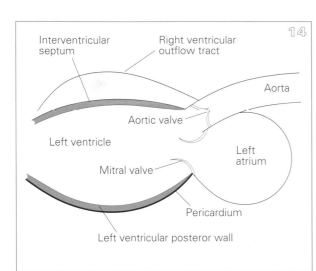

Interventricular septum
Right ventricular outflow tract
Aorta
Aortic valve
Left ventricle
Left atrium
Mitral valve
Pericardium
Left ventricular posteror wall

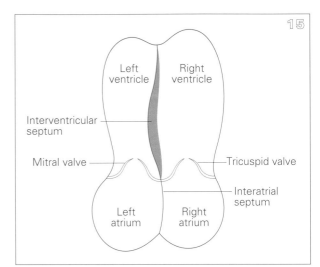

Left ventricle
Right ventricle
Interventricular septum
Mitral valve
Tricuspid valve
Interatrial septum
Left atrium
Right atrium

- HCM (**20**, gross hypertrophy of the interventricular septum is arrowed).
- Left ventricular thrombus (**21** thrombus at the apex is arrowed; **22** thrombus is arrowed).
- Aortic stenosis (**23**, calcified aortic valve arrowed).
- Vegetation on aortic valve (**24**, echogenic mass on the aortic valve is arrowed).
- Aortic dissection (**25**, aortic dissection flap is arrowed).

Figure **26** is a diagrammatic representation of common examples shown on parasternal long-axis view. Figure **27** is a diagrammatic representation of common examples shown in the four-chamber view.

M-mode echocardiography

The M-mode picture is derived by taking a cross-sectional view from the 2D parasternal long-axis view. The three main views include sections at the level of the aortic valve, at the level of the tips of the mitral valve, and at the level of the papillary muscle. The cross-sectional view at the level of the mitral valve tips is by far the most common view which is shown in examinations because it allows the examiners to test the readers on abnormalities on the mitral valve and the left ventricle (**28**).

Examples commonly shown in M-mode echocardiography:
- Pericardial effusion.
- Left atrial myxoma (**29**, echogenic mass prolapsing through the mitral valve orifice in diastole is arrowed).
- Mitral stenosis (**30**, thickened anterior mitral valve leaflet is arrowed; reduced excursion of the mitral valve in diastole is shown [1]).
- Vegetation on mitral valve (**31**, echogenic mass on the posterior mitral valve leaflet is arrowed).
- Mitral valve prolapse (**32**, hammocking of the posterior mitral valve leaflet in diastole is arrowed).
- HCM (**33**, systolic anterior motion of the mitral valve is shown [1]).

Importance of carefully inspecting mitral valve leaflets to diagnose cardiac abnormalities on the M-mode echocardiogram

On an M-mode echocardiogram, the normal mitral valve has an anterior leaflet which has a characteristic 'M'-shape and a posterior leaflet which has a semi 'U'-shape. In diastole, the anterior leaflet moves forward and the posterior leaflet moves backward, and in systole both leaflets appose. With the exception of pericardial effusion, careful inspection of the mitral valve will enable the reader to diagnose all the abnormalities which are commonly tested.

Figure **34** is a diagrammatic representation of the mitral valve in relation to cardiac lesions on the M-mode echocardiogram.

The mitral valve in relation to cardiac lesions on the M-mode echocardiogram

Abnormality	Mitral valve abnormality
Mitral valve prolapse	Normal appearance in diastole, however, in mid systole there is prolapse of one or both leaflets
Mitral stenosis	There is loss of the M-shape of the anterior leaflet Mitral valve excursion is reduced and there is anterior movement of the posterior leaflet in diastole
Atrial myxoma	There is obliteration of the mitral valve cavity by an echogenic mass in diastole
Vegetation on mitral valve	Echogenic mass on one or both leaflets
HCM	The mitral valve moves forward towards the septum in systole (a phenomenon termed systolic anterior motion of the mitral valve (SAM). In addition, the left ventricular cavity is small and there is septal hypertrophy
Aortic regurgitation	As the regurgitant jet flows back into the left ventricle it 'tickles' the anterior leaflet, causing a fluttering appearance

AMVL: Anterior mitral valve leaflet
PMVL: Posterior mitral valve leaflet

Acid–base Disturbance

Acidosis

The main source of acid (H^+ ions) in the body is tissue respiration. Carbon dioxide produced by cellular respiration is converted to carbonic acid, which dissociates to generate H^+ (acid) and HCO_3^- ions (buffering base). The retention of CO_2, increase in H^+ or reduction in HCO_3^- may result in an acidosis.

$$CO_2 + H_2O \leftrightarrow H_2CO_3 \leftrightarrow H^+ + HCO_3^-$$

Three types of acidosis are recognized:
- Respiratory acidosis.
- Metabolic acidosis with a high anion gap.
- Metabolic acidosis with a normal anion gap.

Respiratory acidosis is characterized by a fall in arterial pH (<7.35) due to CO_2 retention. Metabolic acidosis may result from the retention of fixed or organic acids causing a reduction in the bicarbonate level (which is the main buffering agent for H^+ in the blood) without any change in the chloride situation. In these situations, it is termed metabolic acidosis with a high anion gap. Alternatively, metabolic acidosis may occur as a consequence of bicarbonate loss from the gastrointestinal tract or the kidneys. In these situations, chloride is retained, resulting in a hyperchloraemic acidosis or a metabolic acidosis with a normal anion gap. The anion gap is calculated by subtracting the sum of the sodium and potassium concentrations from the sum of the chloride and bicarbonate concentrations. The normal anion gap is between 10–18 mmol/l. The hallmark of metabolic acidosis of either type is a low arterial pH and a low bicarbonate level.

Regulation of arterial pH is controlled by the kidneys and the lungs. Acidosis can be compensated for either by removing CO_2 from the body (lungs) or by retaining bicarbonate ions (kidneys). Respiratory acidosis is compensated for by the kidneys, which retain bicarbonate ions. In compensated respiratory acidosis the pH is normal, or almost normal, and the bicarbonate level is high. In compensated metabolic acidosis the arterial pH is normal, or almost normal, and the pCO_2 is low. Respiratory acidosis is compensated by the respiratory system through a centrally mediated mechanism which results in hyperventilation and a consequent reduction in the pCO_2. Causes of respiratory and metabolic acidosis are given (*Table*).

Alkalosis

Alkalosis may be respiratory or metabolic in origin. In respiratory alkalosis, there is a high pH due to hyperventilation, causing a low pCO_2. Metabolic alkalosis is usually due to increased loss of H^+ from the kidney or gastrointestinal tract, or to increased ingestion of alkaline agents. It is characterized by a high bicarbonate and a high pH. Respiratory alkalosis is rare and is usually acute. Chronic cases, usually due to chronic hyperventilation, are compensated for by increasing bicarbonate excretion by the kidneys. Metabolic alkalosis – which is much more common than respiratory alkalosis – is compensated for by respiratory hypoventilation, which results in an increase in pCO_2 and hence an increase in H^+.

Causes of respiratory and metabolic acidosis

Respiratory acidosis
- Hypoventilation from any cause, e.g. obesity, thoracic cage deformities and neuromuscular disorders
- Obstructive airways disease
- Acute asthma

Metabolic acidosis (high anion gap)
- Diabetic ketoacidosis
- Uraemic acidosis
- Salicylate poisoning
- Lactic acidosis: shock,
                     liver failure,
                     metformin therapy,
                     glucose-6-phosphate
                         dehydrogenase deficiency,
                     leukaemia
- Methylene poisoning
- Ethylene glycol poisoning

Metabolic acidosis (normal anionic gap)
- Severe diarrhoea
- Pancreatic fistula
- Ureterosigmoidostomy
- RTA
- Acetazolamide therapy

Causes of respiratory and metabolic alkalosis

Respiratory alkalosis:
- Hyperventilation
- Hysteria
- Encephalitis
- Brainstem lesions
- Aspirin toxicity

Metabolic alkalosis:
- Vomiting
- Diuretics
- Antacids
- Hypokalaemic states (these increase renal loss of H^+ by the distal convoluted tubule)

Examination Questions

For the Answers to the Examination Questions, see pages 239–249.

Examination Question 1

A 50-year-old shipyard worker presented with a single episode of haemoptysis comprising of approximately one egg-cup-full of fresh blood. He gave a two-year history of progressively increasing breathlessness and a persistent cough. He had never experienced any chest pain. He stopped smoking two months previously after a chest infection which took several weeks to resolve, but before that was smoking 20–30 cigarettes/day. He kept pigeons in his teenage years, but had not had any direct contact with birds since. The only other past medical history of note was a four-year history of mild hypertension for which he was taking propranolol 80 mg three times daily.

On examination, he was centrally cyanosed and had early finger clubbing. The respiratory rate was 23 per min. On examination of the respiratory system the chest expansion was symmetrical, but generally reduced. The trachea was central. On auscultation of the lung fields there were fine end-inspiratory crackles at both lung bases. Precordial examination was normal, with the exception of a loud pulmonary component to the second heart sound.

Investigations are shown.

1. What is the cause of the haemoptysis (3 marks)?
A. Mesothelioma.
B. Carcinoma of the bronchus.
C. Extrinsic allergic alveolitis.
D. TB.
E. Pulmonary embolus.

2. What is the cause of his breathlessness (3 marks)?
A. Chronic obstructive airways disease.
B. Therapy with propranolol.
C. Extrinsic allergic alveolitis.
D. Cryptogenic fibrosing alveolitis/diffuse pulmonary fibrosis.
E. Asbestosis.

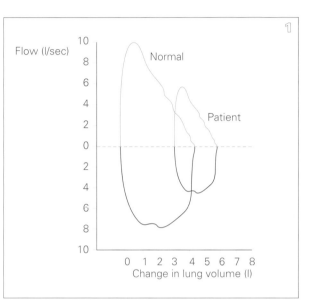

FBC	Hb 14 g/dl
	WCC 9×10^9/l
	Platelets 190×10^9/l
	MCV 91 fl
ESR	64 mm/h
Biochemistry	Sodium 132 mmol/l
	Potassium 3.7 mmol/l
	Urea 7 mmol/l
	Creatinine 91 µmol/l
Arterial blood gases	pH 7.44
	pO_2 7.1
	pCO_2 3.4
	Bicarbonate 21
	O_2 saturation 75%
Chest X-ray	Irregular, linear shadowing at both lung bases
Sputum microscopy	No abnormalities
Flow loop (**1**)	

Examination Question 2

A 16-year-old girl collapsed at school while playing hockey. According to the physical training tutor, she was unconscious for a few seconds and then was completely rousable and did not realize what had happened. The episode occurred without any warning symptoms. There was no history of trauma or head injury during the game, or any ill health before the game. There was no history of epilepsy. She had experienced two previous syncopal episodes at the age of 8 and 11 years. On the first occasion she had witnessed a road traffic accident, and on the second occasion she collapsed after receiving a hoax telephone call. She had been completely well since the last syncopal episode. She was not taking any medication. She had a younger brother, aged 14 who was well. Her parents were well. Her mother had a past history of syncopal episodes during her adolescence for which no cause had been found. Her maternal aunt was found dead in her bed at the age of 15, for which no cause was found at post-mortem.

On examination, the patient was 1.55 m tall and weighed 48 kg. Her heart rate was 65 beats/min and irregular. The blood pressure was 110/65 mmHg. Examination of the precordium was completely normal. There were no carotid bruits, and all peripheral pulses were palpable. The chest was clear and abdominal examination was normal. Examination of the central nervous system including the fundi was completely normal

Investigations are shown.

The following day, the patient was being seen by the consultant cardiologist and his team on the ward when she had a syncopal episode. The tracing from the ECG monitor is shown (**2b**).

FBC	Hb 14 g/dl
	WCC 12 × 10⁹/l
	Platelets 300 × 10⁹/l
Blood glucose	5 mmol/l
ECG (**2a**)	
Biochemistry	Sodium 136 mmol/l
	Potassium 3.5 mmol/l
	Urea 4 mmol/l

1. What are the two abnormalities on the 12-lead ECG (4 marks)?
A. Sinus tachycardia.
B. Short PR-interval.
C. Delta wave in the QRS-complex.
D. Non-sustained polymorphic ventricular tachycardia.
E. Supraventricular tachycardia with aberrant conduction.
F. Ventricular bigemini.
G. Long QT-interval.
H. Ventricular ectopics.

2. What is the best explanation for the syncopal episode during the hockey match (2 marks)?
A. Atrial fibrillation.
B. Supraventricular tachycardia.
C. Ventricular ectopics.
D. Ventricular fibrillation.
E. Cerebral hypoperfusion due to torsades de pointes.
F. Sinus arrest.
G. Cerebral hypoperfusion.

3. What is the diagnosis (2 marks)?
A. Wolff–Parkinson–White syndrome.
B. Lown–Ganong–Levine syndrome.
C. Hypertrophic cardiomyopathy.
D. Ischaemic heart disease.
E. Acquired LQTS.
F. Congenital LQTS.
G. Drug overdose.

4. What is the underlying abnormality in this disorder (2 marks)?
A. Myocardial disarray.
B. Accessory conduction pathway.
C. Premature coronary artery disease.
D. Abnormal sodium/potassium channels in cardiac myocytes.
E. Fibrofatty replacement of the myocardium.
F. Myocardial fibrosis.

5. How would you manage this patient immediately (2 marks)?
A. Intravenous isoprenaline.
B. Intravenous atropine.
C. Intravenous adenosine.
D. A beta blocker.
E. Intravenous magnesium.
F. Intravenous adrenaline.
G. Atrial pacing.

6. Which other important investigation would you perform (3 marks)?
A. Cardiac enzymes.
B. Echocardiogram.
C. Electrophysiological studies.
D. Family screening.
E. Serum cholesterol.
F. Serum potassium.
G. Serum magnesium.

Examination Question 3

1. What is the mode of inheritance in the family shown (**3**) (3 marks)?
A. Autosomal recessive.
B. Autosomal dominant.
C. X-linked recessive.
D. X-linked dominant.
E. Y-linked.

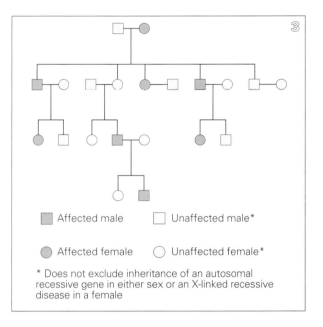

Affected male □ Unaffected male*

Affected female ○ Unaffected female*

* Does not exclude inheritance of an autosomal recessive gene in either sex or an X-linked recessive disease in a female

Examination Question 4

A 16-year-old boy was admitted to hospital with a three-day history of abdominal pain and jaundice. One week before admission he had developed a sore throat, accompanied by fever and myalgia. He had experienced two similar episodes of jaundice and abdominal pain preceded by a sore throat and fever at the ages of 6, 12 and 14, and on each occasion he made an uncomplicated recovery. There was no history of recent travel abroad. He was the only child in the family.

On examination, he had a temperature of 39°C (102.2°F). He was mildly jaundiced and had tender cervical lymphadenopathy. Examination of the throat revealed a purulent exudate. Examination of the lungs was normal. On examination of the abdomen there was a palpable spleen 5 cm below the costal margin.

Investigations were shown.

FBC	Hb 11 g/dl
	WCC 6 × 10⁹/l
	Platelets 100 × 10⁹/l
Monospot test	Negative
Biochemistry	Bilirubin 33 μmol/l
	ALT 23 u/l
	Alkaline phosphatase 120 u/l
Urine	Urobilinogen ++++
	Nil else

1. What is the diagnosis (3 marks)?
2. List two tests which you would perform to confirm the diagnosis (6 marks).

Examination Question 5

A 70-year-old man was awoken with retrosternal chest pain radiating into his left arm in the early hours of the morning. The pain was persistent for 5 hours, and unrelieved by taking antacids before finally subsiding. The following day he consulted his daughter over the telephone, who persuaded him to make an urgent appointment with his general practitioner. There was a past history of mild hypertension and hypothyroidism. The latter was diagnosed over a year ago after the patient presented with lethargy and was treated with 25 µg of thyroxine; however, the drug was stopped by the patient within three months because he felt well again. He was a non-smoker and consumed alcohol on a very infrequent basis. Over the past two months he had felt lethargic and saw another doctor who diagnosed depression. He lived alone. He had been widowed three years previously. He took antacids for infrequent indigestion.

On visiting his general practitioner, an ECG was performed (5). The patient was referred to the local hospital immediately for further evaluation. On arrival at hospital he appeared pale, but was well perfused. His heart rate was 50 beats/min, and blood pressure was 150/95 mmHg. The heart sounds were normal and the chest was clear. There was no clinical evidence of cardiac failure. Neurological examination was normal.

Further investigations are shown.

FBC	Hb 9.6 g/dl
	WCC 4×10^9/l
	Platelets 150×10^9/l
MCV	108 fl
Biochemistry	Sodium 132 mmol/l
	Potassium 3.8 mmol/l
	Urea 3 mmol/l

	Day 1	Day 3
Creatinine kinase	300 u/l	170 u/l
LDH	300 u/l	600 u/l

TSH	21 mu/l
Thyroxine	30 nmol/l
Thyroid microsomal antibodies	Positive 1/3,000
Morning cortisol	800 ng/l
LH	8 u/l (normal 1–10 u/l)
FSH	5 u/l (normal 1–7 u/l)
Prolactin	550 mu/l

1. List three abnormalities on the ECG (5 marks).
A. ST-segment depression in I, II, V3–V6.
B. Inverted T-wave in aVl.
C. Sinus tachycardia.
D. Anterior myocardial infarction.
E. Inferior myocardial infarction.
F. Left ventricular hypertrophy.

2. Give two reasons for the elevated creatinine kinase (4 marks).
A. Anterolateral myocardial infarction.
B. Non-Q-wave anterolateral infarction.
C. Inferior myocardial infarction.
D. Hypothyroidism.
E. Kleinfelter's syndrome.
F. Intramuscular injection.

3. What is the most likely cause of the abnormal thyroid function tests (1 mark)?
A. Secondary hypothyroidism.
B. Tertiary hypothyroidism.
C. Autoimmune hypothyroidism.
D. Hashimoto's hypothyroidism.
E. Sick euthyroid syndrome.

4. Which two investigations would you perform to investigate the cause of this patient's anaemia (3 marks)?
A. Serum B_{12} level.
B. Serum folate.
C. Gastric parietal antibodies.
D. Intrinsic factor antibodies.
E. Schilling test.
F. Serum ferritin.
G. Hb electrophoresis.

Examination Question 6

A 58-year-old man presented with a three-month history of lower back pain. He had also noticed weakness in his legs when climbing stairs, and had considerable difficulty in raising himself from a chair. More recently, he was excessively thirsty and was waking frequently at night to pass urine. He had lost over 4 kg in weight since the onset of his illness. Before this he was well. He was married with two children. He had been smoking over 20 cigarettes per day for more than 30 years. He consumed 3 units of alcohol per day.

On examination, he was thin. The blood pressure was 160/90 mmHg. He had wasting of his thigh muscles. Power in both the arms and legs was slightly diminished, but sensation and reflexes were preserved.

Investigations are shown.

The patient was given 8 mg dexamethasone for three days, and repeat 9.00 am and midnight serum cortisol was over 1,000 nmol/l.

FBC	Hb 11 g/dl
	WCC 13×10^9/l
	Platelets 480×10^9/l
	MCV 89 fl
Blood film	Normal
ESR	44 mm/h
Biochemistry	Sodium 140 mmol/l
	Potassium 3 mmol/l
	Urea 8 mmol/l
	Bicarbonate 30 mmol/l
	Glucose 10 mmol/l
	Calcium 2.7 mmol/l
	Phosphate 1.5 mmol/l
	Albumin 36 g/l
LFT	Normal
Serum cortisol at 9.00 am	>1,000 nmol/l
Serum cortisol at midnight	>1,000 nmol/l

1. What is the cause of this patient's lower limb weakness (5 marks)?
A. Diabetic amyotrophy.
B. Steroid-induced myopathy.
C. Hypokalaemia.
D. Eaton–Lambert syndrome.
E. Metastatic spinal cord compression.

2. What is the most likely cause for the back pain (5 marks)?
A. Bone metastases.
B. Fractured vertebra.
C. Myeloma.
D. Infiltration of the lower spinal nerves by carcinoma.
E. Osteoporosis.

3. List two possible diagnoses (10 marks)?
A. Cushing's disease.
B. Conn's syndrome.
C. Cortisol-secreting adenoma.
D. Ectopic ACTH production from a bronchial carcinoma.
E. Pseudo Cushing's syndrome secondary to alcohol abuse.

4. Which two tests would be most useful in making the diagnosis (10 marks)?
A. Serum ACTH.
B. Chest X-ray.
C. CT scan of the adrenals.
D. Petrosal venous sampling.
E. Lying and standing renin and aldosterone levels.

Examination Question 7

A 36-year-old woman presented with a four-week history of intermittent upper abdominal pain and vomiting. Her bowel movements were unaffected and were normal. There was no blood or mucus in the stool. Her appetite was reduced. She had lost 2 kg in weight. She has a past medical history of ulcerative colitis which was diagnosed at the age of 14 years, and was stable on sulphasalazine. In the past, she had received several courses of steroids for acute exacerbation of her colitis. Her only other drug history was that she was currently on the contraceptive pill. She had been married for 10 years and had two children, aged 7 and 3 years. She smoked 15 cigarettes per day and consumed 1–2 units of alcohol per week.

On examination, she appeared unwell. Her tongue was dry and there was loss of skin turgor. She had mild lower-limb pitting oedema. The heart rate was 98 beats/min and blood pressure was 100/65 mmHg. The temperature was 36.8°C (98.2°F). The abdomen was slightly distended, and there was generalized tenderness. The liver was palpable 4 cm below the costal margin, and was tender. There was no evidence of a palpable spleen or any other palpable masses in the abdomen. Percussion of the abdomen revealed shifting dullness. Rectal examination was normal. Examination of the respiratory and cardiovascular system was normal.

Investigations are shown.

FBC	Hb 13 g/dl
	WCC 8 × 10⁹/l
	Platelets 190 × 10⁹/l
Electrolytes	Sodium 131 mmol/l
	Potassium 3.1 mmol/l
	Urea 7.2 mmol/l
	Creatinine 100 µmol/l
LFT	Bilirubin 20 µmol/l
	AST 24 u/l
	ALT 21 u/l
	Alkaline phosphatase 150 u/l
	Albumin 29 g/l
Chest X-ray	Normal heart size
	Clear lung fields

1. What two investigations would you request to ascertain the cause of the presentation (8 marks)?
2. What two underlying diagnoses would you consider in this patient (4 marks)?

Examination Question 8

A 69-year-old woman presented with pain in her shoulders and upper back, polydipsia and polyuria.

Investigations are shown.

FBC	Hb 9 g/dl
	WCC 14 × 10⁹/l
	Platelets 140 × 10⁹/l
	MCV 89 fl
Biochemistry	Sodium 129 mmol/l
	Potassium 3.4 mmol/l
	Urea 26 mmol/l
	Creatinine 290 µmol/l
	Calcium 2.8 mmol/l
	Phosphate 1.9 mmol/l
	Total protein 98 g/l
	Albumin 34 g/l

1. What is the diagnosis (1 mark)?
2. List three investigations which will help confirm the diagnosis (4 marks).
3. Give four reasons for the raised urea (4 marks).
4. Give three reasons for the anaemia (5 marks).
5. Suggest two possible reasons for the low sodium (2 marks).
6. Give one possible cause for the low potassium (2 marks).
7. Give the most feasible explanation for the polydipsia and polyuria (2 marks).

Examination Question 9

1. Which of the following statements about this
12-lead ECG (**9a**) are correct (5 marks)?
A. Ventricular tachycardia.
B. Left axis deviation.
C. Voltage for left atrial enlargement.
D. LBBB.
E. Right axis deviation.
F. Voltage criteria for right ventricular hypertrophy.
G. RBBB.
H. Voltage criteria for right atrial enlargement.
I. Voltage criteria for left ventricular hypertrophy.
J. Dissociated P-waves.
K. Capture beats.
L. Delta waves.

Examination Question 10

A 17-year-old boy was referred to the local paediatrician because he had not grown very much in the past four years. Apart from feeling more lethargic than his school friends, he gave no other history of note. He measured 1.53 m. He had never needed to shave. His younger brother aged 16 measured 1.73 m and had already started shaving. There were no other siblings. Both parents were well. The father was 1.76 m tall and the mother was 1.63 m tall.

On examination, he was slightly pale. He did not have any facial hair. He was below the third centile for height and was just at the 10th centile for weight. He did not have any evidence of secondary sexual characteristics, and his testes were small. The blood pressure was 115/70 mmHg.

Investigations are shown.

FBC	Hb 10 g/dl
	WCC 7×10^9/l
	Platelets 200×10^9/l
	MCV 102 fl
Biochemistry	Sodium 138 mmol/l
	Potassium 4.3 mmol/l
	Urea 4 mmol/l
	Calcium 2.2 mmol/l
	Phosphate 1.1 mmol/l
	Albumin 38 g/l
	Glucose 4.3 mmol/l

1. List two possible diagnoses (4 marks).
2. Give one confirmatory test for each diagnosis (3 marks).

Examination Question 11

A 17-year-old female was admitted with a six-week history of malaise and joint pains. She had pain affecting her neck, left shoulder and the small joints of both her hands. She had intermittent fever associated with profuse sweating. She was born in Kenya and travelled to England for further studies two years ago. She had not travelled abroad since. She was well while in Kenya, although she had had two mild attacks of malaria at the age of 5 years and 12 years. She was a non-smoker and a tee-totaller. Two days before coming into hospital she developed some sharp infra-mammary chest pain which was worsened by movement, deep inspiration and on lying flat. There was no history of cough or sputum production. Her appetite was slightly reduced and she had lost 2 kg in weight.

On examination, she appeared unwell. She had a temperature of 39.2°C (102.6°F) and a widespread rash shown in **11a**. The heart rate was 110 beats/min and blood pressure 110/65 mmHg. She had small, non-tender, palpable lymph nodes in the anterior cervical triangle. On examination of the cardiovascular system she had a very soft systolic murmur at the left lower sternal angle, and a soft third heart sound. The chest was clear. Abdominal examination revealed a palpable spleen 3 cm below the costal margin. She had a few shotty lymph nodes in the inguinal region.

Cervical spine movements were slightly limited due to pain. Her hands were swollen and tender. The left shoulder was painful to abduct, but there was no obvious swelling of the joint. Examination of the central nervous system and fundoscopy was normal.

Investigations are shown.

FBC	Hb 10 g/dl
	WCC 17 × 10⁹/l
	Platelets 470 × 10⁹/l
	MCV 82 fl
Malaria parasite	Absent
ESR	86 mm/h
CRP	54 g/l
Biochemistry	Sodium 134 mmol/l
	Potassium 3.8 mmol/l
	Urea 5 mmol/l
	Creatinine 70 µmol/l
Blood cultures × 3	Negative
Thyroid function tests	Thyroxine 98 nmol/l
	TSH 1.1 mu/l
ECG (**11b**)	
Chest X-ray	Normal
Echocardiogram (**11c**)	
Rhesus factor	Absent
Urinalysis	Trace of protein
	No blood

1. What is the cause of the patient's chest pain (2 marks)?
A. Pleurisy.
B. Pulmonary embolus.
C. Pericardial effusion.
D. Acute pericarditis.
E. Musculoskeletal.
F. Myocarditis.
G. Endocarditis.

2. What two further tests would you perform (5 marks)?
A. Antinuclear antibody.
B. Repeat blood cultures.
C. Blood film for malaria.
D. Anti-streptolysin O titres.
E. X-ray of hands.
F. X-ray of left shoulder.
G. X-ray of cervical spine.
H. Cervical lymph node biopsy.
I. Mantoux test.
J. CT scan abdomen.
K. Serum ACE level.
L. Transbronchial lung biopsy.
M. *Brucella* titres.

3. What is the most probable diagnosis (5 marks)?
A. Sarcoidosis.
B. Adult-onset Still's disease.
C. Systemic lupus erythematosus.
D. Familial Mediterranean fever.
E. Brucellosis.
F. Rheumatic fever.
G. Rheumatoid arthritis.
H. Infective endocarditis.
I. Malaria.
J. Lymphoma.

Examination Question 12

A 13-year-old girl was admitted with a two-day history of lower abdominal pain and blood-stained diarrhoea. Three days later, she developed pains in her ankles and right elbow and felt nauseous. Positive findings on examination were a purpuric rash affecting the arms and legs, periorbital oedema, and a blood pressure of 150/95 mmHg.

Investigations are shown.

1. What is the most probable diagnosis (3 marks)?
A. Haemolytic–uraemic syndrome.
B. IgA nephritis.
C. Henoch–Schönlein purpura.
D. Systemic lupus erythematosus.
E. Polyarteritis nodosa.

2. List two investigations which would be most useful in confirming the diagnosis (5 marks).
A. Skin biopsy.
B. Renal biopsy.
C. Blood cultures.
D. TT.
E. Serum fibrinogen level.
F. Serum IgA level.
G. Serum ANF level.
H. Serum ANCA.

FBC	Hb 10 g/dl
	WCC 12 × 10^9/l
	Platelets 136 × 10^9/l
	MCV 70 fl
ESR	35 mm/h
Clotting	PT 13 s (control 13 s)
	APTT 34 s (control 36 s)
Biochemistry	Sodium 138 mmol/l
	Potassium 5.9 mmol/l
	Creatinine 130 µmol/l
Urinalysis	Blood ++
	Protein ++

Examination Question 13

A 60-year-old man presents with general malaise and drowsiness. On examination, the blood pressure was 120/70 mmHg.

Investigations are shown.

1. What is the diagnosis (3 marks)?
2. List two investigations which you would perform to confirm the diagnosis (4 marks).

Sodium	108 mmol/l
Potassium	4 mmol/l
Urea	3 mmol/l
Creatinine	56 µmol/l
Bicarbonate	23 mmol/l
Random blood sugar	4.2 mmol/l
Urine glucose	Not detected
Urine ketones	Not detected

Examination Question 14

A 68-year-old woman presented with lethargy, mild weight loss, weakness, and progressive pain and stiffness of her shoulders and thighs. On examination, she had tender shoulder and thigh muscles and a fever of 38°C (100.4°F).

Investigations are shown.

1. What is the diagnosis (2 marks)?
2. List two investigations you would perform to confirm the diagnosis (2 marks).

FBC	Hb 11 g/dl
	WCC $13 \times 10^9/l$
	Platelets $160 \times 10^9/l$
ESR	85 mm/h
Rheumatoid factor	1/640
Biochemistry	AST 86 u/l
	ALT 296 u/l
	Alkaline phosphatase 100 u/l
	Bilirubin 12 µmol/l
	LDH 1500 u/l

Examination Question 15

A 56-year-old woman presented with a four-day history of breathlessness, cough and a high fever. She gave a long history of indigestion and intermittent dysphagia to solids and fluids. On several occasions undigested food would be regurgitated back shortly after she had eaten. She would often wake at nights with episodes of coughing and spluttering. There was no history of weight loss.

On examination, she had a temperature of 39°C (102.2°F). The respiratory rate was 30/min, and the heart rate was 102 beats/min. Chest expansion was moderate and symmetrical. On auscultation of the lung fields there were coarse bilateral basal crackles.

The chest X-ray demonstrated bilateral lower-lobe consolidation.

1. What is the cause of this patient's illness (5 marks)?
A. Hiatus hernia.
B. Benign oesophageal stricture.
C. Achalasia.
D. Pharyngeal pouch.
E. Bronchiectasis.

2. Which investigation would be most useful in identifying the cause of her presentation (5 marks)?
A. Oesophagoscopy.
B. Barium swallow.
C. Oesophageal manometry.
D. Bronchoscopy.
E. CT scan of the thorax.

Examination Answers

Examination Answer 1

1. Maximum mark = 3
A. Mesothelioma. (1 mark)
B. Carcinoma of the bronchus. (3 marks)
C. Extrinsic allergic alveolitis. (0 marks)
D. TB. (0 marks)
E. Pulmonary embolus. (0 marks)

2. Maximum mark = 3
A. Chronic obstructive airways disease. (0 marks)
B. Therapy with propranolol. (0 marks)
C. Extrinsic allergic alveolitis. (0 marks)
D. Cryptogenic fibrosing
alveolitis/diffuse pulmonary fibrosis. (0 marks)
E. Asbestosis. (3 marks)

Total possible marks = 6

The main features of this case are a long-term smoker who presents with haemoptysis. He has worked in the shipyard, an occupation which was historically associated with asbestos exposure. He has objective evidence of lung fibrosis; he is hypoxic, his chest X-ray shows linear shadowing in the lower zones and the flow loop is consistent with shrunken lungs. In the context of this case the most likely cause for lung fibrosis and breathlessness is asbestosis. The history of keeping pigeons may implicate extrinsic allergic alveolitis as a possible cause; however, it has been a long time since he was exposed to avian antigens. Furthermore, extrinsic allergic alveolitis classically causes upper zone reticulonodular shadowing on the chest X-ray, whereas asbestosis is associated with shadowing in the lower zones.

While there are several causes of haemoptysis, the two most probable causes in this case are mesothelioma and bronchial carcinoma. Both malignancies are associated with asbestos exposure. The chest X-ray does not mention obvious pleural thickening or pleural effusion which are classic features of mesothelioma; therefore an underlying bronchial carcinoma would need to be excluded. Smoking and asbestos exposure together increase the risk of bronchial carcinoma several fold. With the exception of extrinsic allergic alveolitis, all the possibilities mentioned may also cause haemoptysis; however, the history is atypical for pulmonary embolus and tuberculosis would be lower down in the differential diagnosis than lung malignancy.

Examination Answer 2

1. Maximum mark = 4
A. Sinus tachycardia. (0 marks)
B. Short PR-interval. (0 marks)
C. Delta wave in the QRS-complex. (0 marks)
D. Non-sustained polymorphic
ventricular tachycardia. (2 marks)
E. Supraventricular tachycardia
with aberrant conduction. (0 marks)
F. Ventricular bigemini. (0 marks)
G. Long QT-interval. (2 marks)
H. Ventricular ectopics. (1 mark)

2. Maximum mark = 2
A. Atrial fibrillation. (0 marks)
B. Supraventricular tachycardia. (0 marks)
C. Ventricular ectopics. (0 marks)
D. Ventricular fibrillation. (0 marks)
E. Cerebral hypoperfusion due to
torsades de pointes. (2 marks)
F. Sinus arrest. (1 marks)
G. Cerebral hypoperfusion. (1 mark)

3. Maximum mark = 2
A. Wolff–Parkinson–White syndrome. (0 marks)
B. Lown–Ganong–Levine syndrome. (0 marks)
C. Hypertrophic cardiomyopathy. (0 marks)
D. Ischaemic heart disease. (0 marks)
E. Acquired LQTS. (0 marks)
F. Congenital LQTS. (2 marks)
G. Drug overdose. (0 marks)

4. Maximum mark = 2
A. Myocardial disarray. (0 marks)
B. Accessory conduction pathway. (0 marks)
C. Premature coronary artery disease. (0 marks)
D. Abnormal sodium/potassium
channels in cardiac myocytes. (2 marks)
E. Fibrofatty replacement of the
myocardium. (0 marks)
F. Myocardial fibrosis. (0 marks)

(Continues on page 240)

5. Maximum mark = 2
A. Intravenous isoprenaline.   (0 marks)
B. Intravenous atropine.   (0 marks)
C. Intravenous adenosine.   (0 marks)
D. A beta blocker.   (2 marks)
E. Intravenous magnesium.   (1 mark)
F. Intravenous adrenaline.   (0 marks)
G. Atrial pacing.   (0 marks)

6. Maximum mark = 3
A. Cardiac enzymes.   (0 marks)
B. Echocardiogram.   (0 marks)
C. Electrophysiological studies.   (0 marks)
D. Family screening.   (3 marks)
E. Serum cholesterol.   (0 marks)
F. Serum potassium.   (2 marks)
G. Serum magnesium.   (2 marks)

Total possible marks = 15

The combination of a family history of premature sudden death, long QT and polymorphic ventricular tachycardia associated with syncope is diagnostic of idiopathic LQTS. The condition is familial in up to 90% of cases, and can be inherited both as an autosomal dominant and recessive trait. The rarer variant (autosomal recessive), is associated with congenital nerve deafness and known as the Jarvell–Lange–Neilsen syndrome. The more common autosomal dominant form is often known as the Romano–Ward syndrome.

In congenital LQTS, defects within transmembrane ion channels produce abnormalities in cardiac repolarization, leading to an increased propensity for syncope due to fatal ventricular arrhythmias in situations causing increased sympathetic activity. Syncope may be precipitated by physical exertion, intense emotion and sudden loud auditory stimuli. The classic arrhythmia is a form of polymorphic ventricular tachycardia termed 'torsades de pointes', which may degenerate to ventricular fibrillation, causing sudden death. Thus far, abnormalities have been demonstrated in genes encoding both potassium and sodium ion transport channel proteins which are located on chromosome 11, 3, 4 and 7 (see below).

Myocardial disarray is a feature of HCM, an accessory conduction pathway would indicate Wolff–Parkinson–White or Lown–Ganong–Levine syndromes; fibrofatty replacement of the myocardium would indicate arrhythmogenic right ventricular cardiomyopathy; and myocardial fibrosis is a finding common to all cardiomyopathies and ischaemic heart disease.

Treatment is aimed at reducing the effects of the sympathetic nervous system on the conduction tissue. The immediate treatment of choice to prevent further ventricular tachycardia (VT) is beta blockers, which may be given intravenously in the first instance. In situations where this produces a profound bradycardia a permanent pacemaker is also implanted. There is some evidence that intravenous magnesium may arrest ventricular arrhythmias in the acute state, even when the serum magnesium level is normal. Patients who continue to have ventricular arrhythmias despite heavy beta blockade, are implanted with an automatic cardioverter defibrillator. It is worth noting that therapy with isoprenaline, a sympathomimetic agent which is useful in acquired LQTS, is contraindicated in congenital LQTS.

Screening of first-degree relatives is very important in this condition. In approximately 60% of cases the diagnosis of idiopathic LQTS is made during screening of first-degree relatives of affected patients. Low serum magnesium and potassium are causes of acquired LQTS which should always be excluded. In this case, there is no obvious cause for an electrolyte deficiency. No marks are awarded for electrophysiological studies because the diagnosis and the potential for VT is obvious.

Acquired causes of LQTS are usually due to drugs and electrolyte disturbances (*Table*). In such cases, treatment involves correction of the electrolyte disturbance and withdrawal of the offending drug. Rectifying serum electrolytes and drug levels can take several days, and prevention of polymorphic VT relies on shortening the QT-interval by atrial pacing at a rate of 60–70 beats/minute.

Genetics of LQTS
Congenital LQTS is a recognized but rare cause of sudden death in young adults. Death is due to polymorphic tachycardia (torsades de points) degenerating into ventricular fibrillation. Syncope is common in affected

---

Acquired causes of long LQTS

Drugs
Class Ia and Ic anti-arrhythmic agents
Tricyclic antidepressants, neuroleptic agents
Erythromycin
Ketoconazole
Certain anti-histamines
Cisapride

Electrolyte disturbances
Hypokalaemia, hypomagnesaemia
Hypocalcaemia

Cardiovascular diseases
Myocardial infarction
Complete heart block
Sick sinus syndrome
Mitral valve prolapse

Others
Subarachnoid haemorrhage
Liquid protein diet

patients, and is due to transient cerebral hypoperfusion from VT. Common stimuli of polymorphic VT include physical exertion, intense emotion and auditory stimuli. Genes encoding sodium and potassium ion channels cause disease. To date, there are four different loci on chromosomes 3, 4, 7 and 11. On chromosome 7, there is a mutation in the HERG gene (potassium channel abnormality). Other mutations include the SCN5A (chromosome 3; sodium ion channels) and KVLQT1 (chromosome 11; potassium ion channels).

Examination Answer 3

1. Maximum mark = 3
A. Autosomal recessive. (0 marks)
B. Autosomal dominant. (3 marks)
C. X-linked recessive. (0 marks)
D. X-linked dominant. (0 marks)
E. Y-linked. (0 marks)

Total possible marks = 3

Examination Answer 4

1. Maximum mark = 3
Hereditary spherocytosis. (3 marks)
Glucose-6-phosphate dehydrogenase
deficiency. (2 marks)
Pyruvate kinase deficiency. (2 marks)
Hereditary elliptiocytosis. (1 mark)
Infectious mononucleosis. (1 mark)
CMV infection. (1 mark)
Acute *Toxoplasma* infection. (1 mark)

2. Maximum mark = 6
Blood film. (3 marks)
Red cell fragility studies. (3 marks)
Direct Coomb's test. (2 marks)
Assess parental blood. (2 marks)
Glucose-6-phosphate dehydrogenase
level. (2 marks)
Pyruvate kinase level. (2 marks)
IgM antibodies to EBV. (1 mark)
IgM antibodies to CMV. (1 mark)
IgM antibodies to *Toxoplasma*. (1 mark)
Sabin–Feldman dye test for *Toxoplasma*. (1 mark)

Total possible marks = 9

The history of recurrent episodes of abdominal pain and jaundice precipitated by a sore throat in a young boy with anaemia, splenomegaly and a raised urinary urobilinogen is suggestive of an inherited haemolytic anaemia. The most likely diagnosis is HS, although other possible causes of this picture include hereditary elliptiocytosis, glucose-6-phosphate dehydrogenase deficiency, pyruvate and kinase deficiency. The history of a purulent sore throat and haemolysis could be explained entirely by infectious mononucleosis; however, it would be unusual for a young boy to have three episodes of EBV infection. In this case, the sore throat has been the precipitant for increased haemolysis in an individual with a red cells which are vulnerable to haemolysis. Marks have been awarded for infectious causes of sore throat, haemolysis and splenomegaly; however, these will not score as highly as marks for a hereditary anaemia.

Hereditary spherocytosis (**4**) is an autosomal dominant disorder of red cells. It is due to a defect in the membrane protein spectrin, which results in membrane loss as the cell passes through the spleen. The surface-to-volume ratio is reduced and the cells become spherocytic. Spherocytes are eventually destroyed by the spleen. The disorder may present as neonatal jaundice; however, most patients have a low-grade haemolysis with an intermittent increase in the rate of haemolysis during infections. During these episodes the patient may become very anaemic and appear jaundiced. Some individuals are asymptomatic and some may present in middle age with complications from gall stones. Aplastic crises may occur following infection with parvovirus, and megaloblastic anaemia may occur due to folate deficiency.

Leg ulcers are well recognized. The blood film will demonstrate spherocytes. When incubated in solutions of increasing hypotonicity or in their own plasma for over 24 hours, the cells demonstrate an increased rate of haemolysis. There is evidence of a haemolytic anaemia (raised bilirubin, reduced haptoglobins, increased urinary urobilinogen). Treatment of anaemia is with splenectomy.

Examination Answer 5

1. Maximum mark = 5
A. ST-segment depression in I, II, V3–V6. (3 marks)
B. Inverted T-wave in aVl. (1 mark)
C. Sinus tachycardia. (1 mark)
D. Anterior myocardial infarction. (0 marks)
E. Inferior myocardial infarction. (0 marks)
F. Left ventricular hypertrophy. (0 marks)

2. Maximum mark = 4
A. Anterolateral myocardial infarction. (1 mark)
B. Non-Q-wave anterolateral infarction. (2 marks)
C. Inferior myocardial infarction. (0 mark)
D. Hypothyroidism. (2 marks)
E. Kleinfelter's syndrome. (0 marks)
F. Intramuscular injection. (0 marks)

3. Maximum mark = 1
A. Secondary hypothyroidism. (0 marks)
B. Tertiary hypothyroidism. (0 marks)
C. Autoimmune hypothyroidism. (1 mark)
D. Hashimoto's hypothyroidism. (1 mark)
E. Sick euthyroid syndrome. (0 marks)

4. Maximum mark = 3
A. Serum B_{12} level. (2 marks)
B. Serum folate. (0 marks)
C. Gastric parietal antibodies. (1 mark)
D. Intrinsic factor antibodies. (1 mark)
E. Schilling test. (1 mark)
F. Serum ferritin. (0 marks)
G. Hb electrophoresis. (0 marks)

Total possible marks = 13

The patient presents with a subendocardial (non-Q-wave) anterolateral myocardial infarction. The blood results suggest that he has primary hypothyroidism. The very high titre of anti-microsomal antibodies indicates atrophic autoimmune hypothyroidism or Hashimoto's hypothyroidism. Hypothyroidism is a well-recognized cause of secondary hypercholesterolaemia (see *Table A* for other causes) and ischaemic heart disease. Other cardiac manifestations of the condition include pericarditis, dilated cardiomyopathy and pericardial effusion. In this case, the raised creatinine kinase level could be explained by myocardial infarction and hypothyroidism. Other causes of raised creatinine kinase are listed (*Table B*). Kleinfelter's syndrome is associated with hypothyroidism, but the normal LH level (usually high in Kleinfelter's syndrome) is against the diagnosis.

Hypothyroidism may cause normochromic normocytic anaemia, macrocytic anaemia or microcytic anaemia. The latter is usually seen in menstruating women who develop menorrhagia as a consequence of hypothyroidism. Macrocytosis in hypothyroidism may be directly due to hypothyroidism or associated pernicious anaemia, which is common in patients with autoimmune hypothyroidism. Pernicious anaemia is best diagnosed by a Schilling test, but the presence of gastric, parietal and intrinsic factor antibodies would also support the diagnosis in the context of the case. Coincidental folate deficiency may also cause macrocytosis.

Table A. Causes of secondary hypercholesterolaemia

Alcohol abuse	Obesity
Diabetes mellitus	Chronic liver disease
Hypothyroidism	Myeloma
Primary biliary cirrhosis	Nephrotic syndrome

Table B. Causes of a raised creatinine kinase

Normal variant in the Negroid population (up to 300 u/l)
Muscle injury or trauma
Septicaemia
Leptospirosis
Polymyositis
Muscular dystrophy
Hypothyroidism
Cholesterol-lowering statin and fibrate drugs

Examination Answer 6

1. Maximum mark = 5
A. Diabetic amyotrophy. (0 marks)
B. Steroid-induced myopathy. (5 marks)
C. Hypokalaemia. (0 marks)
D. Eaton–Lambert syndrome. (0 marks)
E. Metastatic spinal cord compression. (0 marks)

2. Maximum mark = 5
A. Bone metastases. (5 marks)
B. Fractured vertebra. (0 marks)
C. Myeloma. (0 marks)
D. Infiltration of the lower spinal
nerves by carcinoma. (0 marks)
E. Osteoporosis. (0 marks)

3. Maximum mark = 10
A. Cushing's disease. (0 marks)
B. Conn's syndrome. (0 marks)
C. Cortisol-secreting adenoma. (5 marks)
D. Ectopic ACTH production
from a bronchial carcinoma. (5 marks)
E. Pseudo Cushing's syndrome
secondary to alcohol abuse. (0 marks)

4. Maximum mark = 10
A. Serum ACTH. (5 marks)
B. Chest X-ray. (5 marks)
C. CT scan of the adrenals. (0 marks)
D. Petrosal venous sampling. (0 marks)
E. Lying and standing renin
and aldosterone level. (0 marks)

Total possible marks = 30

The patient presented with lower back pain and clinical symptoms of a proximal lower limb myopathy. The latter is confirmed clinically. He is diabetic and hypertensive. Routine blood results demonstrate a low potassium and elevated bicarbonate. The differential diagnosis at this point is between Cushing's disease (ACTH-secreting basophil adenoma from the pituitary), cortisol-secreting adrenal adenoma, or ectopic ACTH production. The diagnosis is narrowed down to a cortisol-secreting adrenal adenoma and ectopic ACTH by the failure of suppression of cortisol following high-dose dexamethasone. (See Answer **70**, page 94.)

The short history of the presenting complaint and history of smoking favour ectopic ACTH production by carcinoma of the bronchus. These patients produce large amounts of ACTH and present primarily with weakness and myopathy associated with hypokalaemia rather than a Cushingoid appearance.

The proximal myopathy is due to steroid excess, and the accompanying muscle weakness is compounded by the hypokalaemia. The hypokalaemia *per se* does not cause myopathy unless it is very long standing. The diabetes would account for the polydipsia and polyuria, but amyotrophy is unlikely to account for the proximal myopathy in a patient with such a short history and the absence of neuropathy. Eaton–Lambert syndrome may complicate oat cell bronchial carcinoma. It is characterized by proximal myopathy, fatigability and depressed reflexes or absent reflexes. It is due to a deficient release of acetylcholine from the nerve terminals. The diagnosis does not explain the normal reflexes or the diabetes and hypertension.

The patient has back pain and, in the context of an underlying carcinoma, this may be suggestive of bony metastases to the spine. Further support for this comes from the elevated serum calcium. Spinal cord compression however, is not plausible in the absence of spasticity in the lower limbs, the absence of a sensory level, and the presence of normal reflexes. In cord compression the reflexes are brisk. Infiltration of the spinal nerves by carcinoma is also unlikely because this would normally cause root pain and weakness of muscles supplied by the nerve affected, as well as altered sensation in the affected dermatomes.

Osteoporosis is a recognized complication of corticosteroid excess, and fractured vertebrae are a recognized complication of osteoporosis; thus, it is possible for either to be the cause of lower back pain in this situation. The bone biochemistry in osteoporosis, however, is normal (with the exception of raised alkaline phosphatase in the presence of a fracture). In this case the calcium and phosphate are elevated. Myeloma would explain the raised ESR, raised calcium and the back pain; however, in the context of the abnormal dexamethasone suppression test this diagnosis is unlikely.

Examination Answer 7

1. Maximum mark = 8

Liver ultrasound and Doppler studies.	(4 marks)
Liver biopsy via internal jugular vein.	(4 marks)
Liver biopsy.	(3 marks)
Hepatic venography.	(3 marks)
Liver ultrasound.	(2 marks)
Isotope liver scan.	(2 marks)
Ascitic tap for cytology and protein estimation.	(2 marks)
ERCP.	(2 marks)
Ascitic tap.	(1 mark)
Abdominal X-ray.	(0 marks)
Urinary protein estimation.	(0 marks)
Anti-mitochondrial antibodies.	(0 marks)
Smooth muscle antibodies.	(0 marks)
Antinuclear antibody.	(0 marks)

2. Maximum mark = 4

Hepatic vein thrombosis.	(3 marks)
Sclerosing cholangitis complicated by cholangiocarcinoma.	(1 mark)
Carcinoma of the colon with hepatic metastases.	(1 mark)
Chronic active hepatitis.	(0 marks)
Cirrhosis of the liver.	(0 marks)

Total possible marks = 12

The patient has a long history of relatively quiescent ulcerative colitis and presents with a short history of intermittent upper abdominal pain, vomiting, tender hepatomegaly and ascites. There is no history of weight loss preceding the illness. However, she is a smoker and on the oral contraceptive pill, both of which are recognized risk factors for venous thrombosis. Ulcerative colitis itself is associated with an increased risk of venous thrombosis due to increased fibrinogen levels and the elevated plasma viscosity. The most likely diagnosis in this patient is hepatic vein thrombosis. Although portal vein thrombosis may also occur in ulcerative colitis, the abnormal LFT and hepatomegaly would be against the diagnosis. The differential diagnosis comprises carcinoma of the colon with hepatic metastases, CAH, cirrhosis of the liver and sclerosing cholangitis. Carcinoma of the colon is 10 times more common in a patient with long-standing ulcerative colitis than in the general population; however, it is unusual for a patient with relatively well-controlled colitis to present with extensive metastatic liver disease without a prodrome of ill health or bleeding per rectum. Primary sclerosing cholangitis is strongly associated with ulcerative colitis. Some 75% of all cases with primary sclerosing cholangitis occur in patients with ulcerative colitis. The activity of the colitis is inversely related to the severity of sclerosing cholangitis. It is usually asymptomatic in the early stages, the only indicator being a raised alkaline phosphatase. Pruritis, jaundice, abdominal pain and weight loss are features of advanced cholangitis. Rapid deterioration may occur when sclerosing cholangitis is complicated by a cholangiocarcinoma. If this patient's presentation were due to primary sclerosing cholangitis or cholangiocarcinoma complicating sclerosing cholangitis, one would expect a higher bilirubin level and alkaline phosphatase level, particularly if the associated cirrhosis was severe enough to cause hepatocellular failure, as is suggested by the low albumin and ascites. Chronic active hepatitis is also recognized in ulcerative colitis, but the normal transaminase level is against the diagnosis.

The investigation of choice is liver US with Doppler studies on hepatic venous flow. Liver biopsy and hepatic venography are also useful in making the diagnosis. A liver isotope scan may demonstrate preservation of the Riedel's lobe.

Some marks are awarded for investigation of the ascites. In malignant ascites, cytology may be positive and the protein count is elevated. In ascites due to cirrhosis or hepatic failure, the protein count is low. ERCP would be useful in excluding the possibility of sclerosing cholangitis.

All of the complications mentioned above may also complicate Crohn's disease; however, primary sclerosing cholangitis, cholangiocarcinoma and the predisposition

---

Complications of ulcerative colitis

Gastrointestinal
Haemorrhage
Toxic dilatation
Perforation
Carcinoma of the colon
Oral and anal ulcers

Hepatobiliary
Fatty infiltration of the liver
CAH
Cirrhosis of the liver
Sclerosing cholangitis

Dermatological
Erythema nodosum
Pyoderma gangrenosum *Ophthalmic*
Episcleritis
Scleritis
Anterior uveitis

Rheumatological
Seronegative arthritis of the small joints
Ankylosing spondylitis

Haematological
Predisposition to venous thromboses

to venous thromboses is much more common in ulcerative colitis. Perianal ulcers are much more common in Crohn's disease and in addition, patients with Crohn's disease have a higher incidence of gall stones than those with ulcerative colitis The complications of ulcerative colitis are shown (*Table*). With the exception of ankylosing spondylitis and hepatobiliary disease, all the complications of ulcerative colitis are relieved by proctocolectomy.

Examination Answer 8

1. Maximum mark = 1
Multiple myeloma. (1 mark)

2. Maximum mark = 4
Serum immunoelectrophoresis. (1 mark)
Urinary Bence–Jones protein estimation. (1 mark)
Bone marrow aspirate/biopsy. (2 marks)
Skeletal survey. (1 mark)

3. Maximum mark = 4
Dehydration. (1 mark)
Hyperuricaemic nephropathy. (1 mark)
Hypercalcaemia causing nephrolithiasis. (1 mark)
Tubular obstruction by light chain. (1 mark)
Renal amyloid. (1 mark)
Chronic pyelonephritis. (1 mark)
'Myeloma kidney'. (1 mark)
Renal vein thrombosis. (1 mark)

4. Maximum mark = 5
Marrow infiltration. (2 marks)
Marrow suppression due to renal impairment. (2 marks)
Anaemia of chronic disease. (1 mark)
Folate deficiency. (1 mark)

5. Maximum mark = 2
Pseudohyponatraemia from myeloma. (1 mark)
Tubulointerstitial nephritis. (1 mark)
Chronic pyelonephritis. (1 mark)
Analgesic nephropathy. (1 mark)

6. Maximum mark = 2
Proximal RTA. (2 marks)

7. Maximum mark = 2
Nephrogenic diabetes mellitus from hypercalcaemia. (2 marks)

Total possible marks = 20

The diagnosis of myeloma is based on the very high globulin count (albumin subtracted from total protein content), anaemia, renal failure and hypercalcaemia.

The question tests your understanding of the renal and biochemical complications of myeloma.

The causes of anaemia, renal failure and other biochemical abnormalities in myeloma are covered in the answers above. (See also Answer **13**, page 26.)

Examination Answer 9

1. Maximum mark = 5
A. Ventricular tachycardia. (0 marks)
B. Left axis deviation. (1 mark)
C. Voltage for left atrial enlargement. (1 mark)
D. LBBB. (0 marks)
E. Right axis deviation. (0 marks)
F. Voltage criteria for right ventricular hypertrophy. (1 mark)
G. RBBB. (1 mark)
H. Voltage criteria for right atrial enlargement. (1 mark)
I. Voltage criteria for left ventricular hypertrophy. (0 marks)
J. Dissociated P-waves. (0 marks)
K. Capture beats. (0 marks)
L. Delta waves. (0 marks)

Total possible marks = 5

The criteria for left and right atrial and ventricular hypertrophy are discussed in Answer **98**, page 128. Bundle branch block is characterized by a wider QRS complex (more than 120 ms; three small squares on the ECG). In right bundle branch block the QRS complex in lead VI has a rsR pattern and in left bundle branch block the QRS complex in lead VI has a qS pattern (**9b**)

Examination Answer 10

1. Maximum mark = 4
Malabsorption. (2 marks)
Coeliac disease. (2 marks)
Hypothyroidism. (1 mark)
Constitutional delay. (0 marks)
Familial short stature. (0 marks)

2. Maximum mark = 3
Duodenal/jejunal biopsy. (2 marks)
Anti-gliadin antibodies. (1 mark)
Anti-reticulin antibodies. (1 mark)
Thyroid function tests. (1 mark)
Growth hormone. (0 marks)
Gonadotrophins. (0 marks)
Dynamic pituitary function tests. (0 marks)

Total possible marks = 7

This is a difficult question. There is evidence of short stature, delayed puberty, and a macrocytosis. These three features can be best explained by malabsorption. The commonest cause of malabsorption in the Western world is coeliac disease. The macrocytosis in this respect is due to folate deficiency. It is unusual, however, not to also have biochemical evidence of osteomalacia. The differential diagnosis here is hypothyroidism, which may explain the short stature, delayed puberty and macrocytosis; however, the problem has been present for approximately four years and one would expect a history of performing poorly at school or the presence of dry skin on examination. In addition, many children with hypothyroidism are relatively overweight in relation to the height.

GH deficiency or gonadotrophin deficiency could explain short stature and delayed puberty, but do not explain the macrocytosis. As with hypothyroidism, children with GH deficiency are relatively plump.

Examination Answer 11

1. Maximum mark = 2
A. Pleurisy. (0 marks)
B. Pulmonary embolus. (0 marks)
C. Pericardial effusion. (0 marks)
D. Acute pericarditis. (2 marks)
E. Musculoskeletal. (0 marks)
F. Myocarditis. (0 marks)
G. Endocarditis. (0 marks)

2. Maximum mark = 5
A. Antinuclear antibody. (3 marks)
B. Repeat blood cultures. (1 mark)
C. Blood film for malaria. (2 marks)
D. Anti-streptolysin O titres. (0 marks)
E. X-ray hands. (2 mark)
F. X-ray left shoulder. (1 mark)
G. X-ray cervical spine. (1 mark)
H. Cervical lymph node biopsy. (2 marks)
I. Mantoux test. (1 mark)
J. CT scan abdomen. (2 marks)
K. Serum ACE level. (1 mark)
L. Transbronchial lung biopsy. (0 marks)
M. *Brucella* titres. (0 marks)

3. Maximum mark = 5
A. Sarcoidosis. (1 mark)
B. Adult onset Still's disease. (5 marks)
C. Systemic lupus erythematosus. (3 marks)
D. Familial Mediterranean fever. (0 marks)
E. Brucellosis. (0 marks)
F. Rheumatic fever. (0 marks)
G. Rheumatoid arthritis. (0 marks)
H. Infective endocarditis. (0 marks)
I. Malaria. (1 mark)
J. Lymphoma. (1 mark)

Total possible marks = 12

Diagnosis of adult-onset Still's disease

Requires each of:
1. Quotidian fever >39°C (102.2°F)
2. Leucocytosis >15 × 10^9/l
3. Arthralgia/arthritis
4. Macular/maculopapular rash

Plus two of:
(a) Serositis (pleuritic/pericarditic)
(b) Splenomegaly
(c) Generalized lymphadenopathy
(d) Negative rheumatoid factor
(e) Negative anti-nuclear factor

The characteristics of the chest pain are consistently with acute pericarditis, which is confirmed on the ECG.

The patient has malaise, fever, arthralgia, a rash, lymphadenopathy, arthritis and splenomegaly.

The differential diagnosis is between adult-onset juvenile chronic arthritis or Still's disease, SLE, and lymphoma. The high CRP is against the diagnosis of SLE. While lymphoma is quite possible, the seronegative arthritis, neutrophil leucocytosis, high fever and maculopapular rash are best explained by Still's disease. Adult Still's disease is rare. It affects young adults aged between 16 and 35 years. The characteristics are identical to those of juvenile chronic arthritis in younger patients. The diagnosis is essentially clinical, and the clinical criteria are outlined below (*Table*). Anti-nuclear factor (ANF) is negative in Still's disease. Generalized lymphadenopathy is relatively common, and lymph node biopsy shows only reactive changes. If both these tests are negative, then adult Still's disease is the most likely diagnosis.

Infective endocarditis is unlikely with three negative blood cultures. The echocardiogram (**11c**) reveals a normal aortic and mitral valve, and right-sided endocarditis is most unusual in young, previously healthy individuals unless there is a history of intravenous drug abuse. Rheumatic fever may be suspected in a woman living in East Africa with a murmur, fever, arthritis and pericarditis; however, there is no history of streptococcal infection, and her symptoms are relatively long-standing for rheumatic fever. In this case, the murmur is likely to represent hyperdynamic circulation due to the fever; soft systolic murmurs and third heart sounds are relatively common in young individuals with fever. Malaria is unlikely after two years of being completely asymptomatic while in England. While *Plasmodium malariae* infections can be chronic, they do not present with frequent high fever and sweats of sudden onset. Brucellosis partly fits the clinical presentation; however, it is important to remember that it has been eradicated in the UK through pasteurization of milk. Sarcoidosis may mimic Still's disease, but the absence of ocular, respiratory and skin signs make it less probable. Familial Mediterranean fever is most unlikely for two reasons. First, it has a predilection for Jews and Arabs; second, it usually causes a monoarticular arthropathy.

In this case, ANF and lymph node biopsy are necessary to exclude SLE and lymphoma, respectively.

Examination Answer 12

1. Maximum mark = 3
A. Haemolytic uraemic syndrome.   (0 marks)
B. IgA nephritis.   (0 marks)
C. Henoch–Schönlein purpura.   (3 marks)
D. Systemic lupus erythematosus.   (0 marks)
E. Polyarteritis nodosa.   (0 marks)

2. Maximum mark = 5
A. Skin biopsy.   (3 marks)
B. Renal biopsy.   (2 marks)
C. Blood cultures.   (0 marks)
D. TT.   (0 marks)
E. Serum fibrinogen level.   (0 marks)
F. Serum IgA level.   (1 mark)
G. Serum anti-nuclear factor level.   (0 marks)
H. Serum ANCA.   (0 marks)

Total possible marks = 8

The combination of lower abdominal pain, bloody diarrhoea, purpuric rash and nephritis in a young girl are highly suggestive of Henoch–Schönlein purpura. The condition is a small-vessel vasculitis which occurs most commonly in children aged 4–15 years. It is characterized by gastrointestinal symptoms which comprise abdominal pain, diarrhoea, and rectal bleeding, flitting arthralgia affecting large joints, a purpuric rash characteristically affecting the lower limbs and buttocks and an acute nephritis. Complications include intestinal perforation, haemorrhage and intususception, and acute renal failure.

The diagnosis is usually clinical; however, tissue diagnosis is possible with skin or renal biopsy. Skin biopsy demonstrates a leucoclastic vasculitis with IgA deposition. Renal biopsy reveals mesangial IgA deposition associated with a glomerulonephritis. Renal histology is indistinguishable from IgA nephropathy. In this case, more marks are given to skin biopsy because it is safer and more practical than renal biopsy. Serum IgA levels are depressed in approximately 50% of cases. The management is usually supportive, although there may be a role for methylprednisolone in cases of acute crescentic nephritis.

The condition must not be confused with the haemolytic uraemic syndrome (discussed in Answer **49**, page 70) which is also characterized by diarrhoea and renal failure.

Examination Answer 13

1. Maximum mark = 3
SIADH secretion.   (3 marks)
Hypothyroidism.   (1 mark)

2. Maximum mark = 4
Plasma osmolality.   (2 marks)
Urinary osmolality.   (2 marks)
Thyroid function tests.   (1 mark)

Total possible marks = 7

Syndrome of inappropriate ADH secretion (see *Table* for causes) is the most likely diagnosis when the serum sodium is below 115 mmol/l. Hypothyroidism can cause failure to excrete water, and produce a similar biochemical picture to SIADH. The diagnosis is confirmed by demonstrating a low plasma osmolality and an inappropriately high urine osmolality.

Causes of SIADH

Central nervous system
Head injury
Encephalitis/meningitis
Cerebral abscess
Cerebral neoplasm
Cerebral haemorrhage

Respiratory system
Bronchial carcinoma (particularly oat cell)
TB
Pneumonia (Legionnaire's is the college favourite)
Empyema

Drugs
Chlorpropamide
Chlorpromazine
Carbamazepine
Opiates
Vincristine

Miscellaneous
Guillain–Barré syndrome
Acute intermittent porphyria
Carcinoma pancreas/thymoma

Examination Answer 14

1. Maximum mark = 2
Polymyositis.   (2 marks)
Rheumatoid arthritis.   (0 marks)
Polymyalgia rheumatica.   (0 marks)

2. Maximum mark = 2
Serum creatinine kinase.   (1 mark)
Muscle biopsy.   (1 mark)
Electromyography.   (1 mark)
Anti-jo-1 antibodies.   (1 mark)

Total possible marks = 4

Polymositis versus polymyalgia rheumatica		
	Polymyositis	*Polymyalgia rheumatica*
Muscle tenderness	Common	Common
Muscle wasting	Common	May occur
Proximal myopathy	Present	Recognized
Headaches	Absent	May be present
Skin involvement	Present (30%)	Absent
Raised enzymes	Present (usually)	Absent
ANA	Present (30%)	Absent
Rh factor	Present	Absent
Anti jo-1 Abs	Present (20%)	Absent

The differential diagnosis is between polymyalgia rheumatica and polymyositis (see *Table*). Both present with lethargy and weakness, and both may cause a polyarthropathy and tender muscles; however, elevated muscle enzymes and positive serology for rheumatoid arthritis is more characteristic of polymyositis. In 20%, anti-jo-1 antibodies may be present.

Examination Answer 15

1. Maximum mark = 5
A. Hiatus hernia.   (0 marks)
B. Benign oesophageal stricture.   (0 marks)
C. Achalasia.   (5 marks)
D. Pharyngeal pouch.   (0 marks)
E. Bronchiectasis.   (0 marks)

2. Maximum mark = 5
A. Oesophagoscopy.   (0 marks)
B. Barium swallow.   (5 marks)
C. Oesophageal manometry.   (0 marks)
D. Bronchoscopy.   (0 marks)
E. CT scan of the thorax.   (0 marks)

Total possible marks = 10

A history of dyspepsia, dysphagia, oesophageal reflux and a possible aspiration pneumonia are consistent with the diagnosis of achalasia. Hiatus hernia may cause reflux and occasionally nocturnal cough and aspiration pneumonia; however, dysphagia is not a feature unless recurrent reflux has caused a peptic stricture. Peptic stricture may cause all the symptoms of achalasia; however, there is usually a long history of indigestion before onset of dysphagia. Pharyngeal pouch does not cause retrosternal pain, although dysphagia and regurgitation are common.

A barium swallow is the best method of differentiating between achalasia, peptic stricture, hiatus hernia and pharyngeal pouch. Although it is relatively clear that the diagnosis is achalasia, oesophageal manometry scores less marks than barium swallow or oesophagoscopy because other causes of dysphagia – particularly oesophageal stricture – would have to be excluded before entertaining a diagnosis of achalasia. In achalasia, the barium demonstrates dilatation of the oesophagus and lack of peristalsis. The lower end gradually narrows due to failure of the lower oesophageal sphincter to relax. Oesophageal manometry is useful to measure motility.

Achalasia is a motility disorder affecting the oesophagus. It is characterized by lack of peristalsis and failure of the lower oesophageal sphincter to relax. Pathologically, there is degeneration of the ganglionic cells in the nerve plexus of the oesophageal wall. The aetiology is unknown. The disease often presents in middle age. There is a long history of retrosternal pain, intermittent dysphagia, oesophageal reflux and aspiration. Weight loss is unusual. Diagnosis is by a combination of barium swallow and oesophageal manometry. Treatment is by dilating the lower oesophagus by pneumatic inflation. In unsuccessful cases, surgical division of the lower end of the oesophagus (Heller's operation) is required.

Normal Ranges

		SI units	Traditional units
Haematology			
ESR		0–10 mm in 1st h	0–10 mm in 1st h
Hb	male	130–180 g/l	13–18 g/dl
	female	115–150 g/l	11.5–15 g/dl
MCH		27–32 pg	–
MCHC		32–36 g/dl	32–36%
MCV		76–95 fl	$76–95 \times 10^6/mm^3$
PCV (haematocrit)	male	0.40–0.54 l/l	40–54%
	female	0.35–0.47 l/l	35–47%
Platelet count		$150–400 \times 10^9/l$	$150–400 \times 10^3/mm^3$
RBCs	male	$4.5–6.5 \times 10^{12}/l$	$4.5–6.5 \times 10^6/mm^3$
	female	$3.9–5.6 \times 10^{12}/l$	$3.9–5.6 \times 10^6/mm^3$
Reticulocyte count		0.2–2%	0.2–2%
WCC	total	$4–11 \times 10^9/l$	$4–11 \times 10^3/mm^3$
	neutrophils	$2–7.5 \times 10^9/l$	$2–7.5 \times 10^3/mm^3$
	lymphocytes	$1.5–4.0 \times 10^9/l$	$1.5–4.0 \times 10^3/mm^3$
	monocytes	$0.2–0.8 \times 10^9/l$	$0.2–0.8 \times 10^3/mm^3$
	eosinophils	$0.04–0.4 \times 10^9/l$	$0.04–0.4 \times 10^3/mm^3$
	basophils	$<0.1 \times 10^9/l$	$<0.1 \times 10^3/mm^3$
Clotting			
APTT		30–46 s	30–46 s
BT		2–8 min	2–8 min
Fibrinogen		2–4 g/l	0.2–0.4 g/dl
PT		12–14 s	12–14 s
TT		15–19 s	15–19 s
Endocrinology			
Cortisol	09.00 h	170–700 nmol/l	6.1–25.2 µg/dl
	24.00 h	<140 nmol/l	5.0 µg/dl
GH		<10 µg/l	<10 ng/ml
Oestradiol mid-cycle		500–1,100 pmol/l	500–1,100 pmol/l
Prolactin		<360 mu/l	<360 µu/ml
Renin	lying	2–4 µg/l/h	2–4 ng/ml/h
	standing	5–14 µg/l/h	5–14 ng/ml/h
Testosterone	male	10–35 nmol/l	3–10 ng/ml
	female	0.9–3.1 nmol/l	0.3–1.0 ng/ml
Thyroxine		68–174 nmol/l	4.5–13.6 µg/dl
TSH		0.4–3.6 mu/l	0.4–3.6 µu/ml
Biochemistry			
α-fetoprotein		<10 ku/l	<10 u/ml
ALT		5–30 u/l	5–30 mu/ml
Albumin		34–48 g/l	3.4–4.8 g/dl
Alkaline phosphatase		25–100 u/l	25–100 mu/ml
AST		10–40 u/l	10–40 mu/ml
B_{12} (serum)		160–900 ng/l	160–900 pg/ml
Bicarbonate		22–30 mmol/l	22–30 mEq/l
Bilirubin		2–17 µmol/l	0.12–1.0 mg/dl

		SI units	*Traditional units*
Biochemistry (*continued*)			
Calcium		2.2–2.7 mmol/l	8.8–10.8 mg/dl
Cholesterol		3.6–7.8 mmol/l	139–302 mg/dl
Chloride		100–106 mmol/l	100–106 mEq/l
C-reactive protein		0–10 mg/l	0–1.0 mg/dl
Creatinine		50–120 μmol/l	0.57–1.36 mg/dl
Creatinine kinase	males	17–148 u/l	17–148 mu/ml
	females	10–79 u/l	10–79 mu/ml
Ferritin		15–250 μg/l	1.5–25.0 μg/dl
Folate	serum	3–20 μg/l	3–20 ng/ml
	red cell	160–460 μg/l	160–460 ng/ml
Gamma GT		5–30 u/l	5–30 u/l
Glucose (blood)		2.5–7.5 mmol/l	45–135 mg/dl
Iron (serum)	males	14–32 μmol/l	78–180 μg/dl
	females	10–30 μmol/l	56–168 μg/dl
Osmolality		280–296 mOsm/kg	280–296 mOsm/kg
Phosphate		0.8–1.5 mmol/l	2.5–4.65 mg/dl
Potassium		3.5–5.0 mmol/l	3.5–5.0 mEq/l
Protein		62–80 g/l	6.2–8.0 g/dl
Sodium		135–146 mmol/l	135–146 mEq/l
TIBC		40–80 μmol/l	224–448 μg/dl
Urate		0.12–0.42	2.0–7.0 mg/dl
Urea		2.5–6.7 mmol/l	15.0–40.2 mg/dl (BUN)

Immunology

	SI units	*Traditional units*
IgA	0.8–4.0 g/l	80–400 mg/dl
IgG	7.0–18.0 g/l	700–1,800 mg/dl
IgM	0.4–2.5 g/l	40–250 mg/dl

Arterial Blood Gases

	SI units	*Traditional units*
$PaCO_2$	4.7–6.0 kPa	35–45 mmHg
PaO_2	11.2–14.0 kPa	84–105 mmHg
pH	7.35–7.45	7.35–7.45

Cardiology

		mmHg
Venae cavae	mean	2–8
Right atrium	a-wave	3–6
	v-wave	1–4
	mean	1–5
Right ventricle	systolic	20–30
	end diastolic	2–7
Pulmonary artery	systolic	16–30
	diastolic	4–13
	mean	9–18
PCWP		4.5–12
Left atrium	a-wave	4–14
	v-wave	6–16
	mean	6–11
Left ventricle	systolic	90–140
	end diastolic	6–12
Aorta	systolic	90–140
	diastolic	70–90
	mean	70–110

Index